Toward an Integrated Medicine

Classics From *Psychosomatic Medicine,* 1959–1979

Toward an Integrated Medicine

Classics From *Psychosomatic Medicine*, 1959–1979

EDITED BY A COMMITTEE OF THE
AMERICAN PSYCHOSOMATIC SOCIETY

Ann Maxwell Eward, Ph.D., Chair
Joel E. Dimsdale, M.D.
Bernard T. Engel, Ph.D.
Don R. Lipsitt, M.D.
Donald Oken, M.D.
Joseph D. Sapira, M.D.
David Shapiro, Ph.D.
Herbert Weiner, M.D., Dr. Med. (hon.)

Washington, DC   London, England

Note: The authors have worked to ensure that all information in this book concerning drug dosages, schedules, and routes of administration is accurate as of the time of publication and consistent with standards set by the U.S. Food and Drug Administration and the general medical community. As medical research and practice advance, however, therapeutic standards may change. For this reason and because human and mechanical errors sometimes occur, we recommend that readers follow the advice of a physician who is directly involved in their care or the care of a member of their family.

Books published by the American Psychiatric Press, Inc., represent the views and opinions of the individual authors and do not necessarily represent the policies and opinions of the Press or the American Psychiatric Association.

Copyright © 1995 American Psychiatric Press, Inc.
ALL RIGHTS RESERVED
Manufactured in the United States of America on acid-free paper
98 97 96 95   4 3 2 1
First Edition

American Psychiatric Press, Inc.
1400 K Street, N.W., Washington, DC   20005

Library of Congress Cataloging-in-Publication Data
Toward an integrated medicine : classics from Psychosomatic medicine,
   1959-1979 / edited by a committee of the American Psychosomatic
   Society ; Ann Maxwell Edward . . . [et al.].
         p. cm.
   Includes bibliographical references and index.
   ISBN 0-88048-727-5
   1. Medicine, Psychosomatic.   I. Eward, Ann Maxwell.   II. American
Psychosomatic Society.   III. Psychosomatic medicine.
   [DNLM: 1. Psychosomatic Medicine—collected works.   WM 90 T737
1995]
RC49.T674   1995
616.08—dc20
DNLM/DLC
for Library of Congress   94-35345
                                                                              CIP

British Library Cataloguing in Publication Data
A CIP record is available from the British Library.

Figures courtesy of the New York Academy of Medicine.

Contents

Contributors ix

Foreword xi

CHAPTER 1   Is Grief a Disease? A Challenge for Medical Research   1
George L. Engel, M.D.

CHAPTER 2   Concurrent Plasma Epinephrine, Norepinephrine and 17-Hydroxycorticosteroid Levels During Conditioned Emotional Disturbances in Monkeys   9
John W. Mason, M.D., George Mangan, Jr., Ph.D., Joseph V. Brady, Ph.D., Donald Conrad, M.A., and David McK. Rioch, M.D.

CHAPTER 3   Specific Attitudes in Initial Interviews With Patients Having Different "Psychosomatic" Diseases   27
David T. Graham, M.D., Richard M. Lundy, Ph.D., Lorna S. Benjamin, Ph.D., J. D. Kabler, M.D., William C. Lewis, M.D., Nancy O. Kunish, B.A., and Frances K. Graham, Ph.D.

CHAPTER 4   Relationship Between Psychological Defenses and Mean Urinary 17-hydroxycorticosteroid Excretion Rates: I. A Predictive Study of Parents of Fatally Ill Children   45
Carl T. Wolff, M.D., Stanford B. Friedman, M.D., Myron A. Hofer, M.D., and John W. Mason, M.D.

CHAPTER 5	Review of Consultation Psychiatry and Psychosomatic Medicine: II. Clinical Aspects	71
	Z. J. Lipowski, M.B., B.Ch., D.Psych.	

CHAPTER 6	Influences of Suggestion on Airway Reactivity in Asthmatic Subjects	105
	Thomas Luparello, M.D., Harold A. Lyons, M.D., Eugene R. Bleecker, B.A., and E. R. McFadden, Jr., M.D.	

CHAPTER 7	Blood Pressure Changes in Men Undergoing Job Loss: A Preliminary Report	117
	Stanislav V. Kasl, Ph.D., and Sidney Cobb, M.D.	

CHAPTER 8	Learned Control of Cardiovascular Integration in Man Through Operant Conditioning	143
	Gary E. Schwartz, M.A., David Shapiro, Ph.D., and Bernard Tursky	

CHAPTER 9	Effect of Psychosocial Stimulation on the Enzymes Involved in the Biosynthesis and Metabolism of Noradrenaline and Adrenaline	155
	James P. Henry, M.D., Patricia M. Stephens, Julius Axelrod, Ph.D., and Robert A. Mueller, M.D.	

CHAPTER 10	Differences in Perception Between Hypertensive and Normotensive Populations	171
	Joseph D. Sapira, M.D., Eileen T. Scheib, B.A., Richard Moriarty, M.D., and Alvin P. Shapiro, M.D.	

CHAPTER 11	Operant Conditioning of Heart Rate in Patients With Premature Ventricular Contractions	191
	Theodore Weiss, M.D., and Bernard T. Engel, Ph.D.	

CHAPTER 12	An Integrated Theory of Disease: Ladino-Mestizo Views of Disease in the Chiapas Highlands	221
	Horacio Fabrega, Jr., M.D., and Peter K. Manning, Ph.D.	

CHAPTER 13	Socio-Ecological Stress, Suppressed Hostility, Skin Color, and Black-White Male Blood Pressure: Detroit	245
	Ernest Harburg, Ph.D., John C. Erfurt, B.A., Louise S. Hauenstein, Ph.D., Catherine Chape, M.A., William J. Schull, Ph.D., and M. A. Schork, Ph.D.	
CHAPTER 14	**Depression in Infant Monkeys: Physiological Correlates**	273
	Martin Reite, M.D., I. Charles Kaufman, M.D., J. Donald Pauley, Ph.D., and A. J. Stynes, M.S.	
CHAPTER 15	**Consequences of Social Conflict on Plasma Testosterone Levels in Rhesus Monkeys**	281
	Robert M. Rose, M.D., Irwin S. Bernstein, Ph.D., and Thomas P. Gordon, M.A.	
CHAPTER 16	**From Explanation to Action in Psychosomatic Medicine: The Case of Obesity**	299
	Albert J. Stunkard, M.D.	
CHAPTER 17	**Behaviorally Conditioned Immunosuppression**	363
	Robert Ader, Ph.D., and Nicholas Cohen, Ph.D.	
CHAPTER 18	**Social Support as a Moderator of Life Stress**	377
	Sidney Cobb, M.D.	
CHAPTER 19	**Natural History of Male Psychological Health, IV: What Kinds of Men Do Not Get Psychosomatic Illness**	399
	George E. Vaillant, M.D.	
	Index	**415**

Contributors

Christopher L. Coe, Ph.D.
Professor of Psychology, Department of Psychology, University of Wisconsin, Madison, Wisconsin

Joel E. Dimsdale, M.D.
Professor of Psychiatry, University of California, San Diego, California

Bernard T. Engel, Ph.D.
Chief, Laboratory of Behavioral Sciences, National Institutes of Health, Gerontology Research Center, Francis Scott Key Medical Center, Baltimore, Maryland

Ann Maxwell Eward, Ph.D.
Assistant Professor of Epidemiology, University of Michigan; and Director, Clinical Practice Studies, Butterworth Hospital, Grand Rapids, Michigan

Stanislav V. Kasl, Ph.D.
Professor of Epidemiology, Yale University School of Medicine, New Haven, Connecticut

Kathleen C. Light, Ph.D.
Associate Professor of Psychiatry, The University of North Carolina at Chapel Hill, North Carolina

Don R. Lipsitt, M.D.
Clinical Professor of Psychiatry, Harvard Medical School, Cambridge, Massachusetts

John C. Nemiah, M.D.
Professor Emeritus, Harvard Medical School; and Professor of Psychiatry, Dartmouth Medical School, Hanover, New Hampshire

Donald Oken, M.D.
Consultation-Liaison Services, Department of Psychiatry, Pennsylvania Hospital; and Clinical Professor of Psychiatry, University of Pennsylvania School of Medicine, Philadelphia, Pennsylvania

Richard H. Rahe, M.D.
Professor of Psychiatry and Clinical Medicine, Department of Psychiatry and Behavioral Science, University of Nevada School of Medicine, Reno, Nevada

Morton F. Reiser, M.D.
Albert E. Kent Professor Emeritus of Psychiatry, Yale University School of Medicine, New Haven, Connecticut

Robert T. Rubin, M.D., Ph.D.
Professor of Psychiatry, Neurosciences Research Center, Allegheny-Singer Research Institute, Medical College of Pennsylvania, Pittsburgh, Pennsylvania

Joseph D. Sapira, M.D.
Professor of Medicine, St. Louis University, St. Louis, Missouri

David Shapiro, Ph.D.
Professor of Psychiatry and Psychology, Department of Psychiatry, University of California, Los Angeles, California

Jon Streltzer, M.D.
Professor of Psychiatry, John A. Burns School of Medicine, University of Hawaii at Manoa, Honolulu, Hawaii

Louis Vachon, M.D.
Professor, Division of Psychiatry, Boston University School of Medicine, Boston, Massachusetts

Herbert Weiner, M.D., Dr. Med. (hon.)
Professor of Psychiatry & Biobehavioral Sciences, Neuropsychiatric Institute, University of California, Los Angeles, California

Thomas N. Wise, M.D.
Professor of Psychiatry, Department of Psychiatry, Georgetown University School of Medicine, Fairfax Hospital, Falls Church, Virginia

Foreword

In his foreword to *Psychosomatic Classics* (1972), which included articles from *Psychosomatic Medicine,* 1939–1958, Carl A. L. Binger, the journal's second editor-in-chief, correctly anticipated the most serious challenge that the discipline would have to confront. It turns out to be as true now as it was then. Reviewing the historical development of the field, he wrote,

> It began with a reformer's proselytizing zeal, striving to influence all of medicine and its ancillary sciences. . . . The emphasis was on treating the patient as a whole person. . . . As in all young sciences, new methods were needed. The descriptive ones which ushered in psychosomatic medicine soon proved wanting, although without them there could have been no beginning. Before long, new methods were introduced borrowed from physiology, biochemistry, and dynamic psychiatry, and later from sociology, mathematics and statistics. . . . *Its continued growth will depend upon our fundamental understanding of these sciences, and also of course on our ability to ask the right questions of nature.* (p. viii, emphasis added)

The challenge is, in fact, a dual one: 1) to stay abreast of advancing insights into the nature of the biological, psychological, and social factors that are prerequisite for full understanding of human behavior as well as states of health and disease, and, at the same time, 2) to remember that the primary responsibility of the clinician is to treat patients rather than diseases.

This has not been, nor will it be, a challenge easily met in the face of increasing fragmentation of relevant knowledge and techniques that are at the cutting edge of the life sciences—which is where we are, and should be.

This (second) collection of "psychosomatic classics" from *Psychosomatic Medicine* stands as testimony to the fact that this dual challenge, despite its difficulty, was successfully met during the succeeding years (1959–1979). Clinical patient-oriented interests, dominant in articles by Graham et al. (Chapter 3), Lipowski (Chapter 5), Weiss and Engel (Chapter 11), Sapira et al. (Chapter 10), and Vaillant (Chapter 19), are joined with attention to social as well as biological factors in articles by Kasl and Cobb (Chapter 7), Harburg et al. (Chapter 13),

Stunkard (Chapter 16), and Cobb (Chapter 18). Detailed studies (using contemporary experimental, instrumental, and statistical techniques) on the roles of autonomic, neuroendocrine, and neuroimmune mechanisms involved in psychosocial stress responses are represented both in clinical experimental studies in an article by Wolff et al. (Chapter 4) and in animal model systems relevant to human disease in articles by Mason et al. (Chapter 2), Henry et al. (Chapter 9), Reite et al. (Chapter 14), Rose et al. (Chapter 15), and Ader and Cohen (Chapter 17). The influence of suggestion, learning paradigms, and instrumental and behavioral conditioning techniques on clinically relevant autonomic and immune system responses are represented in articles by Luparello et al. (Chapter 6), Schwartz et al. (Chapter 8), Weiss and Engel (Chapter 11), and Ader and Cohen (Chapter 17). Note that originality in experimental strategies, tactics, and techniques characterize all of these studies. Finally, provocative theoretical articles by Engel (Chapter 1) and Fabrega and Manning (Chapter 12) are included.

It is both wise and appropriate that such work be collected and saved for special attention in one place. The literature currently grows at such a rapid pace that articles more than 5 years old escape attention. When important observations and facts already recorded have to be "rediscovered," it is indeed regrettable.

Finally, I wish that this collection contained an article as prescient as Paul MacLean's "Psychosomatic Disease and the 'Visceral Brain': Recent Developments Bearing on the Paper Theory of Emotion," which appeared in the first *Psychosomatic Classics*. Modern cognitive neuroscience now provides knowledge and techniques that make it possible to know more about the psychophysiological details of the transduction linkage between mental and physiological aspects of responses to psychosocial stress. We should now be in a position to investigate the way or ways in which these mind-brain mechanisms may participate, as MacLean anticipated in determining the qualitative as well as the quantitative characteristics of bodily responses to psychosocial stress.

This serves as a reminder that there is some bad news too. The explosion of knowledge and technical developments since 1979 has expanded the spectrum of disciplinary interfaces relevant to psychosomatic problems. It can now be said that the spectrum extends all the way from molecular genetics at one end through molecular biology, cell biology, neurophysiology, neuroanatomy, neurochemistry, neuropsychopharmacology, all branches of psychology and psychoanalysis, computer science, artificial intelligence, philosophy, sociology, anthropology, political science, and history and the humanities at the other. And each of these interfaces is important. It will be increasingly important to develop ways to train at least a modest cadre of investigators who, in addition to being expert in their own subspecialty area, will be able to work collaboratively across at least one of these interdisciplinary boundaries.

Perhaps the Council of the American Psychosomatic Society in publishing this latest collection of psychosomatic classics is trying to tell us, in looking back, that 1959–1979 were still vintage years—still "the good old days." In looking forward, the society may want to remind us that the present and the years ahead can still be "the good old days"; if—keeping the dual nature of the challenge in mind—we can hold onto the fundamental clinical perspective regarding the whole patient, while absorbing what is new in science, and building on what has already been learned.

Morton F. Reiser, M.D.

CHAPTER 1

Is Grief a Disease?

A Challenge for Medical Research

GEORGE L. ENGEL, M.D.

Prefatory Remarks

Donald Oken, M.D.

Questions about the nature of the grieving process have interest and importance in their own right, and they continue to puzzle, intrigue, and confound us. The grieving process has important ramifications for our understanding of depression and the depressions. But it is hardly this that makes this article a "classic." In addressing the question posed by his deceptively simple title, Engel explored issues that lie at the very heart of psychosomatic medicine. His elegant exposition leads us to look behind the question about grief and to recognize that grief reflects such fundamental matters as how we can define the constructs of *health, normality,* and *disease;* how "causes" of disease may be understood; and how psychological and social factors can qualify as such causes. Engel not only raised these issues, but masterfully explored each and pointed out the directions by which we may come to understand them better. Because it is the special way in which psychosomatic medicine views these matters that constitutes the

---

Volume 23, 1961, pp. 18–22.
   From the Departments of Psychiatry and Medicine, University of Rochester Medical Center, Rochester, N.Y. Presented at the Annual Meeting, American Psychosomatic Society, Mar. 27, 1960, held at Montreal, Canada.
   Received for publication April 14, 1960.

unique core contributions of our field to health science, this article represents a contribution of the most fundamental nature.

Engel's subtitle suggests that this article primarily has implications for research. Certainly, the article does have great value for research: the conceptual beliefs held by all scientists guide and inform their work, limiting or allowing the findings to open doors to genuinely new insights about nature, including human nature; the psychosomatic perspective opens the way to new knowledge that is unattainable when research is carried out within the conventional biomedical paradigm. But Engel is too modest. His clarification of basic psychosomatic issues has value for all who contemplate matters of health and disease in humans, including clinicians, planners, and even the merely intellectually curious who want to understand the basic concepts in this area.

If by a "classic" one simply means something from the past of unusual excellence, then this article certainly qualifies. We tend to think of classic as primarily of historical significance, useful for the present primarily because it explains how we reached our contemporary position, but no longer relevant in its own right. But this article meets the far sterner test for a classic: it has enduring value. The questions Engel honed and explored, and the directions he suggested for addressing them, have every bit as much significance now as when they appeared in this article in 1961. Indeed, in the contemporary period when neurobiological reductionism is so rife, this article has special cogency. I find it invaluable for use in teaching both residents and medical students. Would that physicians outside the psychosomatic field read it, too!

This paper has perhaps more the qualities of a philosophic than a scientific discourse, but for this I offer no apology. I shall present no new data and shall speak of a quite familiar phenomenon, but I shall invite you to view it from a perspective perhaps somewhat different from that to which you are accustomed. In keeping with this philosophic approach I have written this in the form of a Socratic dialogue. I pose the question, "Is grief a disease?"

No doubt this seems a strange question, since grief has not usually been considered in such terms and, on first glance, there seems little reason to do so. Yet, a thoughtful consideration of the issues raised by such a question will, I believe, throw light on some deficiencies in currently held concepts of disease. And the concept of disease held by an investigator, whether or not con-

Is Grief a Disease: A Challenge for Medical Research

sciously utilized, has an important influence on the choice of material and the design of clinical research.[1-3]

Grief is the characteristic response to the loss of a valued object, be it a loved person, a cherished possession, a job, status, home, country, an ideal, a part of the body, etc. *Uncomplicated* grief runs a consistent course, modified mainly by the abruptness of the loss, the nature of the preparation for the event, and the significance for the survivor of the lost object. Generally it includes an initial phase of shock and disbelief, in which the sufferer attempts to deny the loss and to insulate himself against the shock of the reality. This is followed by a stage of developing awareness of the loss, marked by the painful effects of sadness, guilt, shame, helplessness, or hopelessness; by crying; by a sense of loss and emptiness; by anorexia, sleep disturbance, sometimes somatic symptoms of pain or other discomfort, loss of interest in one's usual activities and associates, impairment of work performance, etc. Finally, there is a prolonged phase of restitution and recovery during which the work of mourning is carried on, the trauma of the loss is overcome, and a state of health and well-being re-established.[4, 5]

In what respects does this correspond to other situations that we customarily regard as "disease"? Certainly it involves suffering and an impairment of the capacity to function, which may last for days, weeks, and even months. We can identify a consistent etiologic factor, namely, real, threatened, or even fantasied object loss. It fulfills all the criteria of a discrete syndrome, with relatively predictable symptomatology and course. The grieving person is often manifestly distressed and disabled to a degree quite evident to an observer.

The sceptic quickly raises some pointed questions: *Is not grief simply a natural reaction to a life experience? How can one put it into the same category as the pathological states we call disease?* To this we answer that it is "natural" or "normal" in the same sense that a wound or a burn is the natural or normal response to physical trauma. The designation "pathological" refers to the changed state and not to the fact of the response. That one responds to thermal radiation with a burn is natural or normal. The burn itself constitutes a pathological state and the concept is as appropriately applied to the state of grief as to a wound, burn, or infection.

Or it may be said: *Everyone experiences grief—it's part of life.* But that only emphasizes the ubiquity in life of the significant etiologic factor and the universal vulnerability of human beings to this particular stressful experience. The same may be said of many other disease states to which man is prone—measles, for example. Actually, the statement is not entirely correct. With a short life or under exceptionally favorable circumstances, one may escape both measles and grief.

Our sceptic resumes his argument: *Grief is a self-limited process, requiring no medical attention.* But so too are a great number of disease processes. Actually, many persons suffering primarily from grief do come to physicians but, because of cultural expectations and the role ascribed to or held by the physician, they do not complain to him of grief. Rather, they report some other, often somatic, symptom and the physician may not even learn of the grief. If he does, he may regard it either as not related to the complaint or not his concern. Besides, whether a condition requires medical attention is not relevant to the judgment as to whether it is to be regarded as a disease. The history of medicine provides innumerable examples of conditions that have come in time to be recognized as disease states but which had not been so regarded earlier. Epilepsy, alcoholism, and mental disease are examples. We must not forget that in the prescientific era the roles of physician, magician, and priest were often embodied in the same person. It is the obligation of the physician of today to claim for scientific scrutiny all natural phenomena involving deviations in the individual's state of well-being, of which grief is one.

Grief is a purely subjective, psychological experience that does not involve any somatic changes. But, to my knowledge, no one has ever studied the bodily changes occurring during grief; hence, to begin with, there is no basis for such a statement. But even if it were true, one who holds such a view is, in essence, relegating to an extramedical and extrascientific status any kind of psychological or behavioral disturbance. As a matter of fact, many illnesses are largely subjective—at least, until we as observers discover the parameters and framework within which we can also make objective observations. Hyperparathyroidism, in many of its manifestations, was a purely subjective experience for many patients until we discovered what to look for and which instruments to use in the search. Again, the physician who is familiar with grief will recognize its occurrence through his systematic and ordered observations, even if the patient withholds or denies the necessary information.

No one ever dies of grief. Again, this is an irrelevant argument, even if true; but is it true? The newspapers repeatedly report persons collapsing and dying soon after learning of the death of a loved person. Have these cases been so carefully studied that we can say that the death represented pure coincidence, that the shock phase of the grief contributed in no way to this fatal outcome? I know of no such studies. Literature and folklore are replete with the notion that people fall ill and die "of grief." (I would prefer to say "during grief.") And few of the older physicians, from Hippocrates through the clinical giants of the late nineteenth century, failed to allude to grief as a factor in the causation of disease. While such views hardly constitute scientific evidence, the incidents are so common and the views so widely held that the cautious scientist will not be willing to say, without the benefit of scientific study, that it cannot be so. Actually, many recent investigations indicate that a wide variety of illnesses, including some that are fatal, may begin during a phase of grief. Schmale has recently surveyed a medical population and reviewed the modern as well as some of the older literature from this perspective.[6]

Perhaps one should speak of pathological grief and normal grief and restrict to the former the category of disease. This is a welcome concession, but it does not go far enough. At the outset I intentionally used the term "uncomplicated grief" rather than normal grief. It is normal only in a statistical sense, meaning that it is the common, usual, and predictable response, as is an ecchymosis after a blow or measles after an infection with the measles virus. But it is not normal in the sense of total health. Predictable does not mean invariable and, in any situation, whether it be loss of an object or an exposure to physical trauma or a microorganism, we observe and define conditions under which the response may be different in degree or kind or where it may not occur at all. This is a widely accepted and familiar notion as applied to traditional disease states, but equally appropriate in respect to grief. We are familiar with such responses as the absence of grief, delayed grief, unresolved grief, depression, psychotic or neurotic reactions, pain or other conversion symptoms, and even organic disease occurring in place of or in addition to the usual pattern of grief. As is true of the complications of a wound or an infection, we must also expect that other factors operate to account for these deviations from the usual course. Yet none of these considerations refutes the fact that the experience of uncomplicated grief also represents a manifest and gross departure from the dynamic state considered representative of health and well-being.

Is not grief really just a healthy, adaptive, and reparative process which corrects or overcomes a stress while the above-mentioned responses are the abnormal states that should be called diseases? The element of reparation is indeed to be found in grief, but so too is it found in every other disease; indeed, it always accounts for some of the symptoms and signs of a disease. If the adaptive or reparative processes involved in disease are successful, recovery occurs and the patient reachieves a state of health. If not, continued, progressive, or increased illness or death is the consequence.

Can it not be said that the person is really healthy and that he simply had the misfortune to suffer a loss and is now responding, naturally, with grief? This argument implies that all systems and levels of organization, actually and potentially, must be impaired by the stress before the condition can be considered disease. Actually, not only are health and disease relative concepts, but also at any time parts of the body and person may be more or less healthy, while other parts may be more or less impaired. Indeed, this is the usual situation. It is only in fatal disease, when the victim is near death, that we see total disorganization.

Perhaps by now the sceptic is ready to concede that grief can be considered a disease state. But what is gained by such a position? What are the implications for medical research and practice? They are, in my opinion, important and far reaching:

1. Grief, in all its forms and with all its ramifications, becomes a legitimate and proper subject for study by medical scientists. Research, utilizing the tools of the physical, biological, and behavioral sciences, must be directed to these sufferers no less than to those with other disorders. The occurrence of grief among animals is so well documented as to free the investigator from exclusive dependence on human subjects for such research.
2. The occurrence of grief, preceding or in the course of other illness, somatic and psychologic, as is so often reported by patients or their families, can no longer be passed off as irrelevant or coincidental until such data have been subjected to the same kind of rigorous and systematic exploration and examination that has been applied to other phenomena of disease. That grief in its various forms so often precedes the development of other disease states in itself constitutes no proof of a relationship. But the medical scientist is remiss if he does not subject all antecedent circumstances to examination as to whether they constitute contributing, necessary, or sufficient conditions for the development of a disease state. The obvious derangements in the functioning of the individual suffering from object loss and consequent grief make such inquiry all the more relevant. It is well to be reminded in this era of crash-program applied research that many fundamental discoveries elucidating the pathogenesis and mechanisms of disease states came about through the investigation of just such basic phenomena, often with grounds for anticipating a relationship far less than is the case with grief. One is reminded of the controversies concerning the role of miasmas in the pathogenesis of malaria. The investigation of the climatic and geographic conditions under which malaria occurred eventually provided the basis for elucidation of the disease even though the original theories concerning the miasmas were erroneous.
3. If the actual or threatened loss of an object so consistently disturbs the total adjustment of the organism, then we have identified an etiologic factor of such general importance as to put it in the same class as other major noxa, e.g., physical agents, microorganisms, etc. Until—and not until—much more is known about the biochemical, physiological, and psychological consequences of such losses, no one is justified in passing judgment as to how important this factor is in the genesis of the disease states that seem so often to follow close upon an episode of grief. To dismiss such inquiry as unnecessary or irrelevant

at this stage of our knowledge is an expression of prejudice (in its literal sense, a prejudgment, or forming a judgment without due knowledge or examination). Who now would be so rash as to dismiss the possibilities that biochemical or physiological processes occurring during the grief reaction may not constitute conditions conducive to other somatic changes of more serious consequence?
4. As a corollary of the above, we identify a ubiquitous *psychological stress,* meaning that the concept of objects and of object loss is only meaningful in terms of the existence and operation of the mental apparatus. This means that whatever the consequences of object loss and grief may be, whether manifest ultimately in biochemical, physiological, psychological, or social terms, they must first be initiated in the central nervous system. This imposes upon the medical scientist the necessity to pay more attention to the role of the central nervous system in the maintenance of the functional integrity of the organism as a whole as well as of its various parts. In spite of much lip service to the contrary, most physicians and clinical investigators think and work as if the central nervous system is the seat only of reflexes and of purely intellectual processes and really needs not be considered when studying disease manifest elsewhere in the body. The reluctance and/or inability to consider psychological components of man and his illnesses actually has come to include the nervous system as well. But new knowledge of central integrating and regulating processes, as has been brought forth by recent work on the limbic and reticular activating systems, promises soon to dissipate this barrier.[7]
5. The concept of grief as a disease requires that we keep in view and in perspective aspects of the external environment other than what we have been accustomed to heretofore—namely, the environment made up of the significant psychic objects. This becomes one reason why the persons, job, home, goals, etc., in the life of our patients cannot be disregarded in our consideration of illness, at least not until it has been proven that the vicissitudes of object relations, including grief, the disorder consequent to object loss, plays no role in the pathogenesis of disease.
6. If object loss is a potential stress, then maintenance of objects or replacement of objects must be considered as important variables in sustaining health and adjustment. The physician, the hospital, the clinical investigator, indeed, even the experiment, may come to fulfill the requirements of a necessary and supporting psychic object for a patient. Everyone is aware of the therapeutic influence of the physician on the patient, but how many unwary clinical investigators have been observing physiologic or biochemical changes in their experimental subjects, believing these to be the influence of some drug or other procedure when in fact these changes were secondary to the varying effects of the experimenter's unwitting role as a psychic object for the patient. For many

varieties of clinical investigation it is necessary to regard the experimenter as part of the experiment.[8]

This does not exhaust the Pandora's box opened by such a perspective. Once opened, we cannot easily refute the real, yet unknown influences that must now come under our scrutiny. Yet the human mind, that wonderful instrument of discovery, has a disconcerting capacity to use denial, to turn away from that which is not easily comprehended or which has awesome implications, as I believe is true of this concept. The first response when confronted with news of a grievous loss is, "No, it can't be. I don't believe it; I won't believe it." I would call your attention to the fact that cherished ideas, even if false, are also psychic objects and as such are not easily given up. And only time and much work will establish whose cherished ideas are the false ones.

I close with a quotation ascribed to Albert Szent-Gyorgyi: "Research is to see what everybody else has seen and think what nobody else has thought." To this I would only add that Szent-Gyorgyi wisely refrained from claiming that this necessarily implied that the "new" thought is correct—at least, not until tested. And that is my challenge!

References

1. Engel GL: Homeostasis, behavioral adjustment and the concept of health and disease, in Mid-Century Psychiatry. Edited by Grinker R. Thomas, Springfield, IL, 1953, pp 33–59
2. Engel GL: Selection of clinical material in psychosomatic medicine: the need for a new physiology. Psychosom Med 16:368, 1954
3. Engel GL: A unified concept of health and disease. Perspectives in Biology and Medicine 3(4), 1960
4. Freud S: Mourning and melancholia (1917), in The Standard Edition of the Complete Psychological Works of Sigmund Freud, Vol 14. Hogarth Press, London, 1957, p 237
5. Lindemann E: Symptomatology and management of acute grief. Am J Psychiat 101:14, 1944
6. Schmale AH: Relationship of separation and depression to disease. Psychosom Med 20:259, 1958
7. Jasper HH (ed): Reticular Formation of the Brain. Little, Boston, MA, 1958
8. Engel GL, Reichsman F, Segal HL: A study of an infant with a gastric fistula, I: behavior and the rate of total HCl secretion. Psychosom Med 18:374, 1956

CHAPTER 2

Concurrent Plasma Epinephrine, Norepinephrine and 17-Hydroxycorticosteroid Levels During Conditioned Emotional Disturbances in Monkeys

JOHN W. MASON, M.D.,
GEORGE MANGAN, JR., PH.D.,
JOSEPH V. BRADY, PH.D.,
DONALD CONRAD, M.A., AND
DAVID McK. RIOCH, M.D.

Prefatory Remarks

Herbert Weiner, M.D., Dr. Med. (hon.)

After working approximately 7 years at the Walter Reed Army Institute of Research, Mason perfected techniques for estimating plasma levels of catecholamines and 17-hydroxycorticosteroids (17-OHCS). He joined forces with a distinguished experimental psychologist, Brady, who pioneered the develop-

---

Volume 23, 1961, pp. 344–353.
From the Department of Neuroendocrinology and Department of Experimental Psychology, Walter Reed Army Institute of Research, Walter Reed Army Medical Center, Washington, D.C.
Presented at the Annual Meeting of the American Psychosomatic Society, Mar. 30, 1958.
Received for publication July 8, 1960.

ment of the "conditioned avoidance and emotional" methods—rigorously controllable, quantifiable experimental techniques for eliciting behavioral responses in monkeys—which are designed to teach them to avoid a signaled electrical shock or, by pairing a tone with an unavoidable shock, to elicit "fear." A variation on the theme of unavoidable shock was to add a component of unpredictability to the technique.

In contrast to the work of Cannon and Selye, who measured single variables, Mason was interested in studying unfolding patterns of blood levels of catecholamines and 17-OHCS during three distinct conditions—avoidable, unavoidable, and unpredictable conditions. Mason and his collaborators predicted that distinct patterns would be found in these three situations. By contrast, Selye used experimental "stressors" that were unavoidable and injurious and found an invariant outcome. The results of these experiments bore out the prediction. For example, during the acquisition of avoidant responses, a progressive increase in 17-OHCS levels was observed, but no change in plasma epinephrine content occurred, whereas norepinephrine levels rose quickly and then plateaued. When signaled shocks were unavoidable, similar effects were seen, except that norepinephrine levels fell rapidly after the initial increase. When the preexperimental period of waiting was ambiguous, large increases occurred in the levels of both catecholamines.

These experiments were continued, culminating in Mason's famous 1968 monograph that reported on the use of many other hormone measurements and their unfolding patterns over time with specific, experimental, and stressful experiences.

The use of neuroendocrine approaches in the experimental study of emotional processes has received considerable impetus from the recent development of precise biochemical methods for the measurement of hormone concentrations in blood and urine. In view of the known interaction and interdependence of the hormones of the various endocrine systems, it appears almost axiomatic that one of the ultimate goals of the neuroendocrinologist must be the investigation of the possibility that levels of the many hormones are integrated into characteristic and metabolically purposeful patterns. It is clear that the experimental study of such patterns of endocrine secretion can be achieved only by the accurate measurement of the levels of many hormones at the same time in various types of situations involving reactions to psychological or physical stimuli.

Previous reports from this laboratory have been concerned with the study of pituitary-adrenal cortical responses, as judged by plasma 17-OH-CS levels, to various conditioned emotional stimuli in monkeys.[1,2] In the extension of this work it has recently become possible for us to measure, during such conditioned emotional disturbances, the plasma levels of epinephrine and norepinephrine as well, thus permitting observations of concurrent activity in the anterior pituitary-adrenal cortical system and the sympathetic-adrenal medullary system. Both of these systems are believed to be set into action by generally similar circumstances, that is, conditions involving "threat" or "alarm" to the organism. Clearly, close interrelationships must exist between the central mechanisms integrating the responses of these two systems, but remarkably little direct experimental evidence yet exists that helps define these relationships in terms of the emotional or situational correlates of the release of specific hormones. This report, then, describes a beginning attempt, in the study of this problem, to bring recently developed techniques for the measurement of plasma 17-OH-CS, and epinephrine, and norepinephrine concentrations together with experimental psychological conditioning techniques for the analysis of emotional behavior in the monkey.

Methods

Experiments were conducted with mature rhesus monkeys of both sexes, weighing between 7 and 12 lb. Preliminary experience indicated that conventional procedures for catching and restraining the monkeys, and for performing venipuncture were obviously not applicable to this study because such procedures were in themselves often associated with catecholamine elevations. Consequently, all experiments were performed on animals after they were adapted to an experimental chair-type restraining apparatus previously described as suitable for long-term studies with the monkey.[3,4] Blood samples were obtained by means of an indwelling polyethylene cardiac catheter inserted into the region of the right atrium through the internal jugular vein. The catheter was exteriorized and anchored at the top of the head, and kept patent by a slow infusion of physiological saline solution. This technique is described in greater detail elsewhere.[5] The monkey, seated in the chair, was housed in a sound-resistant cubicle to minimize interference from environmental disturbances. The catheter was extended through the top of the booth into an adjacent room so that blood samples could be withdrawn without handling or confronting the animal. The time required for withdrawal of a 5-ml. heparinized blood sample averaged about 30 sec. Samples were centrifuged immediately, and the plasma was processed and analyzed by the Weil-Malherbe and Bone Method, as described previously.[6,7] Our confidence in the usefulness and reliability of this method was strengthened considerably by a previous series of physiological studies.[8] Plasma 17-OH-CS levels were determined by the Nelson-Samuels Method.[9,10] After withdrawal of the plasma for hormone analysis, the washed red blood cells were reinjected into the donor animal.

For behavioral studies, the chair was equipped with a panel of signal lights, a small loudspeaker for auditory stimuli, a hand lever with which the monkey could operate a microswitch, and footrests wired for administration of electric shock. The conditioning procedures were automatically programed and cumulative recordings of lever-pressing responses were obtained for all experimental sessions. Sessions, usually 30 min. long, were carried out at the same time of day (usually 11 a.m.) with a given animal, and were not repeated more than twice weekly (Tuesday and Friday). Precautions were taken so that the animal was undisturbed for at least 2 hr. before each session.

Conditioned Avoidance Procedure

The conditioned avoidance procedure used in these experiments has been previously described in some detail.[1] Briefly, it involves training the animal to press the lever in order to postpone or avoid a shock that would otherwise be delivered automatically every 20 sec. Blood samples were withdrawn immediately before and 10 and 30 min. after the start of a session. The catecholamine levels of each sample were determined, while the 17-OH-CS levels were measured only in the control and 30-min. samples. In sessions involving hormone measurements, the shock mechanism was usually disconnected until after the blood sample was withdrawn 10 min. after the start of the session. This precaution served to eliminate the possible complication of a shock just prior to the collection of this sample. In most instances this proved unnecessary because lever response rates were usually much higher than the minimum rate required for successful avoidance.

Conditioned Fear or Anxiety Procedure

The conditioned "fear" or "anxiety" procedure used in these experiments has also been previously described in detail.[1] It involves training the animal by presenting a tone for 3-min., which is terminated concurrently with an electric shock to the feet. Such tone-shock pairings are superimposed during sessions in which the animal is pressing the hand lever for sugar pellets or other rewards of food. In this way the disturbing effects of the superimposed stimulus may be measured by the degree of suppression of lever pressing behavior during the 3-min. tone periods as compared with intervening 3 min. periods without the tone. During sessions involving hormone measurements, shock was not delivered and, after the initial training period, needed only to be applied occasionally to maintain the characteristic behavioral and endocrine responses. The sampling procedures, session duration and frequency, and other experimental details were the same as for the avoidance experiments.

Multiple Schedule Program

Another conditioning situation studied was developed from the conditioned fear procedure but was believed to involve a strong component of uncertainty or unpredictability. The situation can probably be best described by reviewing the complete sequence of experimental events as shown in Figure 2–1. Generally, it may be termed a multiple schedule program in which the animal has different kinds of experimental sessions on different days. A session of Type 1 is initiated by withdrawal of a blood sample, and is followed immediately by presentation of a steady white light indicating that lever responses will be rewarded with food pellets during the 30-min. period. A Type 2 session is initiated the same way, but at the end of 10 min. a clicking noise is superimposed that indicates an impending electric shock at the end of a 10-min. period. During the final 10 min., only the white light remains. Type 3 is also initiated with withdrawal of a blood sample, but this is followed immediately by the clicking noise indicating an electric shock will come in 10 min. A Type 4 session is also initiated by withdrawal of a blood sample. In this case, however, it is followed by no specific signal immediately, such as the light or tone, but there is a 10-min. period during which the animal must wait to see whether he will have in addition session Type 1, 2, or 3 on that particular day. It is during this waiting period that unusual hormone responses occur.

A similar type of multiple schedule procedure was also studied in which 10-min. waiting periods were alternated with avoidance periods and "punishment" periods of equal duration. The punishment procedure is one in which the animal inflicts a shock upon himself if he presses the lever. In a sense, this is the diametric opposite of the avoidance procedure. Sessions of this type were also initiated by the blood withdrawal procedure; in addition, an overhead light was turned on. These events were followed by a 10-min. waiting, or "$S\Delta$," period during which striking hormone responses occurred.

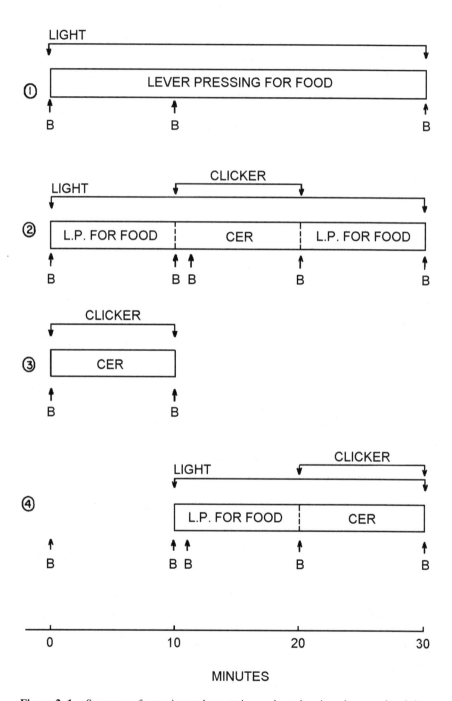

Figure 2–1. Sequence of experimental events in monkey, showing plasma epinephrine elevations during preexperimental waiting period.

Results

The individual plasma norepinephrine and epinephrine levels during 10 conditioned avoidance experiments in 4 monkeys are shown in Table 2–1. There is approximately a twofold increase in mean norepinephrine levels, from 4.6 to 9.1 µg./L., during the first 10 min., and the level drops only slightly to 8.6 µg./L. at the end of 30 min. Although the mean values indicate a slight rise for epinephrine levels at 10 min., examination of individual experiments shows that this is largely due to a response in a single experiment by Monkey M-34. This experiment was the first in which the blood withdrawal procedure was ever carried out in this monkey, and epinephrine elevations did not occur in subsequent avoidance experiments with the same animal. In Figure 2–2 the mean norepinephrine, epinephrine, and 17-OH-CS levels during avoidance in these animals are compared with the mean levels observed in a similar period on control days without conditioning sessions. The mean plasma 17-OH-CS elevation of 10 µg.% in 30 min. closely approximates the maximal rate of rise previously described in the monkey.[2] The pattern, then, for conditioned avoidance appears to be marked 17-OH-CS and norepinephrine elevations with little, if any, change in epinephrine levels.

Table 2–1. Plasma norepinephrine and epinephrine levels during conditioned avoidance sessions

Monkey No.	Norepinephrine (µg./L.)			Epinephrine (µg./L.)		
	0	10 min.	30 min.	0	10 min.	30 min.
M-41	3.7	18.8	16.1	3.1	2.8	5.2
M-34	6.3	10.7	—	1.6	9.2	—
	0.0	7.5	—	0.0	0.0	—
	4.3	8.2	—	0.0	0.0	—
M-40	3.6	8.9	3.7	0.3	1.0	1.4
	2.1	0.0	6.4	0.8	0.8	1.0
	4.0	7.3	8.3	3.1	1.7	0.5
	5.7	10.9	6.1	0.0	1.5	1.6
M-45	8.6	7.2	6.8	0.3	0.6	0.6
	8.1	11.4	12.7	0.0	0.0	0.0
Mean	4.6	9.1	8.6	0.9	1.8	1.5

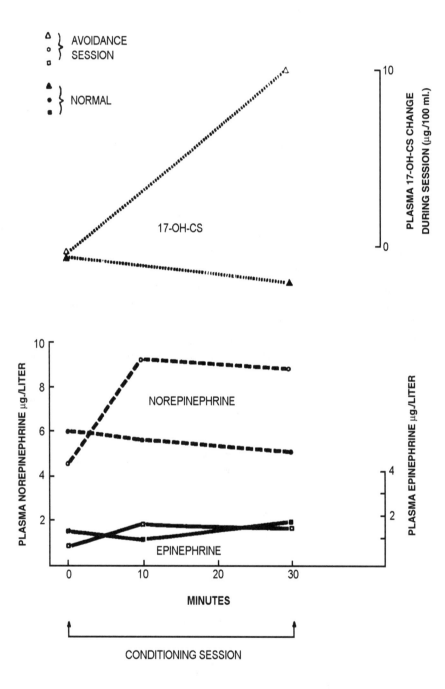

Figure 2–2. Mean plasma 17-OH-CS, norepinephrine, and epinephrine levels during 30-min. conditioned avoidance sessions.

In view of the extremely small changes in plasma epinephrine levels, additional experiments were done in 2 monkeys to test for the possible occurrence of an epinephrine response prior to the 10 min. sample. Figure 2–3 shows that no substantial changes in epinephrine levels were evident in blood samples

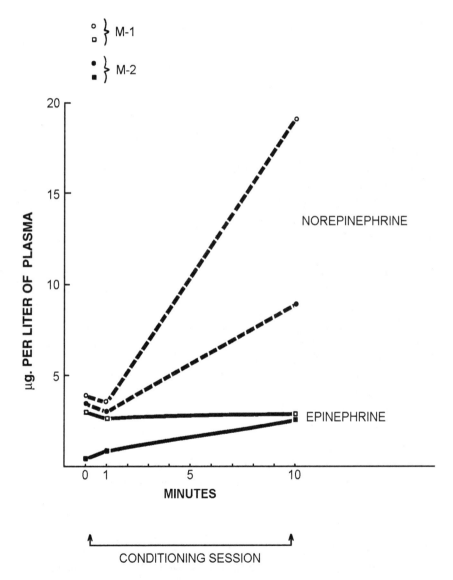

Figure 2–3. Plasma norepinephrine and epinephrine levels during 10-min. conditioned avoidance sessions.

withdrawn 1 min. after the onset of avoidance sessions.

Observations on the effects of conditioned anxiety sessions were limited to a series of experimental and control observations in 1 monkey. The pattern for the mean plasma norepinephrine, 17-OH-CS, and epinephrine levels during conditioned anxiety sessions (Figure 2–4) shows a striking similarity to the pattern observed in the conditioned avoidance experiments. There is a marked plasma 17-OH-CS elevation, a twofold increase in norepinephrine levels at 10 min. with a return to the normal range at 30 min., while epinephrine levels show little, if any, change throughout the session. This animal was studied at an early stage of this work and was not as well shielded from environmental disturbances, as were later animals. It was observed in 3 experiments that the baseline norepinephrine values were high—above 10 μg./L. It was also noticed that, on such days, the monkey did not show the usual hormone responses to the conditioned stimulus. Figure 2–5 shows the mean responses to conditioned anxiety sessions in this animal, if one arbitrarily subgroups the data into those experiments with norepinephrine baseline values above 10 μg./L. compared with those having baselines below 10 μg./L. A twofold elevation occurs when the baseline is below 10 μg./L., while no elevation is observed when the initial baseline value of norepinephrine exceeds 10 μg./L. Epinephrine levels are remarkably constant in both subgroups.

The relative stability of epinephrine levels in our experiments up to this point greatly intensified our interest in the occasional instances where marked epinephrine elevations occurred. The experiment illustrated as Session 4 in Figure 2–1 was one of the first in which large elevations in epinephrine were observed. Figure 2–6 shows the mean plasma norepinephrine and epinephrine levels from successive sessions of this type, indicating the epinephrine levels rose from almost no detectable amount to 8 μg./L. during the 10 min. period that the animal was presumably waiting to receive the specific signal that would indicate which of several types of experimental session was to ensue on that particular day. In samples taken 1 ½ min. after presentation of the specific signal, mean epinephrine levels fell precipitously from 8 μg./L. to 0.5 μg./L. and remained low for the remainder of the session. Norepinephrine levels also rose sharply during the waiting period, dropped moderately with the food signal, but rose again with the conditioned anxiety stimulus.

In a somewhat related experiment, extremely large epinephrine and norepinephrine responses are shown during a 10 min. waiting period prior to the onset of a multiple schedule procedure involving random admixtures of conditioned avoidance, punishment, and rest (*S68*) periods (Figure 2–7). It is of interest that epinephrine and norepinephrine levels decline again after the first specific signal, even though in this case, it was the flashing red light indicating avoidance.

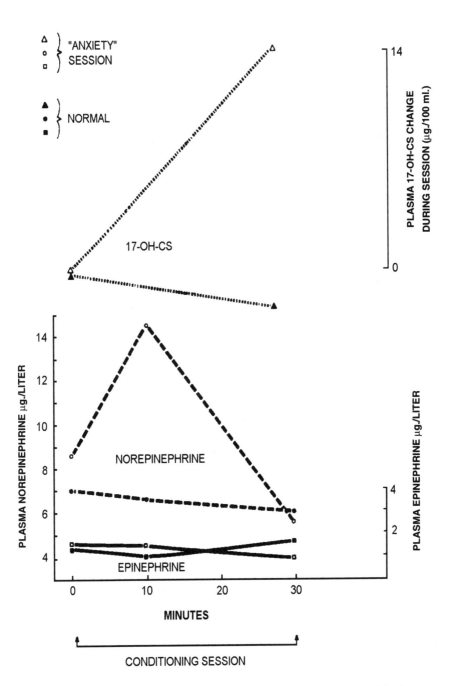

Figure 2–4. Mean plasma 17-OH-CS, norepinephrine, and epinephrine levels in the monkey, during conditioned anxiety or CER sessions.

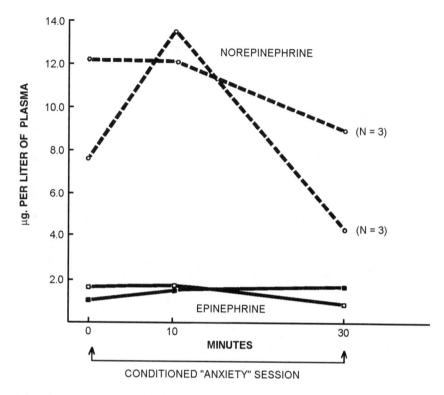

Figure 2–5. Effect of initial baseline level on plasma norepinephrine response to a conditioned anxiety stimulus in a monkey.

Discussion

These studies, involving biochemical measurement of plasma 17-OH-CS, norepinephrine, and epinephrine levels in the conscious monkey, indicate that the level of norepinephrine in peripheral blood increases substantially during a variety of emotional disturbances. In fact, the most common response pattern observed throughout these experiments was characterized by elevations in plasma norepinephrine and 17-OH-CS levels, suggesting a rather broad, nonspecific character for the norepinephrine response.

On the other hand, there appeared to be a greater degree of specificity in the conditions leading to increased epinephrine secretion. While norepinephrine and 17-OH-CS elevations occurred in virtually all of the conditioned emotional disturbances investigated in this study, the instances in which marked epinephrine

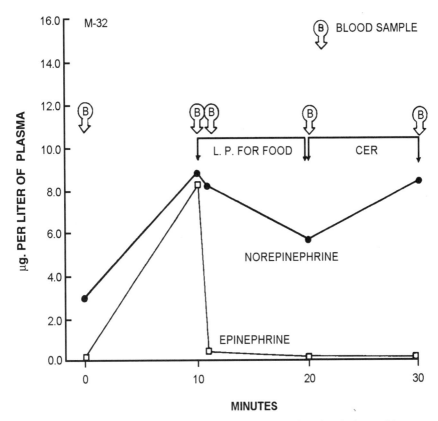

Figure 2–6. Mean plasma epinephrine and norepinephrine elevation during ambiguous preexperimental waiting period.

elevations occurred—that is, levels above 2.5 µg./L., were relatively rare and perhaps bear brief enumeration at this point. Two monkeys, including M-34, as shown in Table 2–1, have shown substantial epinephrine elevations during their first experience with the blood withdrawal procedure involving the intracardiac catheter. This finding prompted us to sham-bleed subsequent monkeys several times initially in order to eliminate this effect. Two monkeys tested in the waiting period conditioning situation showed large epinephrine elevations (Figure 2–6). One monkey on the multiple schedule procedure showed marked epinephrine elevations (Figure 2–7). One monkey trained on avoidance showed a moderate epinephrine elevation when his lever was removed and the red light avoidance signal presented. In a recent experiment, a monkey with a long history of avoidance showed marked epinephrine elevations when he was given occasional free or undeserved shocks during an avoidance session. Although similar

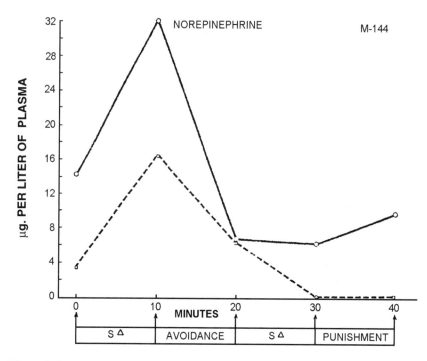

Figure 2–7. Plasma epinephrine and norepinephrine levels in monkey on multiple schedule conditioning procedure.

shocks prior to avoidance training produced little change in epinephrine levels, their occurrence following long experience with successful avoidance behavior appears to take on a new and powerful significance to the animal.

Although the experiments just enumerated involve some diversity of conditions, it appears that certain common elements are present that may bear closer examination in terms of their special relevance to epinephrine release. One striking feature of these situations is that they all possess an appreciable degree of uncertainty, novelty, or unpredictability. The animal has been faced with a threatening situation for the first time, has had the stability or predictability removed from a previously mastered situation, or has been confronted with a conditioned stimulus that has inherent ambiguity. In an effort to relate these observations to adaptive aspects of behavior, it might be suggested that predictability is an important element in the animal's anticipation of mastery or failure in a threatening situation and that these findings are quite compatible with formulations such as those of Funkenstein's, based upon indirect assessment of catecholamine secretion.[11] The present data, however, suggest some modification of the viewpoints derived from earlier clinical work in this field.

So far, in our experience with the monkey it appears that, while norepinephrine level increases may occur in the face of constant epinephrine levels, epinephrine elevations commonly occur with norepinephrine elevations. In fact, the rises in norepinephrine accompanying epinephrine elevations are usually greater than those observed when epinephrine levels remain constant. Under the particular conditions of the present studies, then, it appears that elevations may occur in norepinephrine alone, or of norepinephrine and epinephrine, but not of epinephrine alone. Many additional observations will be needed, however, in further evaluation of this aspect of the problem. The situations involving norepinephrine release alone are characterized as relatively stereotyped, predictable situations in which the conditions associated with the administration of the noxious stimulus to the animal are unambiguous and familiar.

While such elements as the unpredictability, complexity, or difficulty associated with the adaptive task appear to be of special significance in these experiments, it is clear that they must be considered in close relationship to other factors, particularly those concerned with motivational processes. All conditioning sessions in which marked epinephrine elevations were observed involved the threat of a painful stimulus. That the anticipation of pain alone, however, is not sufficient to excite epinephrine release is clear from the regular avoidance and CER situations in which no such response was observed. Yet it appears likely that the anticipation of a noxious stimulus plays a contributory role, in combination with other elements in the situation, which is critical in the production of epinephrine release.

An additional factor of possible importance, as suggested in these experiments, is the anticipation of adaptive or coping activity by the animal. Most of the situations involving epinephrine release appear to entail the necessity for an anticipatory set associated with a high probability that the animal will be required to do something, i.e., act upon the environment to deal with the environmental threat. Since the metabolic effects of epinephrine in the redistribution of blood to skeletal muscles, heart, and brain and in the rapid mobilization of energy resources appear obviously directed at the support of increased muscular activity, the selective occurrence of epinephrine release when the probability of strenuous, coping activity is high would have attractive teleological support. Furthermore, the powerful catabolic effects of epinephrine, necessitating costly and time-consuming reparative metabolic processes in the aftermath of its release, would furnish an additional reason that a highly selective, economical type of control for epinephrine secretion might serve a useful physiological purpose. The present experiments suggest that, if the anticipation of coping activity is important, it must be considered as interrelated to other elements in the situation such as unpredictability and the nature of the threat.

Perhaps the most general conclusion to be drawn from the present studies is the demonstration of the potential value of including a neuroendocrine approach in interdisciplinary studies directed at the differentiation of emotional states. These experimental results furnish a biological basis for distinguishing between two apparently distinct hyperalerting responses that tend to be frequently and uncritically subsumed under the general heading of anxiety or distress. The challenge that remains for future investigation is to define more completely the precise behavioral or situational factors that characterize the two apparently distinct categories of emotional response delimited in these experiments. Our present efforts are being directed largely to the exploration of a variety of experimental situations of the vigilance or monitoring type in which it may be possible to vary independently and quantitatively some of the variables discussed as having possible relevance to epinephrine release. It should be clear that any interpretations at this point have value only insofar as they help to generate future experiments and lead us in the direction of simpler, more operational formulations which may eventually permit predictive studies.

Summary

In studies involving biochemical measurement of plasma 17-OH-CS, norepinephrine, and epinephrine levels during conditioned emotional disturbances in monkeys, elevations in 17-OH-CS and norepinephrine levels were observed in a variety of experimental situations. The regulation of epinephrine secretion, however, appeared to have a more selective basis.

In relatively stereotyped, predictable situations such as avoidance and CER, patterns of 17-OH-CS and norepinephrine elevation, with little or no change in plasma epinephrine levels, were observed.

In first experience situations and rather complicated, multiple-schedule conditioning procedures, a pattern of marked 17-OH-CS, norepinephrine, and epinephrine elevations was observed. These experiments suggest that several interacting elements may be necessary for marked epinephrine release during anticipatory responses. An effort has been made to identify some of these elements in terms of both environmental and biological factors that appear to be common to those situations in which marked epinephrine elevations were observed. It is suggested that the element of uncertainty or unpredictability, in combination with such factors as the threat of a noxious stimulus and the anticipation of coping activity, may be a particularly critical factor in the determination of epinephrine release during emotional disturbances.

References

1. Mason JW, Brady JV, Sidman M: Plasma 17-hydroxycorticosteroid levels and conditioned behavior in the rhesus monkey. Endocrinology 60:741, 1957
2. Mason JW: Psychological influences on the pituitary-adrenal cortical system, in Recent Progress in Hormone Research, Vol 15. Acad Press, New York, 1959, pp 345–389
3. Mason JW: A restraining chair for the experimental study of primates. J Appl Physiol 12:130, 1958
4. Mason JW, Harwood CT, Rosenthal NR: Influence of some environmental factors on plasma and urinary 17-hydroxycorticosteroid levels in the rhesus monkey. Am J Physiol 190:429, 1957
5. Mason JW: In preparation
6. Weil-Malherbe H, Bone AD: The chemical estimation of adrenaline-like substances in blood. Biochem J 51:311, 1952
7. Mangan GF, Mason JW: The fluorimetric measurement of plasma epinephrine and norepinephrine concentrations in man, monkey and dog. J Lab Clin Med 51:484, 1958
8. Mangan GF, Mason JW: Fluorimetric measurement of exogenous and endogenous epinephrine and norepinephrine in peripheral blood. Am J Physiol 194:476, 1958
9. Nelson DH, Samuels LT: A method for the determination of 17-hydroxycorticosteroids in blood: 17-hydroxycorticosterone in the peripheral circulation. J Clin Endocrinol 12:519, 1952
10. Harwood CT, Mason JW: A systematic evaluation of the Nelson-Samuels plasma 17-hydroxycorticosteroid method. J Clin Endocrinol 16:790, 1956
11. Funkenstein DH: Mastery of Stress. Harvard, Cambridge, MA, 1957

CHAPTER 3

Specific Attitudes in Initial Interviews With Patients Having Different "Psychosomatic" Diseases

DAVID T. GRAHAM, M.D.,
RICHARD M. LUNDY, PH.D.,
LORNA S. BENJAMIN, PH.D.,
J.D. KABLER, M.D.,
WILLIAM C. LEWIS, M.D.,
NANCY O. KUNISH, B.A., AND
FRANCES K. GRAHAM, PH.D.

Prefatory Remarks

Joseph D. Sapira, M.D.

In 1952, Grace and Graham published a specificity hypothesis in *Psychosomatic Medicine*. The hypothesis stated that for each psychosomatic disease a specific attitude developed toward the stressful stimuli and physiologic response of that disease. Ten years later, Graham et al. published this article consisting of two studies characterized by careful science and the simultaneous investigation of the same seven diseases that were being studied by Franz Alexander's group in Chicago. (This article additionally includes multiple sclerosis, idiopathic cyclic edema in females, and migraine—only migraine then being considered a psychosomatic disease by most.)

Because this article and the work of Alexander's group (published 6 years later in 1968) represent the only two simultaneous evaluations of all seven diseases, certain comparisons are inevitable. First, the positive results of both studies are not strictly comparable because the work presented in this article was concerned with conscious attitudes easily discernible at the interview, whereas Alexander's group studied the inferred psychodynamic formulations derived from up to three interviews. Second, Graham et al. used both an informed interviewer and a "blind" interviewer (naive to the hypothesis being tested), whereas Alexander used only informed interviewers. Third, Graham et al.'s work used both medical and nonmedical raters (who usually did not differ in accuracy), whereas Alexander's group used both analytic and nonanalytic physicians (who did differ in diagnostic accuracy).

The similarities of the two studies were that 1) both were diagnostically accurate for individual diseases at about the 50% level, which was statistically significant; and 2) both of these studies, although long awaited by workers in the field, had relatively little impact; medical textbooks did not and do not include their results. (This shows that some people will not change their minds no matter how good the data are.) Finally, neither study generated subsequent comparable work, although this article is remarkable by current standards for containing its own replication study. In fact, the methodology and design concepts of this work may represent its other major legacy in addition to content.

A specificity-of-attitude hypothesis for psychosomatic disease, proposed by Grace and Graham,[3] states that there is a specific relation between the attitude which a person develops towards a stressful stimulus and the physiological changes which occur in response to the stimulus. An attitude is defined as the perception of the stimulus situation and the response tendency aroused by it, that is, as what an individual feels is happening to him and what he wishes to do about it. Attitudes said to be associated with 18 diseases have been described. The present paper reports two studies of the relation between disease and attitude as revealed by initial interviews with hospitalized patients.

Patients from the medical service were interviewed concerning events that had occurred prior to the onset or to an exacerbation of their diseases. The recorded interviews were edited to remove references identifying diseases and were then submitted to judges who selected from a list of the previously described 18 attitudes the three attitudes most similar to those expressed in the interview. Judges also ranked all 18 attitudes in the order of their applicability to each patient. The first study employed interviews with 16 patients having eight diseases. The results were reproduced in a second study of 20 patients having 10 diseases. Both studies investigated whether an attitude predicted to be associated with a disease was more applicable to patients having the disease than to patients who did not have the disease.

Procedure

Interviewers

Half of the interviews were conducted by an internist who is in the practice of psychosomatic medicine and is an author of the specificity hypothesis. The remaining interviews were conducted by a psychologist. He was experienced in nondirective therapy but had had no previous association with the School of Medicine or with patients having psychosomatic disease. The psychologist served as a "blind" interviewer. He knew in what form material was desired, but since he did not know the hypothesized attitude-disease relations, they could not influence his conduct of the interview.

Interviews

The purpose of the interview was to locate events occurring close to the onset or exacerbation of a disease and to obtain a statement from the patient of his attitude towards the events. Before the study began, a semi-structured interview technique was developed. The interview lasted for 1 hour. In an introductory period the patient's permission to record the interview was secured and was followed for approximately 10 min. by inquiry concerning symptoms. The patient was then asked what was happening in his life at the time of the most recent attack or at the onset of the disease. This question was used to shift the discussion to personal problems and relationships, and for approximately

20 min. the patient was encouraged to take the lead in bringing out any problem areas. A detailed inquiry into precipitating events and the attitudes associated with them constituted the remainder of the interview. The interviewer was directed to establish the chronological relationship between events and symptoms and, if an attitude was not expressed spontaneously, to question for it. Such questions were restricted to those of a general nature: "How did you feel about that? What were the consequences for you? What seemed to you to be happening?" The use of attitude expressions by the interviewer or the restating of patients' statements in attitude terms was prohibited.

Interviews were edited by the internist interviewer to remove references to symptoms, types of treatment, and illnesses among relatives. A set of rules was devised to make this task as routine as possible. A second reader checked the original editing for any missed references or unnecessary deletions.

Subjects

Ward and private patients on the medical service of the Wisconsin General Hospital served as subjects. In the first study, eight diseases were represented: essential hypertension, bronchial asthma, duodenal ulcer, eczema, hyperthyroidism, multiple sclerosis, rheumatoid arthritis, and ulcerative colitis. The second study included these same diseases plus migraine and metabolic edema (idiopathic edema of females). These were in each instance the primary disease, the major reason for hospitalization. Every patient had a secure diagnosis, made by members of the Department of Medicine. Diagnostic criteria included the following: for essential hypertension, more than half of the diastolic blood pressure readings greater than 100 in the absence of other disease affecting blood pressure; for bronchial asthma, episodic wheezing; for duodenal ulcer, epigastric pain and X-ray confirmation; for eczema, lesions which were chronic, red, itching, and lichenified; for hyperthyroidism, elevated radioiodine uptake and the typical clinical signs; for multiple sclerosis, diagnosis by a neurologist; for rheumatoid arthritis, the criteria for either "classical" or "definite" rheumatoid arthritis listed in the 1958 Revision of "Diagnostic Criteria";[4] for ulcerative colitis, X-ray or proctoscopic evidence; for migraine, high intensity, pulsatile, episodic headache; for metabolic edema, episodic edema not necessarily related to menses and occurring in the absence of cardiac, renal, hepatic, or other disease processes known to be associated with edema.

There were 2 patients with each disease in each of the two studies. One patient with each disease was interviewed by the internist, and one by the psychologist. Of the 36 patients, 21 were female, 15 male; 35 were white, 1 Indian. Ages ranged from 18–78 years with a mean of 41.

Selection of patients for the psychologist interviews was determined by the availability on a given research day of a patient having a disease desired for the study. Diseases were arranged in a priority order, on the basis of probable scarcity, and patients with the highest-listed diseases were selected. The only other requirements were that patients should speak English and that, in the judgment of the medical resident, they should not be obviously psychotic or depressed. In the second study the additional restrictions of superficially normal hearing and age between 18–59 were imposed. The size of the medical service was such that the need to choose among patients meeting these criteria did not arise. No effort was made in either study to select patients known to have emotional problems.

In selecting patients for the internist interviewer, the same procedure was followed for 7 of 8 patients in the first study and for 6 of 10 in the second study. Interviews with the remaining 5 patients, who were also on the in-patient medical service, were arranged in response to consultation requests.

Judges

Four individuals judged the attitudes expressed in each interview. One judge was an internist trained in psychosomatic medicine and a professor of medicine. A second judge was a practicing psychoanalyst and a professor of psychiatry. The third was a postdoctoral fellow in psychology whose previous work had been in experimental psychology, and the fourth was a psychology student who had completed one semester of graduate work.

To provide a common basis for the judging task, judges listened to a recording of 15-min. excerpts from initial interviews with 6 patients, the tapes obtained earlier. The judges rated the attitudes expressed by the 6 trial patients and discussed any questions that arose concerning the nature of the judging task. They were then given the typed and edited complete transcript of 1 patient on the training tape. This case served as practice and as a check on the clarity of the judging instructions. It was not included in the results of the study.

Interviews of patients in the study were then presented to judges in a predetermined order. The order was assigned randomly except that no more than two interviews by the same interviewer were to be given in succession and that no more than two interviews with patients having the same disease were to be given in succession. Judges knew that two interviewers were being employed in the study although their names were deleted from the records. They did not know how many or which diseases were being investigated nor whether patients without psychosomatic disease were part of the study.

The first three judges rated the 16 interviews of the first study over a 4-

month period. They were not informed of results until completion of that study. The second study began approximately 3 months later, and again the three judges were not informed of results until completion of the judging. The fourth judge entered the study after the second one had started and was informed of the patient's disease after judging each interview. Interspersed among the 20 interviews of the second study were three additional interviews obtained for a special study of metabolic edema. Judgments about these are not included in the present study.

Judgments

In the first study, judges were asked to complete for each case a record form on which they were asked to (1) check whether a precipitating event was identified in the interview; (2) check whether the event was a "significant" one; (3) briefly describe the precipitating event(s); (4) check if no attitude or none of the listed attitudes was expressed during the interview; (5) select and rank, from a list of 18 attitudes, the three statements which best describe the patient's attitude towards a precipitating event; (6) document the choices by quoting the patient's words which most clearly expressed the three attitudes; (7) rate the patient's insight into the relationship of life problems to the disease; (8) rate the patient's willingness to discuss emotional problems. After all interviews had been judged, the judges were asked to rank all 18 attitudes as to degree of applicability to each patient.

The following changes in procedure were made in the second study. Judges ranked all 18 attitudes at the same time that they completed other parts of the record form. They also rated on a 6-point scale their degree of certainty as to the applicability of the first three attitude choices.

Attitudes

The 18 attitudes, including the possible alternative statements in parentheses, were presented to the judges in the form in which they are listed below. The disease predicted to be associated with each attitude has been added.

1. *Urticaria.* Felt he was taking a beating and was helpless to do anything about it (was being knocked around, hammered on, being mistreated or unfairly treated).
2. *Ulcerative colitis.* Felt he was being injured and degraded and wished he could get rid of the responsible agent (was being humiliated, screwed; wanted the situation to be finished, over and done with, disposed of).

3. *Eczema.* Felt he was being frustrated and could do nothing about it except take it out on himself (felt interfered with, blocked, prevented from doing something, unable to make self understood).
4. *Acne.* Felt he was being picked on or at and wanted to be let alone (being nagged at).
5. *Psoriasis.* Felt there was a constant gnawing at him and that he had to put up with it (a steady boring, a constant nagging or irritation or annoyance).
6. *Bronchial asthma.* Felt left out in the cold and wanted to shut the person or situation out (felt unloved, rejected, disapproved of, shut out, and wished not to deal with the person or situation, wished to blot it or him out, not have anything to do with it or him).
7. *Hyperthyroidism.* Felt might lose somebody or something he loved and took care of and tried to prevent loss of the loved person or object (tried to hold on to somebody loved and taken care of).
8. *Vomiting.* Felt something wrong had happened, usually something for which the patient felt responsible, and wished it hadn't happened (was sorry it happened, wished could undo what happened, wished things were the way they were before, wished he hadn't done it).
9. *Duodenal ulcer.* Felt deprived of what was due him and wanted to get even (didn't get what he should, what was owed or promised, and wanted to get back at, get revenge, do to him what he did to me).
10. *Constipation.* Felt in a situation from which nothing good could come but kept on with it grimly (felt things would never get any better but had to stick with it).
11. *Essential hypertension.* Felt threatened with harm and had to be ready for anything (felt in danger, anything could happen at any time from any side; had to be prepared to meet all possible threats, be on guard).
12. *Migraine.* Felt something had to be achieved and then relaxed after the effort (had to accomplish something, was driving self, striving, had to get things done, a goal had to be reached; then let down, stopped the driving).
13. *Multiple sclerosis.* Felt he was forced to undertake some kind of physical activity, especially hard work, and wanted not to (had to work without help, had to support self and usually others; wanted not to and might or might not express wish for help or support).
14. *Metabolic edema.* Felt he was carrying a heavy load and wanted somebody else to carry all or part of it (had too much on his shoulders, too much responsibility; wanted others to take their share of it).
15. *Rheumatoid arthritis.* Felt tied down and wanted to get free (felt restrained, restricted, confined, and wanted to be able to move around).
16. *Raynaud's disease.* Wanted to take hostile physical action (wanted to hit or

strangle, wanted to take action of any kind, had to do something).
17. *Regional enteritis.* Felt had received something harmful and wanted to get rid of it (had been given or received something damaged or inferior, felt had been poisoned, wanted the situation to be finished, over and done with, disposed of).
18. *Low backache.* Wanted to run away (wanted to walk out of there, get out of there).

Results

The hypothesis that particular attitudes are associated with particular diseases was tested by determining whether the attitudes which judges selected as characteristic of patients were, in fact, the attitudes predicted by the hypothesis. To characterize a patient, each judge was allowed to select three attitudes, since a single selection would probably have resulted in frequencies too low for satisfactory statistical treatment.

Judges selected the "correct" attitudes, that is, the attitudes predicted to be associated with a patient's disease, proportionately more often than they selected the *same* attitudes when patients had other diseases. Table 3–1 shows the aver-

Table 3–1. Predicted choices of attitudes compared to the mean percentage of unpredicted choices of the same attitudes

Study	Predicted choices (mean %)	Unpredicted choices (mean %)	P-value of difference[*]
	Blind interviews		
I	28.1	17.1	<.050
II	45.0	20.8	<.025
I and II	37.5	19.3	<.005
	Nonblind interviews		
I	38.4	20.2	<.050
II	62.5	13.1	<.005
I and II	52.1	16.3	<.000

[*]P values give the probability that the mean of differences for four judges, between the average proportion of attitude choices in patients with the associated disease (predicted choices) and the average proportion of attitude choices in patients without the associated disease (unpredicted choices), was greater than zero (t-test, 3 df). An arc sine transformation of the proportions was used.

age percentage of predicted choices made by the four judges in choosing the eight attitudes under study in the first experiment or the ten attitudes in the second experiment. Table 3–1 also shows the average percentage of choices of attitudes under study when patients did *not* have the associated disease (unpredicted choices). The difference between proportions of attitude choices in patients with the associated disease and proportions of attitude choices in patients without the associated disease was a significant one in each of the two studies and for both blind and nonblind interviews. Significance was determined by a t-test of whether the mean difference, for four judges, between the proportion of predicted choices and the proportion of unpredicted choices exceeded zero.

The significant results were not produced by only one judge. Table 3–2 shows that, considering both studies together, three of the four judges made predicted choices significantly more often than unpredicted choices on the blind interviews. All four of the judges made significantly more predicted choices on the nonblind interviews. Judges differed little among themselves in their numbers of predicted attitude choices, and they agreed significantly on the particular

Table 3–2. Comparison of each judge's predicted and unpredicted choices of the same attitudes

Judge[*]	Predicted choices (mean %)[†]	Unpredicted choices (mean %)[†]	P-value of difference[‡]
	Blind interviews		
A	38.9	17.5	.025
B	27.8	18.9	.244
C	44.4	21.1	.021
D	38.9	19.8	.048
	Non-blind interviews		
A[§]	52.9	15.7	.000
B	50.0	15.6	.005
C	55.6	16.6	.000
D	50.0	17.3	.002

[*]Judges A and B are medical judges; judges C and D are non-medical.
[†]Mean percentages are the mean of eight attitudes in Study I and ten attitudes in Study II.
[‡]P-values are based on the bionomial expansion and give the probability of obtaining or exceeding the obtained proportion of predicted choices if the expected proportion equals the proportion of unpredicted choices.
[§]Judge A did not judge an interview in Study I which he felt to be "platitudinous."

patients to whom they felt the predicted attitude applied. The nonmedical judges did as well as the medical.

Similar findings were obtained when, for each patient, all 18 attitudes were ranked from 1 to 18 in the order of their applicability to that patient. The median rank of a particular attitude was lower (i.e., the attitude was more applicable) for patients with the associated disease than for patients with other diseases. The differences in rank were significant for the blind interviews in the second study and for the not-blind interviews in both studies (see Table 3–3).

There were 36 patients representing 10 diseases in the two studies. Table 3–4 shows the percentage choice and median rank of the predicted attitude for each disease as well as the percentage of unpredicted choices and the rank of the same attitude in patients without that disease. The table demonstrates that every attitude was ranked lower, or chosen more frequently, when predicted by the hypothesis than when unpredicted. It would not be justified to assume, with the small number of patients in each disease category, that the predicted attitude-disease relation is more accurate for some diseases than for others.

In addition to selecting and ranking attitudes, the judges supplied various ratings described under the heading "Judgments." These are peripheral to the main investigation and will not be presented in detail. Reference is made to them below when they are relevant to the point under discussion.

Table 3–3. Median ranks of predicted attitudes and of the same attitudes in patients with other diseases

Study[*]	Median[†] rank when predicted	Median[†] rank when unpredicted	P-value of difference[‡]
	Blind interviews		
I	7.0	9.25	NS
II	4.75	9.0	<.025
I and II	4.25	9.0	<.01
	Non-blind interviews		
I	5.0	9.25	<.01
II	2.0	10.0	<.01
I and II	3.5	10.0	<.01

[*]There are eight attitudes in Study I and ten in Study II.
[†]Medians are based on ranks assigned by four judges.
[‡]P-values give the probability that the rank of predicted attitudes was lower than the rank of unpredicted attitudes. They were determined by the Wilcoxon non-parametric test for paired replicates.[5]

Table 3–4. Choice and rank of 10 attitudes when predicted and when unpredicted

Diseases* associated with the attitudes	Choices		Rank	
	Predicted (mean %)	Unpredicted (mean %)	When predicted (median)	When unpredicted (median)
Bronchial asthma	31.2	16.4	6.0	10.0
Duodenal ulcer	31.2	21.9	5.5	8.0
Eczema	43.8	19.5	4.0	7.0
Essential hypertension	66.7	8.6	2.0	13.0
Hyperthyroidism	18.8	16.4	7.0	10.5
Metabolic edema	100.0	23.6	1.0	13.0
Migraine	75.0	15.3	1.5	9.0
Multiple sclerosis	68.8	28.1	1.0	6.5
Rheumatoid arthritis	25.0	11.7	7.0	11.0
Ulcerative colitis	31.2	14.8	6.0	8.0

*Two patients had migraine and 2, metabolic edema; there were 4 patients with each of the remaining diseases.

Statistical Procedures

Selection Probability

It is common practice, when a judge makes m choices from among n objects, to assume that the chance of choosing any one of the objects is m/n. In the present study, this practice would lead to the assumption that any one attitude would have a probability of 1/18 of being selected, or of 3/18 when 3 choices were made from among 18 attitudes without replacement. However, this assumption is valid only if each attitude is as likely to be chosen as any other. Such an assumption is dubious in these studies, since there is reason to believe that patients will more readily express socially acceptable attitudes and that judges may also show bias in identifying attitudes. If the attitudes under study (8 in the first study and 10 in the second) were more or less "popular" than the remaining attitudes, the actual probability of obtaining them would not be 8:18 or 10:18 respectively, in the two studies. To correct for possible differences in popularity between the attitudes under study and the attitudes irrelevant to the study, statistical analysis was restricted to the relevant attitudes. Possible differences among the relevant attitudes were equalized by the design of the experiment, since each could be correct an equal number of times.

The null hypothesis tested was that, under the conditions of choice in the study, a particular attitude (A_i) should be selected when a patient had the associated disease (D_i) in the same proportion as when a patient had some other disease ($\overline{D}_i$). That is,

$$\frac{\text{Choices}_{A_i \text{ with } D_i}}{N_{D_i}} = \frac{\text{Choices}_{A_i \text{ with } \overline{D}_i}}{N_{\overline{D}_i}}$$

where N is number.

These proportions were obtained separately for each attitude and the mean proportions for each judge were used in the statistical analysis. Since the specificity-of-attitude hypothesis would be supported only if proportions of predicted choices significantly exceeded unpredicted choices, and would not be supported if they were unequal but less, probabilities are given for one-tail of the distribution.

As Table 3–1 shows, the average proportion of unpredicted relevant attitudes chosen was slightly larger than the 16.7 per cent which would be expected on the assumption that all attitudes were equally likely choices. The empirical estimate of the expected proportion per relevant attitude is thus a more conservative estimate with which to compare the obtained proportion of correct choices.

Agreement Comparisons

Agreement was measured by the number of predicted attitudes which pairs of judges had selected in common. This number was compared to the overlap expected by chance (predicted choices$_{\text{Judge A}}$ × predicted choices$_{\text{Judge B}}$/number of patients). Differences between obtained and expected overlap of one judge with each of the other judges were evaluated by chi square with two degrees of freedom. (Judge A, $\chi^2 = 10.73$, $P < .005$; Judge B, $\chi^2 = 12.18$, $P < .005$; Judge C, $\chi^2 = 4.61$, $P < .05$; Judge D, $\chi^2 = 8.61$, $P < .01$)

Discussion

The present findings are evidence that psychosomatic diseases can be differentiated by what a patient says in a 1-hour interview. However, the validity of the conclusion depends upon the absence of bias and other confounding influences. Possible sources of bias and the steps taken to avoid it will be discussed. Another question is whether differentiation was due solely to differences in attitudes or whether it also depended on differences in other psychological variables. Supplementary findings relevant to this point are considered, as well as results of a similar interview study carried out by Alexander and collaborators.[2]

The most serious source of bias in any study is an investigator's knowledge of the hypothesis being investigated. In the present study, this was controlled by using an interviewer who did not know the specificity hypothesis. Both his interviews and those obtained by the nonblind interviewer showed significant differentiation among diseases, although there was less differentiation among the patients interviewed blind.

While it is possible that the better results obtained in the not-blind interviews reflect bias, they were obtained under conditions which limited the way in which bias could operate. As noted earlier, the kinds of questions which could be asked were specified, and no direct suggestion was permitted. It is more likely that the greater differentiation among the nonblind interviews was a function of differences in interviewing technique. The interviewer who knew the hypothesis had had long clinical experience with psychosomatic patients and especially with the single-consultation interview, which differs from the first interview of a patient entering psychotherapy in that meaningful material must be uncovered quickly.

There is some indication that the two interviewers did differ in the kind of atmosphere which they established. The judges rated how willing to talk patients were, how willing they were to describe life difficulties, and whether or not they felt that life problems were related to their illness. Although differences were not significant, in both studies the patients interviewed by the not-blind interviewer were rated higher in these respects than those interviewed by the blind interviewer.

It was also necessary to have controls for bias of the judges. The principal control consisted in editing interviews to remove references to diseases and symptoms. Additional protection was afforded by standardization of the judges' task in order to limit interpretation and by using four judges, 2 of whom were nonmedical judges who had had no previous experience with the hypothesis.

Editing of interviews may introduce another type of error, namely the removal of material unfavorable to a hypothesis. To avoid this, only material directly relevant to disease identification was deleted. The propriety of this practice was checked by a second editor. Epidemiological clues such as sex, age, age at onset of disease, and time relations in the course of the disease were not removed. While these clues would make some diseases more probable than others and increase the likelihood of success by medical judges in selecting the most probable disease, it was felt that they could not point to any one disease strongly enough to produce bias in selecting attitude statements. Removal of such clues might have distorted the personality picture presented by the interview.

Evidence from two control judges, who selected and ranked diseases rather than attitudes, supported this line of reasoning. One control judge, a resident in medicine, did select as high a percentage of correct diseases as the percentage of predicted attitudes selected by the regular judges. However, the patients whose diseases he correctly identified were not, in general, the patients who expressed the predicted attitudes. While the judges selecting attitudes showed significant agreement among themselves on their predicted choices, their agreement on diagnosis with the judge who selected diseases was insignificantly *less* than chance expectation ($\chi^2 = 2.22$, df = 3, P < .50). A second control judge, a graduate student in psychology, also selected diseases. As would be expected if disease selection depended upon knowledge of subtle epidemiological clues, correct disease selections by this judge were no greater than chance (P = .318 on the blind interviews, obtained choices < expected choices on the nonblind interviews). The evidence suggests that epidemiological clues were present but that medical judges selecting attitudes did not use them and that non-medical judges lacked the knowledge to use them.

Since the intent of the study was to judge attitudes, judges were instructed to evaluate only what the patient actually said about his feelings and wishes. They were asked not to "go behind the patient's statements to what you may feel is a more fundamental or truer expression of his feelings." The specificity of attitude hypothesis refers to attitudes verbally expressed towards precipitating events. We were not concerned in this study with demonstrating that there are significant life events which precede the onset or exacerbation of diseases, but with showing that *if* such an event occurred and *if* the patient stated his attitude towards it, the attitude would be of a specified kind.

To determine whether or not suitable conditions for testing the hypothesis were present, judges were asked to decide whether a significant event temporally related to symptoms was described in an interview and whether an attitude was expressed towards that event. Of the 36 interviews, there were only 16 which all four judges agreed met these conditions. All 36 interviews were judged as to the relative applicability of the 18 attitudes. However, in judging interviews which did not elicit an event or an attitude, judges necessarily had to draw inferences from whatever material was available. According to the specificity-of-attitude hypothesis, differentiation of diseases should be less when judgments are based on reactions to general life situations and on psychodynamic configurations than when they are based on expressed attitudes to precipitating events.

The available evidence suggests that this is the case. In the 10 interviews in the first study which were judged as exhibiting an attitude towards a precipitating event, there was 40 per cent selection of the predicted attitude. In contrast, the incidence of selection of the predicted attitude was only 21 per cent in judging the remaining 6 interviews. In the second study, there was 58 per cent selection of the predicted attitude from the 6 interviews judged to contain both an event and an attitude, and 52 per cent selection of the predicted attitude from interviews which at least one judge felt did not contain either an attitude or an event. There were two interviews which all four judges agreed did not contain an attitude towards a precipitating event. No judge selected the predicted attitude from either of these. It appears that the attitude hypothesis is more likely to be confirmed when patients directly express attitudes to events than when the attitude or event must be inferred.

Judges also rated on a 6-point scale how certain they felt that their choices were attitudes clearly expressed to a precipitating event. They gave higher "certainty" ratings to their first choices when these were, in fact, the predicted attitudes than when they were not. The difference was significant for one of the judges. This is further evidence that the more unequivocal the statements made by a patient about his attitude to a precipitating event, the more likely the attitude was to be the one predicted by the hypothesis.

A similar interview study of specificity factors in psychosomatic disease has recently been reported by Alexander and Pollack.[2] Alexander has described psychodynamic patterns which he believes are characteristic of particular diseases.[1] The attitude hypothesis is not incompatible with this approach and, for some diseases, there is a recognizable similarity between the attitude and the pattern which Alexander has described. It is of interest, therefore, that the finding of significant differentiation of diseases on the basis of interview material has also been reported by these investigators.

There are a number of differences between the Alexander and Pollack study and the present one, but the basic design in both is the judging of interview material edited to remove disease identification. In the Alexander and Pollack study, the majority of patients were interviewed only once, but second and third interviews were conducted when material from the first interview was inadequate. They also edited the interviews more extensively, permitting only one exacerbation and remission period to remain in the record. "The exacerbation report kept in the record was usually that episode about which the greatest amount of psychological material was elicited." As noted above, such a procedure may not be protected from selection bias.

Direct comparison of the degree of differentiation in the two studies is difficult because of these and other differences in the research designs. The most easily comparable figures are the 44 per cent correct "initial diagnoses" reported by Alexander and Pollack and the 52 per cent correct attitude selections in the present study, for the series conducted by the not-blind interviewer. The Alexander and Pollack study did not employ a blind interviewer. Chance expectation was slightly lower in the Alexander and Pollack study since the task was to make a choice of one from among seven diseases (14.3 per cent), while in the present study, the expected average was about 18 per cent. However, it would appear that the two studies agree roughly in the degree of differentiation. The present study has the advantage that attitudes may be more easily judged than the complex psychodynamic configurations with which Alexander is concerned. Identification of these requires extensive training in psychoanalytic theory, while unsophisticated judges with a relatively small amount of specific training were able to identify attitudes.

To discuss similarities and differences in the theoretical formulations of these two "specificity" approaches would require more extensive treatment than is appropriate here. The main point to be made is that, while they have approached the problem from widely different viewpoints originally, there is agreement, both theoretical and empirical, that differences in psychosomatic diseases are associated with differences in psychological variables. There is also a considerable area of agreement in descriptions of the associated psychological variables.

Summary and Conclusions

A specificity-of-attitude hypothesis, proposed by Grace and Graham,[3] stated that there is a specific relation between the attitude towards a stressful stimulus and the disease which occurs in response to the stimulus. Two interview studies with hospitalized patients investigated whether attitudes predicted to be associated with diseases were more applicable to patients having the disease in question than to patients who did not have the disease. There were 16 patients with eight diseases in the first study, and 20 patients with ten diseases in the second study. Half of the patients, matched for disease, were interviewed by a psychologist unfamiliar with the specific predictions of the hypothesis under investigation. The recorded interviews were edited to remove references identifying diseases and were submitted to two medical and two nonmedical judges. Judges selected from a list of 18 previously described attitudes the three attitudes most similar to those expressed in each interview. They also ranked all 18 attitudes in the order of their applicability to the patient.

The percentage of predicted choices was significantly greater than the expected percentage in both studies, and in both the blind and the nonblind interviews. The averages of correctly predicted choices in the two studies were 28 per cent and 45 per cent for the blind interviews, and 38 per cent and 62 per cent for the nonblind interviews.

Three judges chose the predicted attitudes significantly often from the interviews conducted blind and all four judges chose the predicted attitudes significantly often from the nonblind interviews. Judges showed significant agreement with one another and the nonmedical judges did as well as the medical.

A particular attitude was ranked lower, i.e., was judged more applicable than others, when patients had the associated disease than when they had other diseases. The ranks for predicted attitude-disease associations were significantly lower in the blind interviews of the second study and in the nonblind interviews of both studies.

It was concluded that different psychosomatic diseases are associated with different attitudes. The association was demonstrated even when a naive interviewer and naive judges were employed.

References

1. Alexander FG: Psychosomatic Medicine, Its Principles and Applications. Norton, New York, 1950
2. Alexander FG, Pollack GH: An experimental study of psychophysiological correlations. Paper read at American Psychosomatic Association meetings, 1959
3. Alexander F, French TM, Pollack GH: Psychosomatic Specificity: Experimental Study and Results, Vol 1. Chicago University Press, Chicago, IL, 1968
4. Grace WJ, Graham DT: Relationship of specific attitudes and emotions to certain bodily diseases. Psychosom Med 14:243, 1952
5. Ropes MW, Bennett GA, Cobb S, Jacox R, Jessar RA: 1958 revision of diagnostic criteria for rheumatoid arthritis. Bull Rheumat Dis 9:175, 1958
6. Wilcoxon F: Some rapid approximate statistical procedures. Biometrics (Bulletin) 1:80, 1945

CHAPTER 4

Relationship Between Psychological Defenses and Mean Urinary 17-hydroxycorticosteroid Excretion Rates
I. A Predictive Study of Parents of Fatally Ill Children

CARL T. WOLFF, M.D.,
STANFORD B. FRIEDMAN, M.D.,
MYRON A. HOFER, M.D., AND
JOHN W. MASON, M.D.

Volume 26, 1964, pp. 576–591.
From the Adult Psychiatry Branch, Clinical Investigations, National Institute of Mental Health, National Institutes of Health, U.S. Public Health Service, Bethesda, Md., and Department of Neuroendocrinology, Division of Neuropsychiatry, Walter Reed Army Institute of Research, Walter Reed Army Medical Center, Washington, D.C.
Presented in part at the American Psychosomatic Society Annual Meeting, Apr. 28, 1963, Atlantic City, N.J.
The authors wish to express their deep appreciation and admiration to the parents who participated in this study. We wish to thank Dr. David Hamburg for making this study possible. Mrs. Mary Miller and the nursing staff of the normal volunteer ward provided invaluable help. We gratefully acknowledge the cooperation of the physicians and nurses of the Medicine Branch of the National Cancer Institute. We also wish to acknowledge the untiring technical assistance of Mr. Golden Driver, Mr. Willie Gamble, and Mr. Joseph Murphy in the biochemical work, and of Mrs. June Picone, Doris Drake, and Sylvia Lubatkin for their secretarial help. Dr. Donald Morrison and Miss Karen Pettigrew provided helpful statistical consultation. We wish to thank Drs. Merton Gill, Roger Shapiro, and Earle Silber for reading the manuscripts and offering helpful advice.
Received for publication Feb. 19, 1964.

Prefatory Remarks

Donald Oken, M.D.

Selye's concept of "stress" has been so debased by its misuse and indiscriminate overuse in recent years as to have become almost near meaningless. Now, it is difficult to remember how valuable it once was for psychosomatic and other health research. The latter was particularly true during the period from 1950 to 1965, when several major centers, among them the NIMH, carried out superb programs of psychosomatic research utilizing this concept. The methodological rigor and sophistication which characterized this work was admirable. What made it exceptional, however, was its sophisticated application of reliable measures of operationally well-defined psychological variables, matching these qualities on the biological side.

The present paper reflects these qualities. Its particular interest and enduring value stem from still further merits. First, the stressful situation studied is one from real life. The loss of a loved one is ubiquitous, and one of immense impact. Second, this work examines the influences of an ongoing, rather than transient psychological experience, doing so by studying the differences among individuals rather than intraindividual fluctuations during varying situations. Third, it concentrates on a (still) neglected aspect of psychological function: defenses. Stress research has almost always focused instead on affective arousal. And it reflects a sophisticated understanding of the nature of defenses and their relation to affect. Elsewhere, the tendency is to consider the two as simply reciprocal, defense protecting against emotional distress. If so, measuring defense would be redundant, it being merely the inverse correlate of the affect. As these researchers realized, however, not only do defenses have other purposes, but affect, itself, can have adaptive and defensive functions. Designed with this recognition, their measures of the effectiveness of defense contribute new insights about the psychosomatic aspects of these important psychological processes. Finally, note that this is a predictive study, the most rigorous form of testing for the validity of a hypothesis.

Thirty-one parents of children suffering from fatal illnesses were studied psychologically. Urinary 17-hydroxycorticosteroid (17-OHCS) levels were measured concurrently. Throughout the extended crisis, these parents had characteristic mean 17-OHCS excretion rates along the continuum from high to low excretion.

The hypothesis was tested that the more effectively a parent defends against the threat of loss, the lower will be his mean 17-OHCS excretion rate. Criteria for "effective" defense were derived. Each parent was interviewed, and a prediction of the mean 17-OHCS excretion rate was made according to the criteria and independently of the endocrine data. The methods of interviewing and predicting are briefly described.

The results indicated significant correlation between the predictions and the mean 17-OHCS excretion rates. The 17-OHCS and psychologic data of a representative high and a representative low excretor are presented.

The authors suggest that these chronic differences between individuals in mean 17-OHCS excretion rates and effectiveness of defense are importantly related aspects of the individual's response to threat.

With the development of accurate biochemical methods for the measurement of 17-hydroxycorticosteroid (17-OHCS) levels in blood and urine, it has been established that there is an important relationship between psychological function and adrenal cortical activity in man.[1,2] This finding is in accord with recent neurophysiologic evidence that hypothalamic and certain more distant limbic-system structures exert a significant influence on ACTH secretion from the anterior pituitary.[2–5]

Experimental studies in animals have demonstrated that increased anterior pituitary-adrenal cortical activity is a characteristic response of the animal in stressful circumstances. Studies of the Rhesus monkey by Mason et al.[6] revealed that near-maximal adrenal cortical activation can be produced under circumstances of "conditioned anxiety" or "conditioned avoidance."

Although studies of adrenal cortical function in human subjects under stress have revealed the same general relationship between stressful stimulation and adrenal cortical activation, these studies have revealed considerable variability of response *between* individuals. This is in contrast to the animal studies, in which individual animals responded in a more consistent manner to a given stimulus. Most of the human studies have used the presence of overt emotional distress as an indicator of psychological stress, either in naturally occurring life crises or in experimentally threatening situations. Adrenal cortical activation has been shown to occur in groups of anxious subjects,[7,8] depressed patients,[9,10] normal persons or patients encountering a new experience,[11-13] and normal subjects in stressful laboratory experiments[8,14] or in stressful life circumstances.[8,15] Taken as a whole, these studies have indicated that increased adrenal cortical activity is associated with states of heightened "emotionality" or "distress" or with specific affects such as anxiety and depression.

However, a number of individuals in such studies did not show the expected adrenal cortical response despite their being in apparently stressful circumstances and even when they manifested intense overt distress. Other individuals who showed no overt distress had appreciable increases in adrenal cortical activity. These interesting differences *between* individuals indicate that factors other than the amount of stressful stimulation or the intensity of the manifested emotional response are involved in the psycho-pituitary-adrenal cortical response to stress in human beings.

In the studies of Price et al.[16] on preoperative patients and of Fox et al.[17] on normal college students, the attempt was made to study such individual differences by defining certain qualitative factors that might distinguish between high and low 17-OHCS excretors. "Distress involvement" in the former and "emotional urgency" in the latter were characteristic of the higher end of the continuum.

The study of parents of fatally ill children, the first phase of which has been reported by Friedman et al.,[18] presented the opportunity of studying normal adults who were exposed to the prolonged threat of an impending major object loss. In the first phase of the study it was expected that, during such a severe and extended life crisis, each parent who was exposed to varying degrees of environmental stress and was experiencing varying types and intensity of emotional responses would show corresponding changes in adrenal cortical activity. Such a longitudinal study of these parents might then reveal a relationship between adrenal cortical activation and intensity of stressful stimulation or particular affects such as anxiety, depression, and anger. Instead, it was found that (1) each parent had a *relatively* stable rate of 17-OHCS excretion throughout the experience despite apparent emotional fluctuation, (2) most subjects had mean excretion rates within the range usually defined as "normal" despite the apparent severity of the threat to which they were exposed, and (3) each individual could be ranked along a continuum according to his characteristic mean excretion rate.[18] Thus, the first phase of the study established that the most meaningful differences in 17-OHCS excretion rates were those demonstrated *between* individuals.

These stable physiological differences between individuals became the focus of the second phase of the study, which this paper reports. In this current phase, our observations were directed away from transient intraindividual changes in intensity of stress and in type and intensity of affect and toward the more enduring characteristic differences between individuals in their psychological responses in the chronically threatening situation. The observation that a few subjects with low 17-OHCS excretion rates had effectively denied their children's illnesses focused our attention on psychological defenses. Although defensive activity is only one function of the ego, and there are ego functions other than defenses useful in coping with threat, it was the former type of ego function to which the current study was directed.

The hypothesis was derived that individuals whose defenses are *effective* in keeping psychic tension at low levels will have low mean urinary 17-OHCS excretion rates, and the less effectively a parent defends against the impact of the threat of loss, the higher will be his mean 17-OHCS excretion rate. The aim of the present study was to test the above hypothesis by prediction of the mean 17-OHCS excretion rate of each subject on the basis of an interview assessment of the effectiveness of his defenses.

Methods

Subjects

The subjects were 31 parents (19 mothers and 12 fathers) of children who were referred to the National Cancer Institute for chemotherapeutic treatment of leukemia or other fatal childhood neoplasms. The subjects were selected only on the basis of availability for interviews and adequacy of 17-OHCS excretion data (see below).

Most of the parents came from considerable distances and were admitted as inpatients to a "normal volunteer" ward. Details of the program have been described previously.[18, 19] In brief, the normal volunteer ward was situated two floors above the children's ward and was staffed by nurses who made research observations. Normal volunteers from other mental health-projects also lived on this ward. The parents lived on the ward while their children were in the hospital, ate their meals there, but were free to come and go as they pleased. Since there were usually at least six parents on the ward at any one time, there was considerable opportunity for socializing among them.

The mothers had a mean age of 33 years (range 20–49) and the fathers a mean age of 35 (range 25–48).

Biochemical Methods and Analysis of Biochemical Data

The methods of urine collection and processing have been previously described.[18] Urinary 17-OHCS excretion rates were determined on 1- to 4-day urine collections by the Glenn-Nelson chromatographic method[20] further evaluated by Rosenthal and Mason.[21] Urine collections were selected for biochemical analysis to include as representative a sample as possible for each parent during the course of his child's illness. Total mean excretion rates were then computed for each subject who had more than eight collection periods. For the 31 subjects in the study, the average number of collection periods analyzed was 11. The average number of days represented was 23, since many of the collection periods were 3 days. The mean period of study for these subjects was 4.7 months, while the briefest period was 3 weeks.

The predictive interviews often were held months before the end of a parent's stay in the hospital. The predictor could, of course, assess the behavior of the subject only up to the time of the interviews. Therefore, we have used only those 17-OHCS values up to the time of the interviews to compute the mean used for prediction. This will be referred to as the "observed" mean. The range of observed means was divided into low, middle, and high groups. Because of the previously established sex difference in 17-OHCS excretion,[18] the absolute values for the groups were different for the two sexes. The numerical ranges for the groups are included in Table 4–1. By these criteria, there were 6 high, 13 middle, and 12 low excretors in the sample.

Interview Methods

One of us (C.T.W.), who did not participate in the first phase of the study, independently derived the criteria for prediction.

Prior to beginning the predictive study on the sample of 31 parents, he interviewed 8 parents, not included in the sample of 31, in order to become familiar with the range of behavior he might later encounter in the 31 subjects, to develop the interview method, and to evaluate whether the predictive criteria would be applicable to the kinds of interview data he elicited. He made prelim-

Psychological Defenses and Excretion Rates

Table 4–1. 17-OHCS data and predictions for 31 subjects

Subjects	Age	Months in study	No. days analyzed	Range* (mg./24 hr. for 72-hr. period)	Mean (mg./24 hr.) Observed	Predicted	Interview
				Mothers (*N* = 19)			
High group (6.1–8.0 mg./24 hr.)							
A	34	4	33	10.3–4.8	6.8	6.5	5.4
B	32	7½	23	7.5–5.1†	6.2	6.5	5.7
C	42	4½	30	8.3–4.3	6.1	6.2	6.7
Middle group (4.1–6.0 mg./24 hr.)							
D	32	7	29	7.7–1.9	5.4	4.3	5.7
E	30	2½	18	6.3–4.8	5.1	3.1	5.4
F	39	7	42	8.3‡–3.9	5.0	3.0	4.8
G	30	3	23	7.2†–3.6	4.6	6.0	5.6
H	49	19	9	5.6†–3.8†	4.5	5.2	N.A.
I	40	6	26	5.7‡–3.0†	4.2	4.7	4.0
J	38	2	24	7.0–2.4	4.1	4.2	3.7
Low group (2.1–4.0 mg./24 hr.)							
K	20	4	26	5.1–3.0	4.0	3.1	4.4
L	29	5½	24	4.4–3.0	3.8	3.9	4.3
M	30	4	36	5.8–1.7	3.7	7.5	5.8
N	31	3	27	4.5–2.3	3.7	3.3	4.0
O	29	2	24	5.5–2.1	3.5	6.0	5.5
P	37	4	26	4.1–2.1	3.1	4.6	2.7
Q	30	2	22	6.1†–1.9	3.0	4.5	3.0
R	32	¾	11	4.2†–2.4	3.0	3.5	2.7
S	30	7	46	5.4‡–1.2†	2.5	3.0	1.3
MEAN	33	5.0	26		4.3	4.7	4.5
				Fathers (*N* = 12)			
High group (8.1–10.0 mg./24 hr.)							
AA	35	4	29	29.9–3.2†	10.3	7.9	10.6
BB	48	19	8	14.1†–6.5†	9.1	9.5	N.A.
CC	30	1	15	12.7†–7.6	9.0	9.0	6.3§
Middle group (6.1–8.0 mg./24 hr.)							
DD	33	3	19	12.5‡–4.7‡	7.7	7.7	11.1
EE	38	3	27	10.5†–3.6	7.7	6.7	4.6
FF	40	5½	33	10.6†–4.3‡	7.5	8.0	6.4§
GG	35	¾	13	10.0†–5.6†	7.4	6.3	7.3§
HH	36	2½	16	10.1†–5.0	7.3	5.8	5.3
II	38	2½	14	9.6†–4.2‡	6.8	6.8	9.1§

(continued)

Table 4–1. 17-OHCS data and predictions for 31 subjects *(continued)*

Subjects	Age	Months in study	No. days analyzed	Range* (mg./24 hr. for 72-hr. period)	Mean (mg./24 hr.) Observed	Predicted	Interview
Fathers (*N* = 12)							
Low group (4.1–6.0 mg./24 hr.)							
JJ	25	4	17	7.3†–4.3†	5.7	5.5	6.7
KK	34	1½	11	6.8†–3.2‡	5.5	5.0	5.8
LL	33	4	23	8.4–2.2†	5.2	6.0	4.7
MEAN	35	4.2	19		7.4	7.0	7.0

*Range does not demonstrate tendency for most individual values to fall close to mean. For this, see earlier report.[18]
†24-hr. period.
‡48-hr. period.
§Interview means obtained during follow-up visit.

inary predictions on these 8 "practice" subjects and learned their endocrine data before beginning the formal study of the 31 subjects.

On the basis of this preliminary experience, he decided to interview each parent in the study twice, when possible, for a total interview time of 2–4 hr. Both interviews were relatively unstructured. In the first interview, the subject was asked to describe his experience of having a fatally ill child. The majority of parents were available for a second interview which dealt primarily with their previous life history. The interviewer had little or no other contact with the subjects.

It was not possible to interview every parent in the same stage of his child's illness. Most parents were interviewed when their children were doing relatively well clinically and after the parent had been in the hospital situation long enough to have become settled into a characteristic routine. However, a few subjects had to be interviewed relatively soon after the child was first admitted for treatment, and a few had to be interviewed in the terminal phase of the child's illness. Because of the difficulty in obtaining fathers for study, 4 fathers on whom adequate 17-OHCS data had been previously obtained were asked to return for the interviews 6 months after their children had died. Predictions for these fathers posed a particular problem described below.

All interviews were tape recorded. Initial impressions were written immediately after the interviews, and at a later date both the notes and the tape recordings for each subject were extensively reviewed prior to making the prediction.

Method of Prediction

In arriving at a prediction the interviewer had available to him only the following information. He knew of the conclusions from the first phase of the study relating to the stability, range, and sex difference of the subjects' 17-OHCS excretion rates and of the preliminary hypothesis that a subject's mean 17-OHCS rate was related to the effectiveness of his defenses. He did not know the distribution of the 31 subjects within the range of 17-OHCS excretion rates, nor was he aware of their individual 17-OHCS excretion data or of any previously obtained psychological data.

The predictions were based on a clinical assessment of the effectiveness of each parent's defenses in maintaining psychic tension at low levels. Because of the practical and theoretical problems related to this type of assessment, we shall describe the method in detail in a second report.[22] We use the term "effectiveness" of a defense to refer only to the immediate success of tension reduction by the defense, not to its adaptive value. For example, a parent's complete denial of the existence of illness in his child, despite direct evidence to the contrary, was undoubtedly maladaptive not only in respect to his functioning as a parent but also in respect to its possible long-range consequences to himself. Yet such total denial could be highly effective in minimizing the impact of the immediate evidences of danger. So long as it remained successful, it could be associated with low 17-OHCS excretion.

The criteria of effectiveness which were employed will be detailed in the following paper. Briefly, a parent was considered to be effectively defended if (1) he demonstrated little or no overt distress (affect criterion), (2) he showed little or no impairment of his functioning in the stressful situation (function criterion), and (3) he demonstrated the ability to mobilize further his defenses in superimposed acutely stressful experiences ("defensive reserve" criterion). The criteria for ineffective defense were the converse. The affect criterion included not only a quantitative assessment of the intensity of painful affect but also two qualitative assessments. The first qualitative judgment concerned the extent to which the particular affect was in itself threatening to the individual. The second was whether the affect itself was primarily being used in the service of defense.

The criteria were applied to two types of data. The first was the *observed behavior* of the parent during the interviews. The second was his *report of his behavior* during the previous phases of his child's illness. On occasion there was a disparity between the effectiveness of a subject's defenses as *observed* during the interview and the effectiveness of his defenses as *reported* by him in his review of his experience. In such a case, what the interviewer observed during the interview was given more weight in arriving at a prediction.

A written summary of the relevant information and of the rationale of the prediction was made. A numerical prediction of the 17-OHCS excretion rate was recorded for each subject. This will be referred to as the "predicted" mean. It was arrived at by specifying progressively narrower ranges within which the predictor thought the observed mean would fall. It should be emphasized that, in predicting, the various factors described above were not quantitatively rated and combined mathematically, but rather were assimilated into a single clinical assessment.

Results

Table 4–1 lists the data which will be referred to in reporting the results for the 31 subjects. The subjects are ranked in three groups (high, middle, and low) according to their observed means. The column labeled "range" demonstrates the relatively restricted range of 17-OHCS values for each subject throughout the period of study. However, the fact that many of the 17-OHCS determinations were done on 3-day collections tended by itself to reduce the range for each subject.

Figure 4–1 is a 3 by 3 table showing the results of comparing the predicted means with the observed means for each subject according to the predetermined definitions of high, middle, and low; 23 of the 31 predictions corresponded to the actual group. This result is highly significant by the chi-square method. (Chi square = 27.00; P < .001; df = 4.) The results are also significant when analyzed separately for men and women.

None of the 6 high excretors was predicted to be low, and only 1 of the 12 low excretors was predicted high; 6 of the 8 incorrect predictions occurred in distinguishing low and middle excretors; 6 incorrect predictions occurred in the sample of women.

Additional information is obtained by comparing the observed numerical mean values with the predicted numerical means by determining the coefficient of correlation (r) between these variables. Figure 4–2 is a scattergram of observed versus predicted means for the 19 mothers. Points falling within the shaded area represent predictions that were within 1.0 mg. of the observed mean; 11 of the 19 predictions were within this range. The correlation coeffi-

---

One must interpret the chi-square method with caution when there are small expected frequencies in each category because of possible distortion. However, it is quite unlikely that this invalidates the significance of the results, because of the large chi-square value.

cient was .41 (P < .05). The 2 most deviant predictions were much higher than the observed mean (Subjects M and O, left upper quadrant of Figure 4–2). These 2 individuals are discussed below.

Figure 4–3 is a scattergram of the predicted versus observed means for the 12 fathers; 9 of the 12 predictions were within 1.0 mg. of the observed mean. The correlation coefficient for the fathers was .80 (P < .01). Thus, the predictions were appreciably more accurate for the fathers than for the mothers.

There were two factors which appeared to be related to the lesser accuracy of predictions for the mothers. The first was the methodologic problem of evaluating affect expression in the women. This problem will be discussed in the following paper.

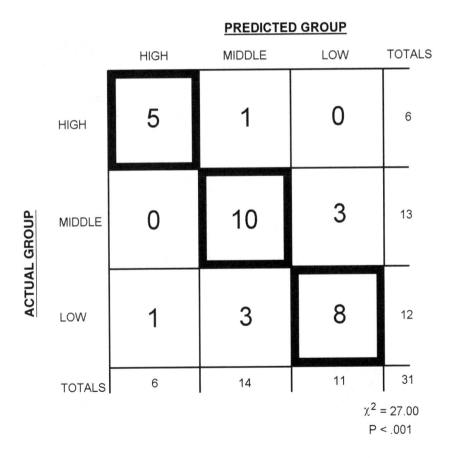

Figure 4–1. Results of predictions for 31 subjects, by groups. Numbers in heavily outlined boxes represent correct predictions.

The second factor involved two particular predictions. There were 2 mothers whose behavior during the interviews was consistent with a high prediction but whose report of their behavior throughout the child's illness was more consistent with a low prediction. In the case of such discrepancy the assessment of the interview behavior was weighted more heavily. Therefore, they were both predicted to be in the higher half of the continuum. They both had observed means in the low range, and these were the 2 most deviant predictions made (Subjects M and O, Figure 4–2).

If the hypothesis relating effectiveness of defense and mean 17-OHCS excretion rates is correct, and if in addition these 2 subjects were less effectively defended at the time of the interview than they had been previously, then one

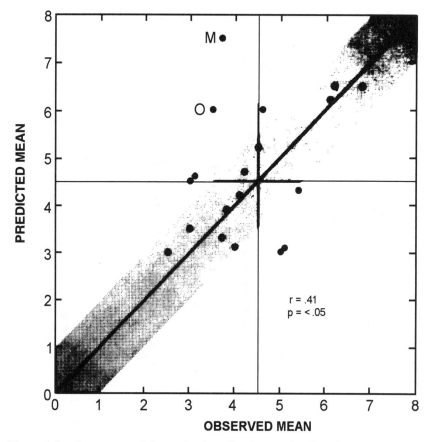

Figure 4–2. Scattergram of observed and predicted means for 19 mothers. Points within shaded area represent predictions within 1.0 mg. of observed mean. Predictions for Subjects M and O were the most deviant (see text).

might expect that their 17-OHCS excretion rates at the time of the interview would be higher than their observed mean rates. This was the case in that both subjects had consistently low values except for the week of the interview, during which both had values for a 72-hr. period in the high-middle range. For this reason it seemed advisable to compute for each parent an "interview" mean, consisting of the value or values obtained during the week in which the interviews occurred. We then compared the predicted values with these interview means. Subject M, who had the highest predicted value, had the second highest interview mean. Subject O, who was ranked fifth by prediction, had the fifth highest interview mean. The individual interview means are listed in Table 4–1. In the majority of cases the interview means were within 0.5 mg. of the observed means.

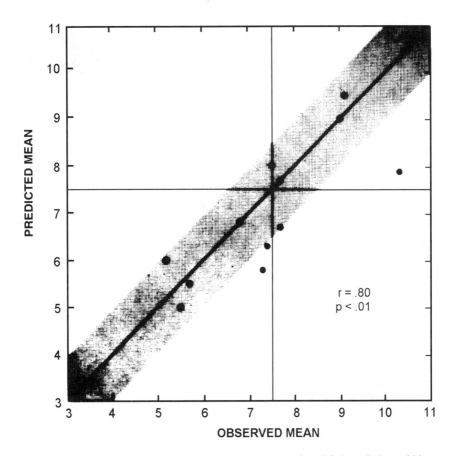

Figure 4–3. Scattergram of observed and predicted means for 12 fathers. Points within shaded area represent predictions within 1.0 mg. of observed mean.

Figure 4–4 is a scattergram of the predicted versus the interview means for 18 of the 19 mothers. (One mother had no urine collections within a month of the interview and was therefore excluded.) The points representing Subjects M and O fall in the correct quadrant of the scattergram (upper right). The correlation of the predictions with the interview means was .58 (P < .01).

Interview means were computed in the same manner for 7 of the 8 fathers who had been interviewed during the course of their children's illnesses. (One father had no collection corresponding to the time of the interview.) The correlation of the predictions with the fathers' interview means was .76 (P < .025). This correlation is of the same order of magnitude as the previous correlation of the predictions with the observed means for the fathers.

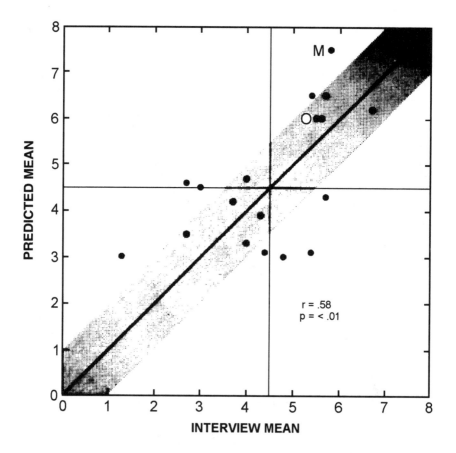

Figure 4–4. Scattergram of interview and predicted means for 18 mothers. Points for Subjects M and O now fall in upper right quadrant (see text).

Four fathers were interviewed on a follow-up visit 6 months after their children had died. We did not include these 4 fathers in the interview mean correlation, since the interviewer excluded the observed behavior and relied only on the subject's report of past behavior in predicting. This was done because the interview observations were made in the period of mourning and were not considered representative of how the subject might have behaved during the period before the child's death. For these 4 fathers, there was a negative correlation (−.67, N.S.) between the 17-OHCS excretion rate during the phase of mourning and the predictions of the pre-loss effectiveness of defense.

All the data above were also analyzed nonparametrically by means of the Spearman rank-order correlation. In all cases the rank order correlations were of the same order of magnitude as the correlation coefficients, although the rank order correlation for predicted versus observed means for women was below significance at the .05 level.

Case Reports

The two cases reported below—a typical high and a typical low 17-OHCS excretor—are presented to illustrate the psychologic data from which predictions were derived.

High 17-OHCS Excretor

Subject A was a 34-year-old mother whose oldest of two adopted children developed a neuroblastoma at 6 years of age. She had adopted the boy at age 2 and had come to regard the child as her own. The fact that her child was adopted did not appear to distinguish her psychological or 17-OHCS response to his fatal illness from those of the other parents. The upper part of Figure 4–5 shows her 17-OHCS excretion data. Her total mean value was 6.8 mg./24 hr. The range was from 10.3 mg./24 hr. over a 4-day collection period to 4.8 mg./24 hr. for a collection period of 3 days. The area represented by the diagonal lines on the figure is the middle range of values for all mothers. None of her values fell below this range. In these respects she was a typical high excretor.

She was a warm, passive, and sensitive woman. Her interview behavior was characterized by considerable distress. Although she was able with difficulty to maintain her composure while relating the details of her experience, she seemed always to be very sad, even when talking about neutral subjects. In contrast, many of the subjects with low excretion rates were able to intellectualize their

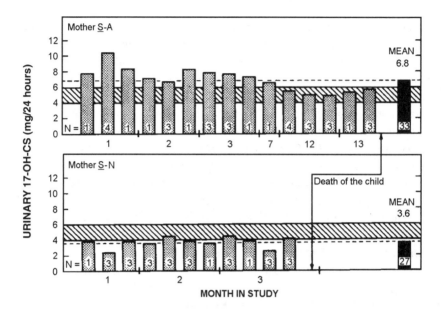

Figure 4–5. At top, 17-OHCS excretion data of mother (Subject A) with high mean excretion rate. At bottom, 17-OHCS excretion data of mother (Subject N) with low mean excretion rate. Black bars and dashed lines represent total mean excretion rates. Shaded bars are individual determinations. Numbers in bars are numbers of collection days for the value. Diagonal area represents middle range for all mothers (4.1–6.0 mg./24 hr.).

experience and present it as if it were a case history. She, however, seemed to be re-experiencing in a painful manner the events she was describing. Thus, her interview behavior fulfilled the affect criterion for ineffective defense. Minimal amounts of probing of emotional issues easily provoked additional distress. Thus, she exhibited little "defensive reserve."

The behavioral evidence of ineffective defense during the interview was corroborated by her report of her experience throughout her son's illness. Even when her son had had a possibly successful surgical removal of the neuroblastoma, when he had been asymptomatic for several months, and when a cure was a realistic possibility, she felt what she called "dread." In her own words, "I just couldn't feel like what I had before. I was living in a dread. I just couldn't feel he'd be completely cured of it." She reported that, when her son developed symptoms which his physician thought were due to a viral infection, she "hoped it was the virus all the time, but . . . I . . . just in the back of my mind, I guess I always had that dread." The predictive significance of this statement was that she was unable to avoid pain by denying, intellectualizing, or isolating her recognition of impending danger. In this respect she was unlike some low excretors who, when faced with the same evidence of an apparently entirely well child, were able to deny that a relapse and death were inevitable. Other low excretors retained an intellectualized awareness of the impending danger but without an associated affective component such as the painful dread of which A spoke. Such low excretors often reported that, during these periods of remission, their thoughts and feelings about their children's illnesses became less frequent and intense and their attention returned to some extent to their more ordinary concerns.

Being unable much of the time to defend against distress, A resorted to physical activity in an attempt to dispel her distressing feelings, as illustrated in the following exchange. She stated, "If I could cry more, I'd slowly get a little bit of feeling off. I've bottled up so much. I get all choked up and just can't express myself." When asked if that made her restless or anxious, she replied, "Yes, I have to keep busy all the time. I can't sit around just doing nothing. I'm always sewing, doing something to keep my hands busy, keep my mind occupied." When asked if this helped, she said, "I don't keep it off my mind, but it helps to pass the time away." Thus, physical activity was also ineffective in decreasing tension.

She demonstrated, in addition, the third criterion of ineffective defense, functional impairment. Her relationship with her husband was impaired. Her sexual relations and degree of satisfaction were quite diminished. She had considerable difficulty in getting to sleep at night and had anxiety dreams about her son. She was consistently overeating and had gained 35 lb., although her appetite had not increased. It is, of course, possible that the compulsive eating was an unsuccessful attempt to counteract her despair. She had also begun to use alcohol in the same compulsive manner.

Thus, she demonstrated much distress, both in the interview and during the course of her child's illness, little "defensive reserve" in the interview, and significant functional impairment throughout the experience. On this basis she was correctly predicted to be a high 17-OHCS excretor.

Low 17-OHCS Excretor

Subject N was a typical low excretor. She was a 31-year-old mother of three whose eldest son developed acute leukemia. The bottom part of Figure 4–5 shows her 17-OHCS excretion data. She had a total mean of 3.6 mg./24 hr., placing her in the low group. Her highest value was 4.5 mg./24 hr., which fell in the lower part of the middle range. There was no overlapping between the range of this low excretor's 17-OHCS values and the range of values of the previous high excretor.

Psychologically, N was a well-organized, highly controlled, obsessional woman with a rather limited range of affect expression and considerable ability to use denial effectively.

She handled the interview in a controlled and factual manner with only occasional moments of distress. When she talked of the initial diagnosis of her son's leukemia or of the possibility of his death, she did become mildly sad, but there was only minimal evidence of anxiety, no expression of guilt, and she seemed able quickly to regain her more typical mood state. Much of the time she actually seemed to be slightly euphoric, particularly when she discussed the religious significance of her son's illness. She stated that God was in complete control, that He was using their family and this disease to bring His message to the world, and that her own awareness that her son might die was not accompanied by painful feeling since her personal life did not matter. She not only denied her distress but also denied the idea that her son's death was inevitable. She believed that he might survive, should God so decide.

Her major concern during the interview was with the question of whether she should go home for a weekend, leaving her son alone in the hospital. She ruminated about the decision in an unemotional way. She was worried that her son might be lonely in her absence, but she did not express concern that a serious crisis might occur while she was away. Such a crisis was a realistic possibility, and she had seen critical episodes of this sort develop suddenly among the other children on the ward. Of importance for prediction was not only the obsessional preoccupation but also the displacement onto less threatening concerns. A forceful attempt by the interviewer to evoke distress by challenging her denial was unsuccessful in overcoming her "defensive reserve."

Throughout her child's illness, N utilized these same defenses. She reported that although she felt tense, frightened, and despairing for a few days after the diagnosis had been made, these feelings suddenly disappeared when she learned that her congregation was praying for her son, and she realized that his fate was in God's hands. From that moment she did not experience any similar intensity of distress and was able to maintain that what happened to her son ultimately did not matter to her since she was simply fulfilling God's plan. She reported an increase in her self-esteem, since her son's illness dispelled her long-standing sense of being unimportant and gave her an important mission. Functionally, she showed no impairment of sleep, appetite, or sexual behavior, and she carried out her role as a mother effectively.

In summary, she showed effective obsessional defenses and an impressive degree of denial both of the external inevitabilities and of her own feelings. Not only did these defenses seem highly effective in minimizing her distress but they actually seemed to permit her to experience a degree of pleasurable mood that was not observed in the group of high excretors. She was correctly predicted to be a low 17-OHCS excretor.

Discussion

These results support the hypothesis that the more effectively a parent defends against the impact of the threat of loss, the lower will be his chronic mean 17-OHCS excretion rate.

In regard to selection factors, the parents studied were a representative sample of all parents who brought their children to the National Cancer Institute during the study. Only 4 of the 90 parents who were available to participate in the project refused to do so in its 3-year existence. However, these 90 parents may not have been representative of the class "parents of fatally ill children," since there may have been some selection in the process by which parents brought their children to the National Cancer Institute. It could not be determined how many parents refused to accept the initial referral of their children to the National Institutes of Health. Among such parents might have been individuals, for example, who totally denied the existence of the illness or others who decided that it was better not to seek treatment for a fatal illness. We do not know whether the hypothesis would apply to this type of individual.

Our subjects may have differed somewhat from the usual normal volunteers in psychiatric research projects in that their primary reasons for joining the study were that it enabled them to be near their children and it was economically advantageous. Of less importance as motivations were their interest in learning about themselves and the wish for psychiatric treatment. The parents were not aware on arrival that there was a psychiatric study connected with the treatment of children with leukemia.

It might be supposed that the particular environment of the study grossly altered the 17-OHCS and psychological responses of these parents. We did hope that the program for these subjects might be "therapeutic." It included supportive nursing care and occupational activities and presented the opportunity to discuss problems with psychiatrists and to share experiences with the other parents. However, as previously described,[18] the 17-OHCS and psychological patterns of the inpatient parents as a group did not differ significantly from an outpatient group who were living at home and, therefore, had much less opportunity to participate in the program. Thus, it seems that the inpatient program did not grossly influence these patterns.

Since the assessed effectiveness of defenses did not account for all the interindividual variability in mean 17-OHCS excretion rates, we have investigated other psychological and physiological factors. The following variables showed roughly zero correlation with the 17-OHCS means: (1) length of exposure to the chronically stressful situation, (2) number of other children the parent had, (3) number of previous losses, (4) educational level as a gross index of I.Q., (5) age of parent. For 13 of the mothers we obtained a gross index of physical activity as rated on a three-point scale by the nursing staff. There was a correlation of $-.31$ (N.S.) between this measure of activity and the mean excretion rate. There was a lower-order positive correlation between body weight and mean 17-OHCS excretion rate. For 33 mothers from both phases of the study, the correlation was .32 ($P < .05$). For 21 men the correlation was .26 (N.S.). The investigators were unaware of this correlation until the predictions had been completed.

It appears likely that some of the errors in predicting were related to the incompleteness of the method of assessment. The assessment of effectiveness of defenses was clinical, the criteria were incompletely defined, and factors of predictor bias were not entirely eliminated. Our clinical experience with these parents suggests that more accurate predictions, particularly in respect to the mothers, might have been obtained with a more refined and rigorous method.

This study provides evidence for the intimate relationship of psychological defenses and the adrenal cortical response in this particular chronic stress. Much of the previous work in the psychoendocrine field has concentrated on the stressful stimulus or the emotional response as the most likely variable to relate to adrenal cortical activity. Such studies have demonstrated that stressful situations can elicit emotional responses and increased adrenal cortical activity in monkeys and human subjects. In the Rhesus monkey, Mason et al.[6, 23] have shown that there is marked interindividual uniformity of adrenal cortical response to both unconditioned and conditioned threatening stimuli. Although the degree of the 17-OHCS elevation may vary somewhat from monkey to monkey, almost all monkeys show a definite response in controlled stressful circumstances.

In contrast, such uniformity of adrenal cortical response among human subjects in a stressful situation has not been observed. This greater variability is understandable in view of the fact that ego development in man has provided a powerful organization intervening between stimulus and response. This fact makes imperative the study of specific functions and aspects of the ego such as the defenses which, until recently, have been relatively neglected in psychophysiologic research.

Since our results were obtained on "normal" parents in a chronically stressful situation, it is important to consider whether the "effectiveness of defense" hypothesis would apply more generally to all chronically stressful situations, to acutely stressful situations, and to situations in which severe life crises were absent. Would the hypothesis also apply to a different type of normal subject or to a patient population?

In another psychoendocrine study addressed to the problem of interindividual differences in chronic 17-OHCS excretion rates, Fox et al.[17] reported on 18 healthy college students who were not experiencing any severe life crises and showed a similar range of excretion as our fathers. Their tentative hypothesis suggested that "the more a person reacts emotionally, the higher the level of the 17-hydroxycorticosteroids. The more guarded the individual, the more that control is exercised over feelings, the lower the 17-hydroxycorticosteroids." This seems to be in accord with the findings of the present study.

Sachar et al.[24] studied 4 acute schizophrenics and found that in stages of the illness where the patient was effectively defended, either with healthy or psychotic mechanisms, and distress was diminished, the urinary 17-OHCS output was lower than during stages of "acute turmoil" or "depression." While the study dealt with changes in single individuals over time and not with differences between individuals, it would seem that our findings complement each other.

In a study of acute experimental stress, Oken et al.[25] reported on a group of chronically ill psychiatric patients characterized by depression, inadequacy, and a tendency to avoid and shut out all stressful stimuli. They found that when these habitual avoidance defenses were rendered ineffective in an interview, the blood level rose, lending further support to the possibility that the hypothesis can be generalized. It is possible that evaluation of defenses might help to explain some of the inconsistencies in adrenal cortical response observed in previous studies of subjects in stressful situations.

It is necessary to consider whether the 17-OHCS excretion rate of each of our subjects is a product of the particular threat encountered and the specific defenses mobilized to meet it, or whether these subjects would maintain the same rank on the continuum of mean 17-OHCS excretion rates in other threatening circumstances or in ordinary "non-stressful" life. We would speculate that just as each individual might vary in the effectiveness of his defenses in other stressful circumstances, so too might his mean 17-OHCS excretion rate vary accordingly. For example, a high excretor in the situation of threat of loss might be a low excretor in threatening circumstances for which his defenses were more effective. A definitive answer to this question would require long-term longitudinal study of individuals in various types of stressful situations.

A related question concerns the possibility that there is a specific class of defenses or a particular defense which was associated with low 17-OHCS excretion in our study. It might be supposed on theoretical grounds that denial would be particularly suited for dealing with the threat of loss and the relatively external nature of the source of danger. A number of the low excretion group did demonstrate such a defense. However, several of the low excretors showed little or no denial, and there were individuals in the high range who tried to utilize denial but were not successful. This observation suggests that it was the *effectiveness* of whatever defense was available to the subject, rather than the existence of a particular one, which was the relevant phenomenon.

The answer to this question, however, has remained inconclusive because of the inherent difficulties in the method of evaluating defenses. Defenses operate on an unconscious level. The presence, type, and strength of a defense is inferred indirectly from the perceptions, impulses, affects, and thoughts that are accessible to consciousness or *absent* from it. This being so, there was no way of which we were aware to "measure" defenses. Furthermore, in our sample of subjects, as in most individuals, there was always a variety of defensive activities used, and no subject demonstrated a "pure culture" of denial or isolation, etc.

It may be asked why we have focused particularly on the defensive activities of the ego and have paid less attention to ego functions other than defenses which have their usefulness in coping with threatening situations. We have not wished to imply that it was only defenses which were effective for these parents. However, it appeared to us that the defenses were of relatively great importance in this particular threatening situation because the parents were confronted by the *inevitability* of loss and they were *unable to modify the outcome* in any way. In many other danger situations (threat of *possible* but not inevitable injury, death, object loss, etc.) clear perception, reality testing, logical thinking, planning a course of action, and executing that action can effectively reduce intrapsychic tension. This is so because such a series of ego functions can lead to successful modification of the environment and elimination or circumvention of the danger. Such ego functions enabled the parents to deal with and master certain aspects of the threatening situation, such as the necessity of arranging appropriate treatment for their child and the day-to-day requirements of living with and caring for a sick child. However, it was our impression that these functions were of less use in dealing with the major and unchangeable aspect of the threat, the impending object loss. The extent to which subjects were able to mobilize defenses that were effective against this threat and thereby diminish the dread, anxiety, and pain that it stimulated seemed the major variable that distinguished the lower 17-OHCS excretors from the higher ones.

Implications

There are several broad implications of these results for future psychoendocrine research. First, they describe a different dimension of the psycho-pituitary-adrenal cortical response to naturally occurring environmental threat. Until recently, the main focus of study has been on the relationship between acute changes in adrenal cortical activity and acute changes in emotional state. It now seems likely that, in addition, the chronic "base line" around which these fluctuations occur is profoundly influenced by the defensive organization of the ego. If the function of the pituitary-adrenal cortical system has any relevance for healthy somatic adaptation to the environment on the one hand, or for the development of psychosomatic illness on the other, it may be that these chronic differences between individuals are a more significant factor than the acute changes referred to previously. It may also be that such maintained differences are a factor in the differential susceptibility of individuals to various types of medical illness.

Second, these results indicate that, in the study of man's psychoendocrine response to stress, it is necessary not only to consider the nature of the stressful stimulus and the emotional and physiological responses but also to include in such a stimulus-response model those intervening variables which are subsumed under the general area of ego function and, in particular, the defenses.

Finally, this study illustrates a method for the use of nonquantitative assessment of behavior in psychophysiologic research. The inclusion of qualitative aspects of psychological functioning in such study has seemed to us a desirable step. It can avoid the loss of information which may occur with attempts at quantification that are forced at present to exclude nonmeasurable aspects of behavior. Although quantitation is an ultimate requirement for psychophysiologic research, we suggest that at present the search for significant variables and hypotheses remains the main need.

Concluding Summary

Thirty-one parents of children suffering from fatal illnesses were studied psychologically. Urinary 17-OHCS were measured concurrently. Throughout the extended life crisis during which he was exposed to the threat of major object loss, each parent had a characteristic mean 17-OHCS excretion rate. Subjects could be classified according to their mean 17-OHCS excretion rates as high, middle, or low excretors.

The hypothesis was derived that the more effectively a parent defends against the threat of loss, the lower will be his mean 17-OHCS excretion rate. To test the hypothesis, one of the authors (who did not know the endocrine data) independently derived criteria for assessing the effectiveness of an individual's defenses, interviewed each available subject, and made predictions of each subject's mean 17-OHCS excretion rate based on these criteria. The criteria and method of interviewing are described.

The results supported the hypothesis by showing a significant correlation between the predicted mean excretion rates and the observed means for both fathers and mothers. The predictions for the fathers were considerably more accurate than for the mothers, and this finding is discussed.

The 17-OHCS excretion data and the interview data of a typical high and a typical low excretor are presented to illustrate the relevant differences between individuals of the high- and low-excretion groups and to indicate the way in which the predictions were made.

It is concluded that, for parents subjected to the chronic threat of loss, interindividual differences in mean 17-OHCS excretion rates are related to interindividual differences in the effectiveness of defenses against the impact of the threat of loss. The authors suggest that this relationship between defenses and mean 17-OHCS levels may be a general phenomenon of man's response to all types of threat.

References

1. Hamburg DA: Plasma and urinary corticosteroid levels in naturally occurring psychologic stresses, in Ultrastructure and Metabolism of the Nervous System. Edited by Korey S. Williams & Wilkins, Baltimore, MD, 1962
2. Michael RP, Gibbons JL: Interrelationships between the endocrine system and neuropsychiatry. Internat Rev Neurobiol 5:243, 1963
3. Mason JW: Plasma 17-hydroxycorticosteroid response to hypothalamic stimulation in the conscious Rhesus monkey. Endocrinology 63:403, 1958
4. Mason JW, Nauta WJH, Brady JV, Robinson JA, Sachar EJ: The role of limbic system structures in the regulation of ACTH secretion. Acta Neuroveg 23:4, 1961
5. Mandell AJ, Chapman LF, Rand RW, Walter RD: Plasma corticosteroids: changes in concentration after stimulation of hippocampus and amygdala. Science 139:1212, 1963
6. Mason JW, Brady JW, Sidman M: Plasma 17-hydroxycorticosteroid levels and conditioned behavior in the Rhesus monkey. Endocrinology 60:741, 1957
7. Persky H, Grinker RR, Hamburg DA, Sabshin M, Korchin SJ, Basowitz H, Chevalier JA: Adrenal cortical function in anxious human subjects: plasma level and urinary excretion of hydrocortisone. AMA Arch Neurol & Psychiat 76:549, 1956

8. Bliss EL, Migeon CJ, Branch CHH, Samuels LT: Reaction of the adrenal cortex to emotional stress. Psychosom Med 18:56, 1956
9. Board FA, Waseson R, Persky H: Depressive affect and endocrine functions: blood levels of adrenal cortex and thyroid hormones in patients suffering from depressive reactions. AMA Arch Neurol & Psychiat 78:612, 1957
10. Board FA, Persky H, Hamburg DA: Psychological stress and endocrine functions: blood levels of adrenocortical and thyroid hormones in acutely disturbed patients. Psychosom Med 18:324, 1956
11. Fishman J, Hamburg DA, Handlon J, Mason JW, Sachar EJ: Emotional and adrenal cortical responses to a new experience. Arch Gen Psychiat 6:271, 1962
12. Davis J, Morrill R, Fawcett J, Upton V, Bondy PK, Spiro HM: Apprehension and elevated serum cortisol levels. J Psychosom Res 6:83, 1962
13. Sabshin M, Hamburg DA, Grinker RR, Persky H, Baskowitz H, Korchin SJ, Chevalier JA: Significance of pre-experimental studies in the psychosomatic laboratory. AMA Arch Neurol & Psychiat 78:207, 1957
14. Persky H, Korchin SJ, Basowitz H, Board FA, Sabshin M, Hamburg DA, Grinker RR: Effect of two psychological stresses on adrenocortical function: studies on anxious and normal subjects. AMA Arch Neurol & Psychiat 81:219, 1959
15. Connell AM, Cooper J, Redfearn JW: The contrasting effects of emotional tension and physical exercise on the excretion of 17-ketogenic steroids and 17-ketosteroids. Acta Endocrinol 27:179, 1958
16. Price DB, Thaler M, Mason JW: Preoperative emotional states and adrenal cortical activity. AMA Arch Neurol & Psychiat 77:646, 1956
17. Fox HM, Murawski BJ, Bartholomay AF, Gifford S: Adrenal steroid excretion patterns in eighteen healthy subjects. Psychosom Med 23:33, 1961
18. Friedman SB, Mason JW, Hamburg DA: Urinary 17-hydroxycorticosteroid levels in parents of children with neoplastic disease: a study of chronic psychological stress. Psychosom Med 25:364, 1963
19. Friedman SB, Chodoff P, Mason JW, Hamburg DA: Behavioral observations on parents anticipating the death of a child. Pediatrics 32:610, 1963
20. Glenn EM, Nelson DH: Chemical methods for the determination of 17-hydroxycorticosteroids and 17-ketosteroids in urine following hydrolysis with B glucuronidase. J Clin Endocrinol 13:911, 1953
21. Rosenthal WR, Mason JW: Urinary 17-hydroxycorticosteroid excretion in the normal Rhesus monkey. J Lab Clin Med 53:720, 1959
22. Wolff CT, Hofer MA, Mason JW: Relationship between psychological defenses and mean urinary 17-hydroxycorticosteroid excretion rates. II. methodologic and theoretical considerations. Psychosom Med 26:592, 1964
23. Mason JW, Harwood CT, Rosenthal NR: Influence of some environmental factors on plasma and urinary 17-hydroxycorticosteroid levels in the Rhesus monkey. Am J Physiol 190:429, 1957

24. Sachar EJ, Mason JW, Kolmer HS, Artiss KL: Psychoendocrine aspects of acute schizophrenic reactions. Psychosom Med 25:510, 1963
25. Oken D, Grinker RR, Heath HA, Sabshin M, Schwartz N: Stress response in a group of chronic psychiatric patients. Arch Gen Psychiat 3:451, 1960

CHAPTER 5

Review of Consultation Psychiatry and Psychosomatic Medicine
II. Clinical Aspects

Z. J. LIPOWSKI, M.B., B.CH., D.PSYCH.

Prefatory Remarks

Thomas N. Wise, M.D.

Written over 25 years ago, this review is still the classic essay about consultation-liaison psychiatry for all health professionals interested in the interface between psychiatry and medicine. The taxonomy of problems seen by consultants continues to retain heuristic utility to describe the clinical issues on a consultation service. Lipowski's hope for better studies to determine the prevalence of psychiatric morbidity in medical populations is being realized. Improved diagnostic systems and sophisticated psychometric strategies have better defined the prevalence and nature of psychiatric morbidity in a variety of hospital settings. Effective strategies to treat depression and anxiety in such patients are emerging. Unfortunately, the disparity between the prevalence of patients with psychiatric disorders and actual referral rates remains great. The challenges for consultation psychiatry are to close this gap in a clinically realistic manner and

---

Volume 29, 1967, pp. 201–224.
From McGill University and the Psychiatric Consultation Service, Royal Victoria Hospital and Montreal Neurological Hospital, Montreal, Canada.
Received for publication Aug. 29, 1966.

to practice consultation psychiatry in the ambulatory primary care arena. This article provides the clinical template for the content of this subspecialty of psychiatry.

Studies of prevalence of psychiatric morbidity in the nonpsychiatric areas of general hospitals as well as of frequency and patterns of referrals for psychiatric consultation are critically reviewed. Commoner psychiatric diagnostic and management problems encountered on the medical and surgical wards are classified and discussed. The importance of these problems for psychiatric and psychosomatic theory, as well as their practical implications for training and research, are pointed out.

In Part I of this review[73] an attempt was made to outline the scope, organization, and functions of consultation psychiatry in general hospitals. Part II surveys the types of diagnostic and management problems encountered by psychiatric consultants in the medical and surgical divisions of a general hospital. For clarity of presentation, the writer will first review some studies of the prevalence of psychiatric illness in this type of hospital and the frequency of and trends in referrals for psychiatric consultation. While such a survey may give some information about the *quantitative* aspects of the problem, it can tell little about the manifold *quality* of psychopathological and social phenomena which psychiatrists can observe in a medical setting. To do justice to this broader and theoretically far more important aspect, a synopsis of psychiatric aspects of medical practice in a general hospital will be presented. It is expected that such treatment of the subject will make the review more useful for a wider circle of readers and offer clearer implications for teaching, therapeutic needs, research possibilities, and use of psychiatric manpower.

The writer is aware of the vagueness of the phrase "psychiatric aspects of medical practice" but can offer no better substitute at present. His selection of clinical material is based both on the problems which psychiatric consultants are actually asked to help with and on his judgment that a given class of facts can be more adequately observed, understood, and managed if a psychiatrist's special knowledge and techniques are brought into play. This does not, of course, mean that everything that falls into this category is necessarily "abnormal" and in need of psychiatric therapeutic intervention. To describe what psychiatric consultants see and what they are called upon to deal with would be of only limited interest. More important are the varieties of human behavior and experience that can be observed in a medical setting, which are usually ignored by nonpsychiatric observers and are yet of importance both for over-all medical care and for their theoretical interest to the students of human behavior.

Quantitative Aspects

Psychiatric Morbidity in Hospitals' Nonpsychiatric Areas

Prevalence studies are intended to estimate the number of patients with a mental disorder of recognized severity in a population at one point in time.[96] For practical purposes, however, this means the number counted not at one instant but at any time during the period of survey. Such studies are of value for estimating the need for psychiatric care. Data about the prevalence of psychiatric illness in various nonpsychiatric divisions of general hospitals are still limited and inconclusive. It appears that the most frequently studied population have been the patients attending medical outpatient clinics.[17, 42, 53, 66, 68, 98, 125-127] Culpan and Davies[17] tabulated findings from some previous reports on the number of patients with psychiatric illness in various "medical" populations and arrived at a mean percentage of 27.3. This is a low estimate compared with their own study in which they found that 51% of 100 consecutive new referrals to a medical outpatient clinic and 21% of corresponding referrals to a surgical clinic had psychiatric illness. Stoeckle et al.[127] have recently reviewed surveys of psychiatric illness in medical practice (not confined to general hospitals) and comment that criteria of case selection and definitions used by the various studies make comparisons between them practically impossible. The writer concurs with this opinion. Stoeckle et al. studied the incidence of "psychological distress" in 101 new patients attending the medical clinic at the Massachusetts General Hospital and found it to be 84%. They emphasize the importance of such distress for the timing of the patient's decision to attend the doctor.

Kaufman and Bernstein[53] studied the records of 1000 consecutive patients referred to the outpatient diagnostic clinic at the Mount Sinai Hospital in New

York and found that 81.4% had psychological factors as the basis for their complaints. Thus only 16.6% of the 1000 patients had organic illness without a psychological component. It appears that in 69% of the patients no organic disease was present.

The similar findings of Stoeckle and Kaufman and of others suggest that the prevalence of psychiatric morbidity in outpatient clinic populations is indeed high and may actually be higher than the occurrence of organic disease. The implications of this finding for the organization and staffing of such clinics are apparent. There is clearly a need for the availability of psychiatric consultants in medical outpatient departments and for the provision of community mental health clinics.

Studies of the prevalence of psychiatric morbidity among medical and surgical inpatients are relatively few.[19, 40, 55, 85, 89, 93, 97, 109, 140] Table 5–1 shows the total number of patients studied by each investigator and the percentage of those showing psychiatric disease or distress. The wide range of the reported frequency of psychiatric illness is notable. How meaningful and practically useful are these figures? The only generalizations that can be made at this stage are methodological ones. The following variables appear to be directly relevant to the evaluation of these studies:

1. Type of setting studied—general or private hospital, ward or outpatient clinic, medical or surgical, etc.

Table 5–1. Prevalence of psychiatric morbidity in "medical" populations

	Patients in study	
Investigator	**No.**	**% with psychiatric disease**
Denney et al.[19]	39	72
Denney et al.[19]	54	32
Helsborg[40]	500	41
Kaufman et al.[55]	253	66.8
Mittelman et al.[85]	450	30
Payson[89]	109	72.5
Querido[93]	1630	46.6
Richman et al.[97]	184	36
Schwab et al.[109]	100	15
Zwerling et al.[140]	200	86

2. Demographic characteristics of the patient population (e.g., Denney et al.[19] found twice as much psychiatric morbidity among the medically indigent than in private patients).
3. Case-finding methods—psychiatric interview, self-administered questionnaires, personality scales, or the judgment of a nonpsychiatrist.
4. Presence or absence of a psychiatric unit in the hospital studied. (One could expect that if such a unit were present, some patients would be steered to it directly, thus reducing the incidence of purely psychiatric illness on the medical wards.)
5. Definition of psychiatric disorder or distress. This seems to be the most difficult variable to control, and unless such definitions are operational and rigorously adhered to, the meaning of the survey is doubtful.

The crucial question is: How relevant is the finding of a certain prevalence of psychiatric illness to the needs for psychiatric treatment and, as a result, manpower? For example, one finds in Zwerling's[140] study that as many as 86% of his 172 surgical patients had "psychiatric disorder," but that this included 108 (54%) with character and behavior disorders such as passive-aggressive and emotionally unstable personalities. (These two types accounted for almost 100% of this diagnostic subgroup.) One wonders what the value is of such an overinclusive diagnostic dragnet for any prevalence study and especially for rational planning of psychiatric services. (Perhaps the most urgent and promising task is to focus research endeavors on that *rara avis*—a medical patient defying psychiatric diagnosis.) More realistic and practically useful is the type of survey reported by Querido[93] from Amsterdam. He tried to assess the prevalence of distress—defined as social and/or psychic tensions too heavy for the patient to bear—in a sample of medical patients and predict the chances of each patient's recovery from somatic illness. He found distress in 46.6% of his patients and states that a follow-up investigation showed a significant difference in frequency of recovery between distressed patients and those without distress. A conclusion was reached that distress is a highly significant variable which adversely influences the effectiveness of medical treatment. Predictive studies of this type are likely to offer a realistic basis for planning preventive measures.

In summary, the frequency of psychiatric morbidity in nonpsychiatric divisions of general hospitals is not known with certainty, but there is some evidence that 30–60% of inpatients and 50–80% of outpatients suffer from psychic distress or psychiatric illness of sufficient severity to create a problem for the health professions. Carefully designed (particularly predictive and longitudinal) studies are needed to establish not only the quantity of but also the type, severity, and duration of such illness as a basis for rational planning of services and action.

Referrals for Psychiatric Consultation

What percentage of medical and surgical inpatients are referred for psychiatric consultations? How does the frequency of such referrals compare with the prevalence of psychiatric morbidity? What are the characteristics of the referred patient populations? What seems to influence the decision for and timing of requests for psychiatric consultations? There is some published information which can help answer, however tentatively, these questions.[12, 19, 24, 31, 52, 58, 64, 83, 89, 97, 102, 107–112, 115, 119, 123, 135, 136]

Frequency
Published data giving the total number of patients admitted to the medical and surgical wards over a period of time and the percentage of patients referred for psychiatric consultation are still too few. The several American publications available[12, 19, 64, 83, 89, 107, 123, 135] show the range as being 4–13%, with an average of 9%. A striking exception is the low figure of 2.2% reported by Eilenberg[24] from the Mayo Clinic. However, since the time periods under consideration vary from 3 months[24, 89] to 8 years,[64] it is difficult to talk about general trends. A national survey of all general hospitals is clearly indicated. The two British studies[31, 115] give the percentage of referrals as 0.7 and 1.34 respectively, and these figures contrast strikingly with the American ones. The Norwegian study by Rud[102] gives the figure of 4.9% of patients referred to a psychiatrist over a 3½-year period. It seems clear that such figures are likely to differ from country to country and from hospital to hospital, and to reflect a variety of factors. It is likely that American teaching hospitals, especially those possessing a well-established consultation service, will generally show the highest frequencies of psychiatric referrals.

Comparison with actual prevalence of psychiatric morbidity. Studies such as those by Richman et al.[97] and Denney et al.[19] suggest a discrepancy between estimated psychiatric morbidity and the frequency of referrals. While these studies may reflect no more than purely local conditions, a comparison of the estimates quoted above of psychiatric morbidity among medical and surgical inpatients with the reported frequency of psychiatric referrals strongly suggests that there is a wide disparity between the number of referrals and patients who could presumably benefit from a consultation. Does this mean that the prevalence figures are unrealistically high and thus of little value for the planning of psychiatric services in general hospitals; that nonpsychiatric physicians are woefully unaware of what their patients need; or that they deal with the psychiatric problems without our assistance? There are no ready answers to these questions at the present time. What is also involved here is the wider issue of medical philosophy, namely: Where does a physician's professional responsibility end? Is he expected to take into account and *somehow* deal with psychosocial distress and classifiable personality disorder in all his patients, or call upon his psychiatric consultant to do it for him even if this applies to 60, 70, or 86% of the patients at any given time? Surely a line has to be drawn somewhere if we are not to advocate a medico-social utopia.

Diagnostic Characteristics
The number of published studies giving pertinent data is still small[12, 31, 64, 109, 119, 123, 135] and comparison among them is made difficult by diverse and/or undefined diagnostic terminology used by the authors. Until there is greater uniformity and consistency in the usage of psychiatric classification such surveys will be of limited value. In addition, the samples tend to be small, which limits their usefulness even more. The six American studies which this writer succeeded in finding and which give diagnostic breakdown of the patient populations[12, 64, 109, 119, 123, 135] show that the relative frequency of psychiatric diagnoses differed from study to study, making general conclusions difficult.

The study by Wilson and Meyer[135] calls for special comment as it illustrates the value of consistency in the use of psychiatric diagnostic terms. These authors compared two groups of patients referred to a psychiatric liaison service in each of 2 successive years and found "a high degree of concordance in the diagnoses assigned by the service." One notes that the organic brain syndromes accounted for 21% and 28% of the diagnoses made in the 2 years respectively and were thus the commonest condition referred, followed by personality disorder, psychoneurosis (excluding depression), and depression (neurotic and psychotic). Schizophrenia was found in only 9% of the entire group. In another comparable study,[64] depression and personality disorders were each found in 21% of the referred patients and were thus most frequent. In a third study,[12] psychoneurosis topped the list, but the authors note that the symptom of depressive mood prompted the referral in 30% of the patients. Poe et al.[91] encountered depression in 52% of 192 patients referred for psychiatric consultation. Thus the overall impression from the studies quoted is that the group of depressions is probably the commonest class of psychiatric syndromes referred to psychiatric consultants.

One striking finding is that of the 808 consultation referrals reported in the American studies only 46 (6%) were given that vague but officially approved diagnosis of psychophysiologic reaction. The so-called psychosomatic disorders are mentioned in three studies,[12, 24, 64] and accounted for only 2, 6.1, and 7% respectively of all the consultation requests. The writer's impression from his own consultation service confirms this very low frequency of referrals of "psychosomatic" patients. These findings highlight our medical colleagues' lack of faith in our ability to contribute to the management of this class of patients. It appears that years of psychiatrists' preoccupation with these conditions and the massive volume of published studies have had little impact on medical practice beyond the spread of vague specificity stereotypes. There is little doubt that the bulk of a psychiatric consultant's work on medical and surgical wards consists of clinical problems unrelated to the psychosomatic disorders in the strict sense of the term. This fact can be expected to further divert research interests away from these disorders and consequently influence psychosomatic theory.

One general conclusion that can be drawn from a review of the studies referred to above is that the standard of reporting is generally low and more factual information is badly needed. It should be possible to organize a national survey of data possessed at present by all the psychiatric consultation services in the general hospitals on this continent. Such pooled information would surely encompass thousands of patients referred for consultation over a number of years, and provide meaningful data which are lacking at present. One has to consider that the six American studies quoted here pertain to a total of only a little over 800 referrals—a sample which any psychiatric consultation service in a large hospital could collect in 1 to 2 years. This writer and his group do 350–400 public consultations and about 200 private consultations a year and will publish their findings when these are analyzed.

The three British studies[31, 58, 115] are difficult to compare with the American ones because of different diagnostic terminology. One notes, however, that the British authors also found depression to be the commonest psychiatric syndrome referred to psychiatrists, although Shepherd et al.[115] report a slightly higher percentage of toxic and organic reaction.

Patterns

The reasons for the requests for psychiatric consultation are specified in a number of studies.[12, 24, 31, 52, 58, 64, 123] Here again the lack of homogeneous terminology thwarts any attempts at meaningful comparison. There is a need for an agreement to record and report such data in a standardized fashion; otherwise the published reports will largely remain of limited value, if any, with no general trends discernible. Some writers give "psychiatric problem" or "psychiatric symptoms" as a reason for referral and do not specify whether the request was primarily for diagnosis, management, or disposition. Thus one study[52] reports that 61.4% of referrals were for differential diagnosis, while another[12] does not mention diagnosis at all but gives percentage of referrals for "psychiatric symptoms," "drugs and procedures," and "no organic explanation for symptoms." If any generalization can be drawn from these reports it is that diagnostic uncertainty on the part of the physicians and a need for advice on management of patients are the main reasons for consultation.

There is also little information regarding the type of patient referred irrespective of psychiatric diagnosis. Payson[89] noted that patients from higher social classes, the middle-aged, women with little education, and highly educated men who had low occupational status were all favored in referrals. Wilson and Meyer[136] found that residents selected for psychiatric consultation younger (i.e., those less than 49 years of age) patients with less serious medical illnesses. These authors emphasize what others have already noticed, that "the quietly depressed patient whose behavior is unremarkable" is the one usually unrecognized by both physicians and nurses as he does not disturb them in their work. Patients with organically impaired brain function are often not referred since, as has been suggested,[19] there is pessimism regarding our therapeutic efficacy when the patient's cerebral function is impaired. Schwab et al.[107, 109–112] discuss in a series of papers the characteristics of 100 hospitalized medical patients referred for psychiatric consultation and draw some conclusions regarding referral patterns. They found that their referred patients were characterized by "longstanding illnesses, intractable in quality, and unchanging in symptomatology." It is of note that less than half of these patients had positive physical findings related to their symptoms. These writers suggest that when a patient gives a history of increase in a chronic illness, combined with a high number of adverse events in the past and unsatisfactory home life, there is increased probability that he will be referred. Regarding timing of the referral for consultation, Schwab et al. found that when physical diagnosis on admission is negative, the patient is likely to be referred early; but if he has serious organic disease and abnormal physical findings and laboratory results, referral is late. These investigators make a strong plea for referrals to the psychiatric consultants early in the period of hospitalization if the physician finds evidence of significant psychopathology on admission.

In a separate paper Schwab et al.[108] report that despite common fear among physicians that patients may react adversely to a psychiatric referral, the majority of the patients whom they studied and who had been referred reacted favorably to their physician's decision to arrange for a psychiatric assessment. A more general and theoretical discussion of the factors which influence a physician's decision whether and when to refer a patient for psychiatric consultation can be found in Meyer's articles[81, 82] and in Part I of this review.

Psychiatric Diagnostic Problems on Medical Wards

A psychiatric consultant on the medical and surgical wards is often called to assist in the diagnostic process. Apart from relatively few cases of gross psychiatric disorder, the two questions he is asked most frequently are: (1) Is this particular bodily complaint (or set of complaints) explicable as an expression of psychological ill-health, i.e., is it partly or wholly psychogenic? (2) Is the inner experience of psychic change reported by the patient or his observable behavior explicable as the direct results of, or a psychological reaction to, organic disease? The only method by which the consultant can attempt to answer these questions is the psychiatric interview, possibly supplemented by interviews with other observers. All this is common knowledge, but its theoretical implications are seldom analyzed and discussed. Psychiatrists in training and physicians in general are urged to avoid diagnosis by exclusion, and high value is set on "positive" diagnosis of psychopathology—a salutary goal, but what does it really imply and can it always be achieved in practice? Studies of the prevalence of psychiatric morbidity indicate that it is relatively easy to attach an acceptable "positive" psychiatric diagnosis to as many as 7 or 8 out of every 10 "medical" patients. In the case of somatic symptoms we have at our disposal the unfailing wastebasket called the psychophysiologic reaction. Yet what is the practical value of this labeling and its relevance to the given diagnostic problem? Faced with the question about the determinants of a given somatic symptom (e.g., pain), the consultant can (1) affirm that it is psychogenic, e.g., a symbolic expression of conflict; (2) discuss the diagnosis in descriptive psychiatric and/or psychodynamic terms while evading the question about the symptom itself or stating his inability to explain its nature; (3) attempt to show that the symptom is meaningful and fully accounted for by consideration of the patient's personality dynamics, past history, and current life situation—even though no symbolic meaning has been discerned; (4) express the opinion that further medical investigations are needed to rule out organic basis. The crucial question is: How reliable is the psychiatric interview as a diagnostic tool when applied to the elucidation of somatic symptoms? Sandt and Leifer[104] give a clear answer to this question as it relates to pain, the commonest presenting complaint. According to them psychiatric consultation which depends upon psychological or psychodynamic investigation can only add to the diagnosis but not differentiate psychogenic from physical illness. The writer agrees with this viewpoint but with some reservations. The consultant has the choice of either confining himself to a psychodynamic exploration or expanding it to include a functional inquiry and critical evaluation of the symptom from the medical viewpoint. A psychiatrist's interviewing skills and his ability to secure the cooperation of the patient may allow him to obtain vital information which has eluded the patient's physician and which may help in establishing an organic diagnosis. Should the psychiatrist shirk this opportunity because of a rigid conception of his role as an expert in psychodynamics only? The writer does not believe so. A psychiatric consultant to medicine must surely be more than a peripatetic sketcher of psychodynamic profiles.

The problem of diagnosis could be easier to solve if we had a better understanding of the determinants and psychophysiological mechanisms of somatic symptoms not directly due to organic disease. Szasz,[129] Kepecs,[59] Seitz,[113] Malmo et al.,[77] and others have made important contributions to this problem—an area of clinical research to which psychiatrists working on the medical wards could usefully contribute. An example of such an endeavor can be found in Lipin's paper.[72] This author presents some psychiatric methods of determining the nature of somatic symptoms. He postulates that pain and other somatic sensations may be not only a manifestation of organic or hysterical illness but also of memories of bodily symptoms experienced during a forgotten childhood illness, brought into awareness through association with current experiences. This hypothesis is worth attempting to validate. What we need is a theory of somatic symptoms and practical guides to differential diagnosis based on it.

From the psychological viewpoint, each somatic symptom can be regarded as a perception and/or communication. Thus a person can report a somatic perception, just communicate psychological distress in bodily metaphors, or do both. Pain, weakness, and tingling are all sensations which immediately give rise to cognitive and emotional responses. How the patient feels about his symptom will depend on its *meaning* to him, conscious and unconscious. The meaning in turn depends on the patient's past experience, level of knowledge, personality organization, conflicts and modes of coping with them, and current psychosocial situation. What results may be an extremely complex network of variables which change the quality and intensity of the original sensation and may result in secondary, tertiary, etc., symptoms. These symptoms can be partly physiological concomitants or equivalents of affective arousal (e.g., anxiety), and partly an expression of the symbolic meanings of the original and derivative symptoms and their inclusion in the intrapsychic conflict. These processes are further complicated by the perceived responses of others to the communication of the symptom, by cultural norms, etc. It is clear that what the patient experiences and how he communicates it to his physician is the resultant of multiple psychic processes as well as the doctor-patient relationship. We have yet to learn how to identify and evaluate the relative contribution of these multiple variables to the patient's presenting complaints.

A common pitfall for the beginning and even the experienced consultant is to include the presenting somatic symptoms into a plausible psychodynamic formulation. The symptom is then presented as a bodily expression of an ideational content. The writer recalls reading a senior psychiatric resident's consultation note on a patient presenting with paraplegia:

"This patient shows severe castration anxiety which he displaced from his penis to his legs and hence the paralysis. The diagnosis is conversion hysteria. Psychotherapy is recommended." This was a truly positive diagnosis but, as it turned out, equally positive was the patient's Wassermann reaction. While the resident's remarks about the castration anxiety may have been correct, the causal chain including the patient's paralysis was an artifact, however plausible it appeared. This raises the crucial problem of degrees of relevance in the psychological interpretation of somatic symptoms. The symptom may seem to fit a dynamic formulation, but in fact the latter can be partly or totally irrelevant to it. How can such compromising mistakes be avoided? The reviewer believes that psychiatric residents should be taught to exercise appropriate caution in drawing inference and to temper their interpretative zeal with careful observation and logical reasoning.

Guze et al.[37] offer a schema for comprehensive diagnosis which is worth keeping in mind. They propose that every patient should be examined in terms of four points of reference: (1) factors in the environment (or life situation); (2) heredity and past experience; (3) changes in the function and structure of organs and tissues; and (4) contribution of these changes to subsequent behavioral responses and nature of the latter.

Such schemes are useful as general guidelines, but they do not facilitate a consultant's task when faced with a concrete diagnostic problem. Directly relevant to the consultant's work is the growing literature on the psychiatric aspects of pain,[10, 25, 61, 80, 94, 122, 129, 132] some of which will be dealt with in detail below.

In summary, an attempt to integrate the various theoretical and experimental approaches to the understanding of somatic symptoms is overdue. Such a study might provide practical guidelines for differential diagnosis which are lacking at present. Woolly generalities about comprehensive or positive diagnosis should not conceal our ignorance in this area.

Classification

Psychiatric diagnostic problems encountered on the medical wards may be grouped as follows:

1. Psychological presentation of organic disease
2. Psychological complications of organic disease
3. Psychological reactions to organic disease
4. Somatic presentation of psychiatric disorders
5. "Psychosomatic" disorders

It is clearly impossible to review all the relevant material on this subject—a book would be required for adequate coverage. This review only attempts to outline and organize the facts, viewpoints, and procedures which constitute the field of consultation psychiatry in general hospitals. The above grouping is an empirical one and reflects the actual modes of presentation of diagnostic problems to the consultant. There is obvious overlapping of the different groups, but a more rigidly defined classification would artificially delimit what in nature is intertwining, fluid, and shifting.

Psychological Presentation of Organic Disease

A person suffering from an organic disease can present with complaints expressed in psychological terms; i.e., in terms of disordered cognition, perception, and/or affect. Or the patient may not complain of anything but people around him notice changes in his behavior which physicians sometimes refer to as "personality change." Such change may be either an accentuation of the patient's characteristic personality style (i.e., he appears to be more obsessional, hysterical, or psychopathic), or a display of behavior which is unusual and atypical for the patient. Thus a cautious and pedantic businessman may become reckless or a normally outgoing housewife morose and withdrawn, etc. Such personality change occurring in patients who are over the age of 40 raises the suspicion of cerebral disease, primary or secondary. Chapman and Wolff[13] give a particularly useful account of psychological changes brought about by disease of the neopallium. It is not only cerebral disease that can present with psychological manifestations; e.g., carcinoma of the body and tail of the pancreas is well-known for its tendency to simulate psychiatric illness.[90] The writer saw 3 patients on the same ward within a few months who had been referred to him as sufferers of pure depression but actually suffered from unsuspected pancreatic cancer. In all 3 he postulated the presence of organic disease on the basis of a careful history and evaluation of the presenting symptom of pain, even though the patients did suffer from varying degrees of depression.

Some patients unconsciously deny or consciously conceal significant somatic symptoms and may even present the consultant with their own diagnosis of a psychological illness. The writer is always on guard when a patient tells him from the start: "It's all psychosomatic, doctor." Such introduction calls for particular care in evaluation of the symptoms. Anxiety or depression aroused by subjective awareness of physical ill health and its possible ominous implications may mask the underlying disease. This has been repeatedly observed in the case of brain tumor.[39] Conditions such as epilepsy[16, 46, 76] or pheochromocytoma[21] may give rise to anxiety attacks indistinguishable clinically from those accompanying psychogenic illness. Stengel[122] suggests that it was one of Paul Schilder's main contributions to psychopathology to recognize that the same symptoms, such as depersonalization or body-image disturbances, can be produced by both organic and psychogenic causes. The theoretical implications of this fact should be brought into focus again.

In general, any organic disease may give rise to any type of neurotic or psychotic symptoms, depending on the patient's personality structure; and these symptoms overshadow those of the basic disease. The practical implications of this fact are clear: The psychiatric consultant in a general hospital must have the knowledge of and be constantly aware of the psychological presentation of organic disease which may *mask* the latter and be easily overlooked by physicians.[101]

Psychological Complications of Organic Disease

Psychiatric disorders which fall roughly into the category of acute and chronic brain syndromes can be regarded as a direct result of organic disease on the highest integrative functions of the brain. Their hallmark is the impairment of cognitive functions, either global or relatively selective. The acute syndrome is by definition reversible; the chronic one, irreversible. The two syndromes may, of course, coexist in the same patient. Prolonged observation may be necessary before the extent of apparent irreversibility can be reasonably established. Etiological factors are many[20, 41] since any factor which interferes with the supply, uptake, and/or utilization of oxygen or glucose by the cerebral neurones may bring about an organic brain syndrome. Predisposing factors are inadequately known, particularly the psychological ones.

These syndromes are a strangely neglected subject in the English-language literature. Their terminology, psychopathology, and diagnostic criteria are in need of revision. Various authors use terms such as "delirium," "acute confusional states," "exogenous reaction type," "toxic psychosis," "infective-exhaustive psychosis," etc., to denote the reversible syndrome. Clear definitions and classification are needed before progress can be made in this important area. A few authors[27, 67] have called attention to the general lack of interest in delirium and the frequent failure of both physicians and psychiatrists to recognize it clinically.[95] Psychosomatic investigators have showed hardly any interest in the reversible syndrome. This is surprising since it is a condition in which both organic and psychological changes occur in close temporal proximity, and their interaction would deserve study. Perhaps in the future delirium will come to be regarded as a model of a psychosomatic disorder. Engel and Romano[27] offer one of the best available reviews of delirium in English and point out that many seriously ill hospitalized patients display some degree of it. This claim is borne out by incidence studies carried out in the nonpsychiatric hospitals.[95, 99, 116] It has been found that as many as 50% of patients over 60 years of age may show evidence of delirium on admission to hospital.[99, 116] Willi,[9] using a different terminology, estimates that 5–10% of medical patients in his Swiss hospital suffer from the acute exogenous reaction type. If this estimate is a generally valid one, it follows that only a fraction of such patients are referred to psychiatric consultants. A survey of 10 publications giving relevant figures[12, 24, 31, 38, 58, 64, 95, 115, 123, 135] shows that the two brain syndromes constitute about 17% of all referrals.

A psychiatric consultant can make several contributions in this area: first, diagnosis;[27, 41, 118] second, help with the management;[41] third, clinical research.[38, 79] The consultant is often the only physician sufficiently familiar with delirium and allied states to make a correct diagnosis. This is not an academic matter since medical progress brings with it a new crop of potential causes of organic psychoses. It is enough to mention steroids,[92] open-heart surgery,[65] and psychotropic drugs[28, 50] as representative examples. Withdrawal states from alcohol,[18] barbiturates,[7] and opiates[6] are often treated on the medical wards, and the psychiatric consultant may be called upon to play a key role in their diagnosis and therapy. He can draw attention to some psychological aspects of the care of delirious patients, such as the need for adequate sensory stimulation, human contact, etc. An outstanding example of a consultant's imaginative contribution to such problems is the management of delirium after eye surgery.[134]

With regard to research, psychiatric consultants have a unique opportunity to study all degrees and varieties of delirium. Mendelson et al.[79] illustrate this potential in their study of the psychiatric theory of psychopathological disturbances in poliomyelitis patients confined in a respirator. Suggested problems in need of organized inquiry are: (1) classification of the reversible syndrome which, in the writer's opinion, is at present too crude and muddled; (2) investigation of psychopathological features from the viewpoint of modern psychology, e.g., the concepts of "confusion" and "clouding of consciousness"; (3) psychological predisposing factors in delirium, e.g., degree of ego strength, personality structure, etc.; (4) psychodynamic meaning of delirious productions (generally taken for granted but seldom investigated); and (5) the possible effect of delirium experienced in childhood on psychological development and predisposition to psychiatric disorders.

One can consider delirium and allied states from the theoretical viewpoint as a class of disorders of consciousness. As such they invite comparison with and delineation in psychological and physiological terms from model psychoses, disturbances attending alterations of sensory input, effects of sleep and dream deprivation, psychogenic confusional states, and dissociative reactions. This is surely an intriguing area of comparative psychopathology almost untouched by psychosomatic research. Much of the relevant clinical material can be found on the medical and surgical wards.

In contrast to the English school, German psychiatry has a long tradition of interest in psychiatric disorders complicating organic diseases. Since Bonhoeffer delineated the acute exogenous reaction type more than half a century ago, there has been a massive output of relevant literature recently reviewed by several authors.[9, 15, 30] Bleuler[8] distinguishes three different subtypes of this reaction type: (1) reduction of consciousness, (2) alteration (clouding) of consciousness with confusion, and (3) dysmnesic or Korsakoff's syndrome. He claims that each of these forms has its own psychopathology and pathophysiology. This seems to be a more adequate classification than lumping together diverse states under the heading "acute brain syndrome." The latter offers no room for such disorders as toxic psychosis due to amphetamine or cortisone where "clouding of consciousness" does not usually occur.

In summary, psychiatric complications of organic disease are an area on the borderlands between psychiatry and medicine which has been untapped by psychosomatic research. Accruing evidence indicates the relatively high incidence of these complications in general hospitals and their high priority in a psychiatric consultant's work. They offer wide scope for cooperative investigation likely to be appreciated by our medical colleagues and to open new vistas for psychosomatic research and theory.

Psychological Reactions to Organic Disease

The distinction between psychological "reactions" and "complications" is an arbitrary one and no clear-cut line can be drawn between them. The organic brain syndromes have been traditionally distinguished on the basis of impairment of cognitive functions (i.e., remembering and thinking); but it is generally known that affective disturbances, such as lability of affect, are often present, too.[118] On the other hand, impaired intellectual functioning and judgment as well as confusion may be present in acute schizophrenia.[118] Yet as a general rule lack of evidence of organic dysfunction is usually associated with a final diagnosis of functional mental illness, and vice versa.[118] While allowing for a continuum and intermingling of the "organic" and "psychogenic" consequences of organic disease there is still heuristic merit in separating the predominantly affective and symbolic effects of such disease from those due to demonstrable cerebral insufficiency.[27]

Psychological reactions to physical illness have been variously conceptualized in terms of psychological stress,[26, 45] psychological trauma,[4] crisis,[126] change in body image,[3, 106] or shift in libido economy.[29] Each of these approaches tends to emphasize different facets of the total human response. The writer finds Engel's[26] conception of psychological stress a particularly comprehensive and useful conceptual framework. Engel regards broadly conceived injury or threat of injury to the body a special category of psychological stress. Thus his general outline of responses to such stress can be applied logically to physical illness. These responses can be summarized as follows:

1. Formation of an unpleasant affect, or sequence of affects (anxiety, guilt, hopelessness, helplessness, shame, disgust)
2. Pathological affective states, i.e., long-lasting and/or excessively intense affects associated with manifest bodily changes
3. Employment of ego mechanisms of defense against the unpleasant affect (This results in development of neurotic or psychotic symptoms and character disorders.)
4. Inadequate evaluation and avoidance of external stresses as possible consequence of developments under Item 3
5. Harmful somatic effects of the physiological concomitants of dysphoric affects (e.g., precipitation of anginal pain)
6. Influence of secondary somatic effects (Items 4 and 5) on the psychic functions; this could be called "positive feedback" effect on the original psychological stress.

Bellak[3] proposes a different scheme of psychological reactions to physical illness: (1) "normal" reaction, (2) avoidance reaction, (3) reactive depression, (4) channeling of premorbid pathological anxiety into preoccupation with the physical disease, and (5) psychological invalidism.

Particularly useful clinically is the list of possible psychological responses to serious physical disease, such as cancer, suggested by Senescu:[114] (1) the dependency response or revival of dependent patterns of behavior, (2) the feeling of damage and reduction of self-esteem, (3) the anger response, (4) the guilt response, (5) the loss of gratification or pleasure, and (6) the responses to the physician's attitude and behavior.

Other important contributions to the subject include Kahana's and Bibring's[49] discussion of the meaning of illness and its implications for the patient's behavior and management in terms of different personality types.

A valuable sociological concept is that of illness behavior[78] which refers to ways in which different patients perceive, evaluate, and act (or not act) upon their symptoms. This concept stresses the individual differences in the reaction to disease.

This writer believes that a set of variables influences any patient's psychological response to disease to a varying extent. These include such factors as:

1. Personality structure and unconscious conflicts[4, 49]
2. The meaning and importance for the patients of the affected organ, lesion, actual bodily change, changed proprioceptive sensations, and body image
3. The degree and nature of the inclusion of Item 2 into unconscious conflicts
4. Psychodynamic effect of the beliefs about the cause of disease[2]
5. Cultural[105] and educational[75] factors
6. The state of the patient's current interpersonal relationships
7. The actual extent of mutilation and loss of function and their socioeconomic consequences for the patient
8. Previous experience with disease
9. The patient's state of awareness and cognitive functioning
10. Degree of acceptance by him of the "sick role"[78]
11. The doctor-patient relationship

All these variables have to be evaluated when the consultant wants to obtain an over-all picture of a patient's psychological response to his illness as a basis for therapeutic action. Senescu[114] suggests some practical behavioral criteria for the assessment of pathological reactions to illness.

From the nosological viewpoint, psychological reactions to organic disease spread over the whole spectrum of neuroses, psychoses, and personality disorders. The incidence of more extreme degrees of personality disorganization in response to illness is virtually unknown. Kaufman et al.[55] found the prevalence of psychiatric illness on a medical service to be as high as 66.8%, but one half of these patients suffered from "benign psychiatric disorder." Functional psychosis was found in only 7.5% of the patients; it is not clear what proportion of them suffered from it prior to the onset of organic disease. Some studies[22, 124] indicate that a considerable proportion of patients became depressed as a result of severe illness. More data are clearly needed.

Up to this point the psychological reactions have been dealt with in general terms, and a premature impression might be gained that such reactions are totally independent of the type of organic disease present. There is actually some evidence that certain diseases are more likely than others to precipitate disorders having the features of functional rather than organic psychiatric illness. As examples one may mention viral infections,[36] such as hepatitis,[74] which are often followed by a depression; systemic lupus erythematosus;[87] multiple sclerosis;[35] porphyria;[1] and Cushing's syndrome.[120] The relative importance of the disease in question as an etiological factor in psychiatric illness is difficult to evaluate.[23] Quarton et al.[92] offer a brilliant paradigm for the evaluation of the variables and hypotheses relevant to psychiatric disorders due to ACTH and cortisone. Their schema could well be applied by consultants to other drugs and diseases.

Somatic Presentation of Psychiatric Disorders
The inclusion of the whole gamut of functional psychiatric disorders would be of little practical value. Only those disorders which give rise to diagnostic difficulties in medical settings are described below.

Depression. The depression syndrome is the most common and versatile imitator of organic disease. The range of somatic symptoms accompanying the various types of depression is wide.[14] Fatigue, insomnia, localized and diffuse pain, impotence, paresthesias, and palpitations are some of the commonest complaints noted.[5, 10, 47, 91, 125] As many as 25% of patients suffering from a psychotic depression may present with physical symptoms.[47] Depressed patients seem to form the bulk of those at medical clinics who present with somatic complaints not supported by positive signs of organic disease.[125] The diagnosis rests on characteristic psychological symptoms.[91, 125] The language of emotions is foreign to some patients while others unconsciously or consciously deny any awareness of depressed mood, making diagnosis difficult. The term "depressive equivalent" has been used to describe such depressions.[5] In a doubtful case with negative physical signs a therapeutic trial with antidepressants may be used.

Conversion reaction and hysteria. Nearly 30 years ago Lindemann[71] discussed hysteria as a problem in a general hospital, and his observations are still pertinent. He noted that in conversion symptoms we are dealing with functional physiological alterations, but that knowledge of how "psychogenic factors operate to cause physiologic change is not available yet." There is little that we can add to his remarks today. The whole concept of hysteria has disintegrated in the last two or three decades, prompting a historian of this disease[131] to ask if it has really disappeared in modern life. Psychiatric consultants in the general hospital can reassure the historian that it has not. A typical comment is: "... men, women, and children continue to suffer illnesses diagnosed as conversion hysteria, in numbers similar to illnesses considered far from uncommon."[70] Other consultants also confirm that they see "substantial numbers" of conversion reactions on the medical wards.[137] The same observers discuss operational diagnostic criteria and a conceptual model of conversion reaction.[137-139] They point out that the diagnosis of this reaction cannot be established by either psychiatric or physiological considerations alone but requires assessment of both these aspects. In this writer's experience it is indeed rare that a convincing symbolic meaning of a symptom can be established during a single psychiatric consultation—a degree of probability is usually all one can achieve. A discovery of a symbolic meaning for a symptom does not settle the issue of diagnosis since any organically derived symptom may acquire secondary symbolic elaboration.

While the concept of hysteria has been officially replaced by conversion and dissociative reactions, some authors still claim[34] that hysteria is a syndrome with characteristic clinical features of which conversion symptoms are not an essential part.

The frequency of the different conversion symptoms is not known but it appears at present that pain is the commonest of them.[137] Engel[25] observes that the largest number of patients with "psychogenic" pain belongs to the conversion reaction category. Merskey[80] reports that persistent pain shows common association with hysteria. Yet Slater[117] issues a chilling warning: "The diagnosis of 'hysteria' is a disguise for ignorance and a fertile source of clinical error." In a similar vein, Walters[132] suggests that the term "hysterical pain" be abandoned in favor of "psychogenic regional pain." Thus the controversy continues.

Whether pain and other more circumscribed symptoms are the commonest form of conversion reaction is still an open issue. The more dramatic manifestations believed by some to be extinct are still with us.[62] Lipin[72] describes gross mental disturbances with depersonalization, amnesia, and emotional outbursts occurring during the early weeks following the onset of a major conversion symptom. He emphasizes that when there is no major psychic decompensation at that stage, the symptoms are not likely to be conversion. It is notable that Lipin's interesting observations on the natural history of conversion were made in a neurological hospital. This writer has been struck by the relative frequency with which various types of conversion symptoms can be found on the wards of the neurological hospital where he is consultant. The wards of the general and neurological hospitals are some of the best settings in which to study conversion reactions, affording consultants another opportunity to contribute to psychopathology.

In summary, conversion reaction and hysteria are concepts currently in a state of revision and flux. The relevant phenomena, however they may be named, do exist and pose common and sometimes difficult diagnostic problems for consultants. Conversion symptoms may coexist with and mask organic disease, severe depression, or schizophrenia. Diagnostic criteria could be improved; the definition of conversion reaction in psychodynamic terms tends to impede diagnosis. Physiological mechanisms are still unknown.

Anxiety reaction. Anxiety is a much used and abused term. Three related meanings of it may be distinguished: it is an affect, a clinical syndrome, and a theoretical or explanatory concept. These three meanings are seldom explicitly distinguished and this causes confusion. The clinical syndrome can occur in association with any disease, psychiatric or organic, and it is only when anxiety dominates the clinical picture in the absence of psychosis that the term "anxiety reaction" applies. The syndrome consists of a cognitive aspect, feeling tone, observable behavior, and physiological concomitants. At times only the latter are in evidence—an anxiety equivalent. Somatic complaints are always part of the syndrome and may be the presenting complaint. One of the best descriptions of the syndrome is still that by Freud.[32] Current psychiatric textbooks tend to devote more space to psychodynamic generalizations about anxiety than to description of its clinical features. Kolb[63] gives a useful presentation of diagnostic criteria.

Particularly difficult for the diagnostician are isolated symptoms, such as headache or hyperhidrosis. Hyperventilation is a common concomitant of chronic and acute anxiety and gives rise to a variety of symptoms which may imitate organic disease, from coronary thrombosis to epilepsy.[69] Such symptoms may be unilateral and suggest neurologic disease.[130] The predominantly cardiovascular symptoms in the so-called neurocirculatory asthenia is another diagnostic pitfall.[60] Many patients presenting with painful somatic symptoms, such as headache, suffer from an anxiety reaction.[61]

In conclusion, psychiatric consultants to medicine have an opportunity to see varied symptomatic presentation of anxiety reaction. They encounter anxiety states precipitated by organic disease or resulting from focal epilepsy[16, 46, 76] or pheochromocytoma.[21] They could contribute to the building of a truly psychosomatic theory of anxiety which would integrate descriptive, psychodynamic, and biological approaches. The tendency of anxiety to have primarily autonomic, and that of conversion reaction to have largely nonautonomic, physiological concomitants suggests two different biological modes of response to danger—internal or external.

Schizophrenia. This syndrome is often accompanied by somatic symptoms. Of special practical importance for psychiatric consultants as well as medical practitioners is the fact that many schizophrenic patients go from one medical clinic to another presenting their somatic complaints for diagnostic considerations. The true diagnosis is probably often missed,[88] especially in early and in so-called ambulatory schizophrenia.[43, 84] These patients seem to have a predilection for neuromuscular symptoms, such as backache[61] as well as gastrointestinal and EENT[84] complaints and those referred to the genitourinary tract.[86] The ambulatory or borderline schizophrenic patients often suffer from such somatic symptoms, regard themselves as physically ill, and resent referrals to psychiatrists.[43] Many of them suffer from psychogenic pain and fail to be correctly diagnosed.[25] Engel[25] regards such pain as a delusion and claims that correct diagnosis can be made if the patient is allowed to give his own explanation for the pain. It seems that many of these patients are labeled in medical clinics as hypochondriacs or psychophysiologic reactions. Miller[84] provides some useful diagnostic clues, such as the highly personalized and excessive character of the complaints, their bizarreness, etc. Another writer[133] offers a practical set of suggestive clinical features that permit the diagnosis of early schizophrenia. One should mention especially the disturbances of the body image which may bring such a patient to a plastic surgeon with the request for surgical correction of the shape of his nose or penis. The reviewer recalls a young man, circumcised in infancy, who went from surgeon to surgeon demanding that his prepuce be "replaced" by a new one to allow him to have an erection. Not all these patients are easy to spot early since many come with ordinary somatic complaints, such as headache. Unless a thorough discussion of the presenting complaint is attempted on the first interview, the patient may end up with a full diagnostic work-up and be told that he is really quite well. A psychiatric consultant should be called in early in such cases.

Hypochondriasis. This term has been dropped from the official American classification but it is still used as evidenced by a spate of recent papers devoted to it.[44, 56, 57, 61, 121] The revived interest no doubt stems from the fact that every medical clinic has its hard core of chronic complainers showing relatively fixed somatic complaints in the absence, or as overlay, of organic disease. Some of these patients are frankly delusional and, in any case, give the impression of being persecuted by their symptoms, such as pain.[25] They tend to describe their complaints with an intensity, persistence, and urgency which is in striking contrast to the typically indifferent hysteria.[25] Some of these patients are prepsychotic, and it is of interest that hypochondriasis shows rather common association with frank schizophrenia.[121] It appears, however, that many of these patients never fully decompensate into psychosis; those who do are likely to develop paranoid schizophrenia.

It would seem that the group of patients just described is a fairly homogeneous one, but this is denied by others. Kreitman[66] found that about one-fifth of them were suffering from depression. Kenyon[56, 57] discusses the meaning, history, and current state of hypochondriasis as a clinical entity. He lists 18 different usages of the term and suggests that hypochondriasis is always part of another syndrome, especially an affective one, and that there is no such entity as "primary hypochondriasis."

This writer believes that there may be some merit in retaining the term hypochondriasis to designate a group of chronic complainers with a paranoid personality structure. The writer repeatedly saw such patients as a consultant. He recalls a man who for some 30 years complained of rectal pain which he described "like a big stick trying to push through a small hole" and ascribed it to a rectal examination before an appendectomy. This man was a single and lonely individual with marked but not conscious homosexual interests who decompensated into a schizo-affective psychosis on several occasions. When psychotic, he claimed that his rectal pain was unbearable. This type of chronic patient should be distinguished from one who has transient hypochondriacal complaints as part of a depressive or anxiety reaction. It is well known that medical students suffer from fears of disease and various feelings of ill health; but as Hunter et al.[44] point out, these should be seen as a largely occupationally based nosophobia while hypochondriasis is rare and has serious significance.

Psychiatric consultants to the medical clinics are strategically placed to study this whole problem and to come up with a definitive statement on the issue of hypochondriasis.

"Psychosomatic" Disorders

Little needs to be said about these conditions here. As noted earlier they constitute but a fraction of the cases referred to psychiatric consultants. The focus of medical-psychiatric cooperation has largely shifted away from these disorders. The vast quantity of research carried out on them has left us with a body of valuable observation and such outstanding works as Engel's study of ulcerative colitis or Mirsky's formulation of the necessary conditions for the development of peptic ulcer. The value of our contribution to the therapy of these disorders has fallen far short of the promise of the "great-leap-forward" phase of psychosomatic medicine. We are also perhaps less sanguine in our search for psychogenicity which, as Schilder[106] remarked, is not very likely to solve the problem of organic disease.

What is a "psychosomatic disorder"? In this reviewer's opinion it is a misnomer with a vague meaning. It haunts the consultant like a bad ghost from the past. The consultant has to repeatedly correct the impression that all there is to psychosomatic medicine begins and ends with dependence, repressed anger, and the internalized bad mother symbolically nibbling at the gastric mucosa. Stereotypes die hard! It is an open question if it is methodologically sound to retain the concept of the psychosomatic disorders at all. In any case, those disorders are of importance to psychiatric consultants only insofar as they are presented by patients who have significant psychiatric difficulties, whether or not they antedated and/or followed the onset of the given disorder.

Management Problems on Medical Wards

Psychiatric Aspects

As noted above, up to one-half of requests for psychiatric consultation concern problems of management of patients. A general discussion of this aspect of the consultant's role as well as the more important techniques of dealing with the problems can be found in Part I[73] of this review. What remains is to list and briefly discuss some of the commoner problems to which the consultant may usefully contribute solutions. Such a list can hardly be complete, but it gives substance to the vague term "management problems" and conveys some idea of the scope of psychiatric consultants' work.

1. **Suicidal attempt or threat.** The consultant is called in to evaluate every patient admitted as a consequence of a suicidal attempt or attempting or threatening suicide during his hospitalization. (Some 10–20%[12,31,58] of referrals to consultation may stem from this cause.) Brown and Pisetsky[11] found the suicide rate in a general hospital to be 1.55 per 10,000 admissions. All the general ward patients in their series were chronically or terminally ill and suffered pain, dyspnea, or severe disability. Jumping from windows was the commonest method of suicide. The authors conclude that while suicide cannot be infallibly predicted, good rapport between doctor and patient offers the best possibility of assessing suicidal hazard.

   Stoller and Estess[128] report on 33 patients who committed suicide in the medical and surgical wards. All had severe physical illness and were older men with few relatives. The authors stress the importance of training medical personnel in recognition of depression and adequate reporting by the nurses of their behavioral observations. Early and adequate psychiatric consultation is recommended. A report on a series of patients admitted to a general hospital after a suicidal attempt notes that none made another attempt during the hospitalization.[33]

2. **Grossly disturbed behavior.** Delirium, functional psychosis, agitated dementia, panic state, nondiagnosable outbursts of rage, etc., are examples of this problem. In these cases, thorough familiarity with psychotropic drugs is necessary

if the consultant is to be helpful. A well-sedated patient may remain on the ward with minimum interruption of investigations and treatment, avoiding an emergency transfer to a psychiatric facility.

3. **Excessive emotional reactions.** This problem is characterized by fear, anger, depression, or suspicion related to hospitalization,[81] diagnostic procedures,[51] ward routine (such as rounds),[54] therapy and its effects,[45] and disclosure of the diagnosis.[54]

4. **Refusal to cooperate.** This includes such problems as refusal to undergo recommended surgery or other medical or surgical procedure or therapy, and signing out from the hospital against medical advice.[48] This type of problem is usually related to Item 3 above, but may also be an expression of conflict between the patient and his doctor. In that case, refusal to cooperate is only a symptom of a crisis in relationship.

5. **Delayed convalescence.** Every physician knows the type of patient who displays disability incompatible with objective findings of pathology, or who shows an apparent relapse or new symptoms when discharge is mentioned. These responses may be related to the patient's separation anxiety at the prospect of leaving the hospital on whose personnel he has become dependent; or to his fear, rational or irrational, regarding his state of health; or to his enthusiastic acceptance of the "sick role" for socioeconomic reasons. A psychiatrist is often called in to elucidate the problem and offer practical advice on how to speed up the patient's recovery. Such patients are often resented by the medical staff as weaklings and parasites—which only serves to complicate matters. The consultant may help overcome the stalemate.

6. **Conflict between patient and personnel.** Apart from refusal to cooperate with major aspects of the medical management, a patient may fall into a conflict with any member of the medical or nursing staff with resulting disruption of the therapeutic relationship.[82] Any patient who is demanding, complaining, openly critical of the hospital, unduly flirtatious, or hostile may draw disapproving attention of a doctor or nurse; the result is usually some form of rejection and possibly avoidance of the patient. When this happens, tension affects the entire ward; the patient may demand immediate discharge or try to pick a quarrel with his doctor. In this event, a psychiatrist usually receives an urgent call. The writer was asked to see a man who insisted on smoking at times when it was not allowed, which quickly led to a major crisis on the ward. It turned out that the patient could not tolerate authority, particularly if exercised by women (nurses). He had to assert his masculine and masterful position at any cost. The case was dealt with by explain-

ing the situation to the staff and patiently pointing out to the patient why certain rules had to be observed on the wards for his own and others' comfort and safety. It worked and the conflict was settled.

7. Patient with psychiatric history. Many physicians work on the unspoken assumption that "once a crock, always a crock." If a patient gives history of previous psychiatric hospitalization, especially for schizophrenia, he is likely to be watched with suspicion and fear. Such a patient may be discharged earlier than thorough diagnostic work-up and adequate therapy would justify. All his symptoms tend to be taken with skepticism, and serious organic disease may be overlooked. If such patient has difficulty in communicating, his fate is sealed. The same applies to previous diagnosis of hysteria. Such labels do stick! It is often up to the psychiatric consultant to take a careful history from such patients and point out to the referring physician that psychiatric and organic disorders are not incompatible—a truism often forgotten.

This writer recalls being asked, prior to the patient's hysterectomy, to see a woman because her old chart showed diagnosis of hysteria. During a lengthy and difficult interview, it transpired that the patient had recently developed spells in which she noticed a bad smell. "I am a clean woman!" she protested. A tentative diagnosis of uncinate fits due to an expanding lesion was made by the reviewer. A series of specialist consultations and tests followed and resulted in a conclusion that the patient was "just a hysteric." A few days after the operation she developed tentorial pressure cone and died. A large aneurysm of the internal carotid artery pressing on the tip of a temporal lobe was found at autopsy. The case was instructive for the many people concerned, but the patient was dead!

8. Psychiatric side effects of drugs. This management problem is encountered with drugs such as steroids and can not be elaborated here.

9. Selection and/or preparation of patients. Elective surgery, and other therapeutic procedures, such as hemodialysis,[103] etc., sometimes evoke reactions like those described in Items 3 and 4 above. When there are reasons to expect such undesirable responses, a predictive psychiatric assessment and preparation of the patient are called for.[45, 100]

10. Disposition. Ideally, this problem, which includes transfer of patients to the psychiatric ward and commitment, should occupy a fraction of a consultant's time if his work is efficient.

Summary and Conclusions

In this review an attempt has been made to present the scope of consultation psychiatry in the general hospitals. The evaluation of the importance of this whole area of work for psychiatric practice, teaching, and theory is left to the readers. The widening of the scope of psychosomatic medicine resulting from the diversification of the consultants' work and experience seems to be beyond doubt. A survey of the diagnostic and management problems confronting us in the various parts of the general hospitals has been presented here. The writer has aimed at comprehensiveness rather than intensive treatment of specific areas, each of which would deserve a separate paper. This approach was chosen deliberately with a view to illustrating the manifold quality of the psychosocial and psychopathological phenomena encountered in the medical settings. The writer considered it worthwhile to try and encompass this diversity in one review. He hopes to counteract the current malaise and uncertainty regarding the nature, scope, and goals of psychosomatic medicine. There is no need for defeatism. Fascinating vistas for clinical psychosomatic research are opening up. They should be welcome to all those disillusioned with the meager practical and theoretical results of the decades of search for psychogenic etiological factors in relatively few and elusive diseases. We are now closer to the truly comprehensive conceptions of that great, if too-little-recognized, pioneer of psychosomatic medicine, Paul Schilder. In the preface to his most significant book[106] he wrote: "It would be erroneous to suppose that phenomenology and psycho-analysis should or could be separated from brain pathology. It seems to me that the theory of organism could and should be incorporated in a psychological doctrine which sees life and personality as a unit . . . I have always believed that there is no gap between the organic and the functional."

Consultation psychiatry, despite its modest designation, has practical value for teaching and for collaboration with the rest of medicine. But beyond that it deals with the facets of the human condition which are of importance for the science of man, and such science must be *psychosomatic* in the full sense of the word.

References

1. Ackner B, et al: Acute porphyria: a neuropsychiatric and biochemical study. J Psychosom Res 6:1, 1962

2. Bard M, Dyk RB: Psychodynamic significance of beliefs regarding the cause of serious illness. Psychoanal Rev 43:146, 1956
3. Bellak L: Psychology of Physical Illness. Grune, New York, 1952
4. Beres D, Brenner C: Mental reactions in patients with neurological disease. Psychoanal Quart 19:170, 1950
5. Biloon S, Karliner W: The clinical picture of manic-depressive equivalents. New Eng J Med 259:684, 1958
6. Blachly PH: Management of the opiate abstinence syndrome. Amer J Psychiat 122:742, 1966
7. Blachly PH: Procedure for withdrawal of barbiturates. Amer J Psychiat 120:894, 1964
8. Bleuler M: Akute psychische Veraenderungen bei akuten Koerpererkrankungen. Schweiz Med Wschr 92:1521, 1962
9. Bleuler M, et al: Akute psychische Begleiterscheinungen Körperlicher Krankheiten. Thieme, Stuttgart, 1966
10. Bradley JJ: Severe localized pain associated with the depressive syndrome. Brit J Psychiat 109:741, 1963
11. Brown W, Pisetsky JE: Suicidal behavior in a general hospital. Amer J Med 29:307, 1960
12. Butler RN, Perlin S: Psychiatric consultations in a research setting. Med Ann DC 27:503, 1958
13. Chapman LF, Wolff HG: Disease of the neopallium. Med Clin N Amer, May 1958
14. Cleghorn RA, Curtis GC: Psychosomatic accompaniments of latent and manifest depressive affect. Canad Psychiat Ass J 4 (suppl):13, 1959
15. Conrad K: "Die symptomatischen psychosen," in Psychiatrie der Gegenwart (Bd. 2). Edited by Gruhle HW. Springer, Berlin, 1960
16. Court JH: Anxiety among acute schizophrenics and temporal lobe patients. Brit J Soc Clin Psychol 4:254, 1965
17. Culpan R, Davis B: Psychiatric illness at medical and surgical outpatient clinic. Compr Psychiat 1:228, 1960
18. Cutshall BJ: The Saunders-Sutton syndrome: an analysis of delirium tremens. Quart J Stud Alcohol 26:423, 1965
19. Denney D, et al: Psychiatric patients on medical wards. Arch Gen Psychiat (Chicago) 14:530, 1966
20. Dewan JG, Spaulding WB: The Organic Psychoses. University Press, Toronto, 1958
21. Doust BC: Anxiety as a manifestation of pheochromocytoma. Arch Intern Med (Chicago) 102:811, 1958
22. Dovenmuehle RH, Verwoerdt A: Physical illness and depressive symptomatology, 1: incidence of depressive symptoms in hospitalized cardiac patients. J Amer Geriat Soc 10:932, 1962
23. Eilenberg MD: Psychiatric illness and pernicious anemia. A clinical reevalu-

ation. J Ment Sci 106:1539, 1960
24. Eilenberg MD: Survey of inpatient referrals to an American psychiatric department. Brit J Psychiat 111:1211, 1965
25. Engel GL: "Psychogenic" pain and the pain-prone patient. Amer J Med 26:899, 1959
26. Engel GL: Psychological Development in Health and Disease. Saunders, Philadelphia, 1962
27. Engel GL, Romano J: Delirium, a syndrome of cerebral insufficiency. J Chronic Dis 9:260, 1959
28. Essig CF: Newer sedative drugs that can cause intoxication and dependence of barbiturate type. JAMA 196:714, 1966
29. Ferenczi S: Disease- or pathoneuroses, in Further Contributions to the Theory and Technique of Psycho-Analysis. Hogarth Press, London, 1926
30. Fleck U: Symptomatische Psychosen (1941–1957). Fortschr Neurol Psychiat 28. Heft 1, 1960
31. Fleminger JJ, Mallett BL: Psychiatric referrals from medical and surgical wards. J Ment Sci 108:183, 1962
32. Freud S: The justification for detaching from neurasthemia a particular syndrome: the anxiety-neurosis, in Collected Papers, Vol 1. Basic, New York, 1959, p 76
33. Friedman JH, Cancellieri R: Suicidal risk in a municipal general hospital. Dis Nerv Syst 19:556, 1958
34. Gatfield PD, Guze SB: Prognosis and differential diagnosis of conversion reactions. Dis Nerv Syst 23:623, 1962
35. Geocaris K: Psychotic episodes heralding the diagnosis of multiple sclerosis. Bull Menninger Clin 21:107, 1957
36. Gould J: Virus disease and psychiatric ill-health. Brit J Clin Pract 11:1, 1957
37. Guze SB: A formulation of principles of comprehensive medicine with special reference to learning theory. J Clin Psychol 9:127, 1953
38. Guze SB, Cantwell DP: The prognosis in "organic brain" syndromes. Amer J Psychiat 120:878, 1964
39. Haberland C: Psychiatric manifestations in brain tumors. Akt Fragen Psychiat Neurol 2:65, 1965
40. Helsborg HC: Psychiatric investigations of patients in a medical department. Acta Psychiat Neurol Scand 33:303, 1958
41. Henry DW, Mann AM: Diagnosis and treatment of delirium. Canad Med Ass J 93:1156, 1965
42. Hilkevitch A: Psychiatric disturbances in outpatients of a general medical outpatient clinic. Int J Neuropsychiat 1:371, 1965
43. Hollender M: Ambulatory schizophrenia. J Chronic Dis 9:249, 1959
44. Hunter RCA, et al: Nosophobia and hypochondriasis in medical students. J Nerv Ment Dis 139:147, 1964
45. Janis IL: Psychological Stress. Wiley, New York, 1958

46. Jonas AD: Ictal and Subictal Neurosis. Thomas, Springfield, IL, 1965
47. Jones D, Hall SB: Significance of somatic complaints in patients suffering from psychotic depression. Acta Psychother (Basel) 11:193, 1963
48. Kahana RJ: Teaching medical psychology through psychiatric consultation. J Med Educ 34:1003, 1959
49. Kahana RJ, Bibring GL: Personality types in medical management, in Psychiatry and Medical Practice in a General Hospital. Edited by Zinberg EN. International University Press, New York, 1964
50. Kane FJ Jr, Ewing JA: Iatrogenic brain syndrome. Southern Med J 58:875, 1965
51. Kaplan SM: Laboratory procedures as an emotional stress. JAMA 161:677, 1956
52. Kaufman RM: A psychiatric unit in a general hospital. J Mount Sinai Hosp NY 24:572, 1957
53. Kaufman RM, Bernstein S: A psychiatric evaluation of the problem patient. JAMA 163:108, 1957
54. Kaufman RM, et al: The emotional impact of ward rounds. J Mount Sinai Hosp NY 23:782, 1956
55. Kaufman RM, et al: Psychiatric findings in admissions to a medical service in a general hospital. J Mount Sinai Hosp NY 26:160, 1959
56. Kenyon FE: Hypochondriasis: a clinical study. Brit J Psychiat 110:467, 1964
57. Kenyon FE: Hypochondriasis: a survey of some historical, clinical and social aspects. Brit J Med Psychol 38:117, 1965
58. Kenyon FE, Rutter ML: The psychiatrist and the general hospital. Compr Psychiat 4:80, 1963
59. Kepecs JG: Some patterns of somatic displacement. Psychosom Med 15:425, 1953
60. Keyes JW: Iatrogenic heart disease. JAMA 192:951, 1965
61. Klee GD, et al: Pain and other somatic complaints in a psychiatric clinic. Maryland Med J 8:188, 1959
62. Knight JA: Epidemic hysteria: a field study. Amer J Public Health 55:858, 1965
63. Kolb LC: Anxiety and the anxiety states. J Chronic Dis 9:199, 1959
64. Kornfeld DS, Feldman M: The psychiatric service in the general hospital. New York J Med 65:1332, 1965
65. Kornfeld DS, et al: Psychiatric complications of open-heart surgery. New Eng J Med 273:287, 1965
66. Kreitman N: Hypochondriasis and depression in out-patients at a general hospital. Brit J Psychiat 111:476, 1965
67. Levin M: Delirium: a gap in psychiatric teaching. Am J Psychiat 107:689, 1951
68. Lewis BI: A psycho-medical survey of a private out-patient clinic in a university hospital. Amer J Med 14:586, 1953

69. Lewis BI: The hyperventilation syndrome. Ann Intern Med 38:918, 1953
70. Lewis WC, Berman M: Studies of conversion hysteria. Arch Gen Psychiat (Chicago) 13:275, 1965
71. Lindemann E: Hysteria as a problem in a general hospital. Med Clin N Amer, May 1938
72. Lipin T: Psychic functioning in patients with undiagnosed somatic symptoms. Arch Neur and Psychiat 73:239, 1955
73. Lipowski ZJ: Review of consultation psychiatry and psychosomatic medicine, I: general principles. Psychosom Med 29:153, 1967
74. Lowy F: The neuropsychiatric complications of viral hepatitis. Canad Med Ass J 92:237, 1965
75. Mabry JH: Lay concepts of etiology. J Chronic Dis 17:371, 1964
76. Macrae D: Isolated fear: a temporal lobe aura. Neurology (Minneap) 4:497, 1954
77. Malmo RB, et al: Specificity of bodily reactions under stress, in Life Stress and Bodily Disease. Assoc Research Nervous Mental Disease. Edited by Wolff HG. Williams & Wilkins, Baltimore, MD, 1950
78. Mechanic D: The concept of illness behavior. J Chron Dis 15:189, 1962
79. Mendelson J, et al: Hallucinations of poliomyelitis patients during treatment in a respirator. J Nerv Ment Dis 126:421, 1958
80. Merskey H: The characteristics of persistent pain in psychological illness. J Psychosom Res 9:291, 1965
81. Meyer E: Disturbed behavior on medical and surgical wards: a training and research opportunity, in Science and Psychoanalysis: Psychoanalytic Education, Vol 5. Edited by Masserman JH. Grune, New York, 1962
82. Meyer E, Mendelson M: Psychiatric consultations with patients on medical and surgical wards: patterns and processes. Psychiatry 24:197, 1961
83. Meyer E, Mendelson M: The psychiatric consultation in postgraduate medical teaching. J Nerv Ment Dis 130:78, 1960
84. Miller MH: The borderline psychotic patient: the importance of diagnosis in medical and surgical practice. Ann Intern Med 46:736, 1957
85. Mittelman B, et al: Personality and psychosomatic disturbances in patients on medical and surgical wards: a survey of 450 admissions. Psychosom Med 7:220, 1945
86. Nussbaum K: Somatic complaints and homeostasis in psychiatric patients. Psychiat Quart 34:311, 1960
87. O'Connor JF, Musher DM: Central nervous system involvement in systemic lupus erythematosus. Arch Neurol (Chicago) 14:157, 1966
88. Offenkrantz W: Multiple somatic complaints as a precursor of schizophrenia. Am J Psychiat 119:258, 1962
89. Payson HE, et al: Recognition and referral of psychiatric illness on a university medical inpatient service. Scientific Proceedings of the 117th Annual Meeting of the American Psychiatric Association, Washington, DC, 1961

90. Perlas AP, Faillace LA: Psychiatric manifestations of carcinoma of the pancreas. Amer J Psychiat 121:182, 1964
91. Poe RO, et al: Depression. JAMA 195:345, 1966
92. Quarton GC, et al: Mental disturbances associated with ACTH and cortisone: a review of explanatory hypotheses. Medicine (Balt) 34:13, 1955
93. Querido A: Forecast and follow-up: an investigation into the clinical, social and mental factors determining the results of hospital treatment. Brit J Prev Soc Med 13:33, 1959
94. Rangell L: Psychiatric aspects of pain. Psychosom Med 15:22, 1953
95. Reding GR, Daniels RS: Organic brain syndromes in a general hospital. Amer J Psychiat 120:800, 1964
96. Reid DD: Epidemiological Methods in the Study of Mental Disorders. Geneva, World Health Organization, 1960
97. Richman A, et al: Symptom questionnaire validity in assessing the need for psychiatrists' care. Brit J Psychiat 112:549, 1966
98. Roberts BH, Norton NM: The prevalence of psychiatric illness in a medical out-patient clinic. New Eng J Med 246:82, 1952
99. Robinson WG Jr: The toxic delirious reactions of old age, in Mental Disorders in Later Life. Edited by Kaplan OJ. Stanford University Press, Stanford, CA, 1956
100. Rosenbaum M, Cohen YA: Psychological preparation of the individual for medical and surgical care, in Understanding Your Patient. Edited by Liebman S. Lippincott, Philadelphia, PA, 1957
101. Rossman PL: Organic diseases simulating functional disorders. GP 28:78, 1963
102. Rud F: Psychiatric activities and instruction at a general hospital. J Clin Exper Psychopath 14:139, 1953
103. Sand P, et al: Psychological assessment of candidates for a hemodialysis program. Ann Intern Med 64:602, 1966
104. Sandt JJ, Leifer R: The psychiatric consultation. Compr Psychiat 5:409, 1964
105. Saunders L: Cultural Differences and Medical Care. Russell Sage Foundation, New York, 1954
106. Schilder P: The Image and Appearance of the Human Body. International University Press, New York, 1950
107. Schwab JJ, et al: Differential characteristics of medical in-patients referred for psychiatric consultation: a controlled study. Psychosom Med 27:112, 1965
108. Schwab JJ, et al: Medical patients' reactions to referring physicians after psychiatric consultation. JAMA 195:1120, 1966
109. Schwab JJ, et al: Problems in psychosomatic diagnosis, I: a controlled study of medical inpatients. Psychosomatics 6:369, 1964
110. Schwab JJ, et al: Problems in psychosomatic diagnosis, II: severity of medical illness and psychiatric consultations. Psychosomatics 6:69, 1965
111. Schwab JJ, et al: Problems in psychosomatic diagnosis, III: physical exami-

nations, laboratory procedures, and psychiatric consultations. Psychosomatics 6:147, 1965
112. Schwab JJ, et al: Problems in psychosomatic diagnosis, IV: a challenge to all physicians. Psychosomatics 6:198, 1965
113. Seitz PFD: Symbolism and organ choice in conversion reactions. Psychosom Med 13:254, 1951
114. Senescu RA: The development of emotional complications in the patient with cancer. J Chronic Dis 16:813, 1963
115. Shepherd M, et al: Psychiatric illness in the general hospital. Acta Psychiat Neurol Scand 35:518, 1960
116. Simon A, Cahan RB: The acute brain syndrome in geriatric patients. Psychiat Res Rep Amer Psychiat Ass, May 16, 1963
117. Slater E: Diagnosis of "hysteria." Brit Med J 1:1395, 1965
118. Small IF, et al: Organic cognates of acute psychiatric illness. Amer J Psychiat 122:790, 1966
119. Spencer RF: Medical patients: consultation and psychotherapy. Arch Gen Psychiat (Chicago) 10:270, 1964
120. Starr AM: Personality changes in Cushing's syndrome. J Clin Endocr 12:502, 1952
121. Stenbäck A, Rimon R: Hypochondria and paranoia. Acta Psychiat Scand 49:379, 1964
122. Stengel E: Pain and the psychiatrist. Brit J Psychiat 111:795, 1965
123. Stewart MA, et al: A study of psychiatric consultations in a general hospital. J Chronic Dis 15:331, 1962
124. Stewart MA, et al: Depression among medically ill patients. Dis Nerv Syst 26:479, 1965
125. Stoeckle JD, Davidson GE: Bodily complaints and the other symptoms of a depressive reaction, its diagnosis and significance in a medical clinic. JAMA 180:134, 1962
126. Stoeckle JD, Davidson GE: The use of "crisis" as an orientation for the study of patients in a medical clinic. J Med Educ 37:604, 1962
127. Stoeckle JD, et al: The quantity and significance of psychological distress in medical patients. J Chronic Dis 17:959, 1964
128. Stoller RJ, Estess FM: Suicides in medical and surgical wards of general hospitals. J Chronic Dis 12:592, 1960
129. Szasz TS: Pain and Pleasure. Basic, New York, 1957
130. Tavel ME: Hyperventilation syndrome with unilateral somatic symptoms. JAMA 187:301, 1964
131. Veith I: Hysteria: The History of a Disease. University of Chicago Press, Chicago, IL, 1965
132. Walters A: Psychogenic regional pain alias hysterical pain. Brain 84:1, 1961
133. Weinstock HI: Discussion of schizophrenia in: Early recognition and management of psychiatric disorders in general practice. J Mount Sinai Hosp NY

25:137, 1958
134. Weisman AD, Hackett TP: Psychosis after eye surgery. New Eng J Med 258:1284, 1958
135. Wilson MS, Meyer E: Diagnostic consistency in a psychiatric liaison service. Amer J Psychiat 119:207, 1962
136. Wilson M, Meyer E: The doctors' vs. the nurses' view of emotional disturbances. Canad Psychiat Ass J 10:212, 1965
137. Ziegler EJ, et al: Contemporary conversion reactions: a clinical study. Amer J Psychiat 116:901, 1960
138. Ziegler FJ, Imboden JB: Contemporary conversion reactions, II: a conceptual model. Arch Gen Psychiat (Chicago) 6:279, 1962
139. Ziegler FJ, et al: Contemporary conversion reactions, III: diagnostic considerations. JAMA 186:307, 1963
140. Zwerling I, et al: Personality disorder and the relationship of emotion to surgical illness in 200 surgical patients. Am J Psychiat 112:270, 1955

CHAPTER 6

Influences of Suggestion on Airway Reactivity in Asthmatic Subjects

THOMAS LUPARELLO, M.D.,
HAROLD A. LYONS, M.D.,
EUGENE R. BLEECKER, B.A., AND
E. R. McFADDEN, JR., M.D.

Prefatory Remarks

Louis Vachon, M.D.

This article by Luparello and colleagues was a high-water mark in the investigation of the possible role of psychological factors in asthma. The "paper rose" vignette of MacKenzie a century ago, quoted in most textbooks, is merely a lead-in for a host of questions. Can a purely psychological factor induce the symptoms of asthma? If so, what is the factor, how can it be reproduced in the

---

Volume 30, 1968, pp. 819–825.
From the Departments of Psychiatry and Medicine, State University of New York, Downstate Medical Center, Brooklyn, N.Y.
Supported in part by National Institute of Mental Health Research Career Development Award K3MH 15,620 and Grants MH-13439, National Institute of Mental Health, and 5T1-HE 5485, National Heart Institute, U.S. Public Health Service.
Presented in part at the Annual Meeting of the American Psychosomatic Society, Mar. 30, 1968.
The authors wish to thank Mrs. Frances Klugman for her help in the preparation of the manuscript and Miss Eileen Abramoff for her help with the statistics.
Received for publication Apr. 5, 1968.

laboratory, what response can be expected, and how can it be measured?

Of course, suggestion, a form of learning that includes an emotional component, had been used before, because it is a reasonably simple psychological stimulus, it is reproducible, and it is one that especially can be used in the laboratory. The major advance was the use of whole-body plethysmography as the dependent variable. I think that Marvin Stein, in whose laboratory Luparello was then working, was the first psychiatrist to have reported on psychological observations in humans, in connection with whole-body plethysmography. This instrument, designed to measure noninvasively the resistance of the flow of air in the bronchial tree itself, was just emerging from the laboratory of the pulmonary physiologists. Each research group had to have their instrument custom-made and teach themselves how to use it. When I visited his lab in the early 1960s, Luparello had already had some important publications regarding the effect of hypothalamic lesions on anaphylaxis in rats. We talked about research with asthmatic subjects and the "body box." I remember being somewhat surprised at the conviction with which he said, "The answer will be in there (the body box)." The explanation was to come very shortly.

The first report, reproduced here, and those that followed, had an important and lasting impact. Suggestion, standing in for psychological factors, had an effect, and this effect could be measured and assigned specifically to the bronchial tree itself, rather than to the glottis and/or voluntarily controlled respiratory muscles, a problem that had confounded earlier experiments. With its elegant design, the study discussed in this article provided a solid piece of objective evidence for an important theoretical point.

The effect of suggestion on bronchomotor tone was evaluated in a setting in which accurate, rapid, and reproducible measurements of airway resistance (Ra) could be made. Subjects with asthma, emphysema, and restrictive lung disease, as well as normal subjects, were studied. All subjects were led to believe that they were inhaling irritants or allergens which cause bronchoconstriction. The actual substance used in all instances was nebulized physiologic saline solution. Nineteen of 40 asthmatics reacted to the experimental situation with a significant increase in Ra. Twelve of the asthmatic subjects developed full-blown attacks of bronchospasm which was reversed with a saline solution placebo. The 40 control nonasthmatic subjects did not react.

The investigation of bronchial asthma has been concerned with the role of allergic, infectious, psychological, social, endocrinous, and hereditary factors.[1] Up to now, no single causative determinant has been isolated, and it appears that a variety of factors may be involved in the development and continuance of asthma and in the precipitation of any given acute attack. The effect of psychological stimuli on the precipitation of asthma attacks has been evaluated sporadically over the years. MacKenzie[2] noted bronchospasm in a patient with an "allergy" to roses, when he presented to her an artificial rose. More recently, Dekker and Groen[3] exposed asthmatic subjects to "meaningful emotional stimuli" and were able to measure a decrease in vital capacity in some of the subjects. Each stimulus in that study was specific for a particular subject and represented historical events in the individual's disease process. For example, one subject reported developing asthma attacks at the sight of goldfish in a bowl. When shown an artificial representation of this by the experimenters, the subject developed bronchospasm. Another individual, who had indicated dust as a trigger substance for asthma, reacted with bronchospasm when presented with a sealed glass container filled with dust. Those experiments have demonstrated that certain asthmatics are sensitive to perceptual cues which are capable of affecting bronchomotor tone. However, the heterogeneity of the stimuli employed was such that it was not possible to make meaningful comparisons within the group of subjects. In addition, the respiratory end point chosen was an indirect and relatively insensitive measure of airway obstruction.

The present study was undertaken to overcome these problems and to gain an impression of the prevalence of psychological stimuli as factors in the precipitation of asthma attacks. The independent variable chosen was suggestion, since it could be clearly defined, uniformly applied to all subjects, and easily controlled in a laboratory setting. Changes in airway resistance (Ra) were measured directly by body plethysmography. In addition, it became possible to determine whether the effects of suggestion on bronchomotor tone were unique for asthmatics or were shared by subjects with other lung diseases.

Methods

The data were obtained from 40 asthmatic subjects. The diagnosis of asthma was based on a characteristic history of episodic attacks of reversible bronchospasm associated with a family or personal history or both of allergy, and on an absence of irreversible mechanical defects within the lungs. The subjects were told that they were cooperating in a study related to the control of air pollution and that the experimenters were trying to determine the concentrations at which a variety of substances in the atmosphere would induce attacks of wheezing. It was indicated to each subject that he would be inhaling five different concentrations of an irritant or allergen which the subject had previously indicted as being associated with his asthmatic attacks. The subject was led to believe that he would be exposed to progressively increasing concentrations of this substance, whereas the material actually presented to him, in all instances, was physiologic saline solution. Ra and thoracic gas volume (TGV) were measured in a Collins body plethysmograph, prior to the onset of any test inhalation.[4] Ra and TGV were calculated as the mean of five successive measures of each variable. Resistance was converted to its reciprocal or conductance (Ga) and was expressed as a conductance-thoracic gas volume ratio (Ga/TGV) in order to correct for a variation in lung volume during testing.[5] The normal range for this ratio is 0.13 to 0.35 L./sec./cm. H_2O/L.

After baseline data were obtained, the subjects inhaled over a 30-sec. period ten deep breaths of the suggested "allergen" or "irritant" from a DeVilbiss nebulizer. Following this, Ra and TGV were measured at 1-min. and 4-min. postinhalation intervals, with each measurement representing the mean of 5 determinations at each interval. This procedure was repeated for each new suggested "increased concentration" of the bogus allergen or irritant given to the subject. In the event the subject experienced dyspnea or wheezing, the inhalations were stopped and a placebo in the form of nebulized physiologic saline solution was administered; the subjects were told that they were receiving Isuprel. The Ga/TGV ratios were then determined 3 min. after administering the placebo.

As control subjects, 10 normal individuals, 15 subjects with sarcoid or with tuberculosis (restrictive lung diseases), and 15 individuals with chronic bronchitis were investigated in the same manner, except that they were told the inhalants were 5 different concentrations of industrial air pollutants which cause bronchial irritation and difficulty in breathing.

Results

The data are summarized in Table 6–1. The mean age of the asthmatic subjects was 25.8 years with a standard deviation (S.D.) of 7.4 years. There were 26 women and 14 men. The mean baseline Ra was 2.22 ± 0.27 cm. H_2O/L./sec. This was associated with a TGV of 2.79 ± 0.49 L. which produced a Ga/TGV ratio of 0.18 ± 0.05 L./sec./cm. H_2O/L. Following exposure to the suggested allergen or irritant (i.e., saline solution), the Ga/TGV ratios of the entire group fell to an abnormal level (mean Ga/TGV ratio 0.12 ± 0.05; p = 0.001 by t test). This change was effected by an increase in the Ra to 3.43 ± 1.35 cm. H_2O/L./sec., while the TGV only increased to 3.00 ± 0.74 L. This clearly indicated that the Ga/TGV ratios fell because of a disproportionate rise in Ra.

Correlation between baseline values and postinhalation Ga/TGV ratios in the entire group of asthmatics indicated that the changes produced in this ratio were not a function of the initial value (r = 0.05).

Twelve of the 40 subjects developed full-blown clinical attacks of asthma with dyspnea and wheezing. The mean Ga/TGV ratio of these 12 individuals dropped from a baseline ratio of 0.18 ± 0.03 to 0.07 ± 0.03 L./sec./cm. H_2O/L. following inhalation of the supposed noxious substance (Table 6–2). Following the administration of a placebo, the Ga/TGV ratio rose to 0.13 ± 0.04 L./sec./cm. H_2O/L. (Figure 6–1). An analysis of variance for correlated means reveals significant differences between the baseline values and the lowest G_a/TGV ratios following inhalation of the supposed irritant or allergen, and between this lowest value and that obtained 3 min. following the giving of a placebo. Further analysis by Duncan's New Multiple Range Test showed that there was a significant difference between the baseline levels and the lowest ratio values (p < 0.001) and between the pre- and post placebo administration values (p < 0.001).

Seven of the 40 subjects responded with an increased Ra (Table 6–2) so that their Ga/TGV ratios fell below accepted normal levels. However, the degree of airway obstruction associated with these changes was not of sufficient magnitude to induce signs and symptoms of acute bronchospasm (Ga/TGV ratio baseline values, 0.18 ± 0.05; Ga/TGV postinhalation values, 0.10 ± 0.01). The remaining 21 asthmatic subjects did not respond to the experimental manipulation (Table 6–2), and there was minimal change in their Ra (Ga/TGV ratio baseline values, 0.18 ± 0.05; Ga/TGV ratio postinhalation values, 0.15 ± 0.05; p = N.S.). Figure 6–2 shows the characteristic responses of 2 subjects who reacted to the inhalation of bogus allergens with bronchospasm and the responses of 2 asthmatic subjects who, under similar test conditions, did not react with bronchospasm.

No changes were found in the Ra or Ga/TGV ratios of the normal, restrictive, or bronchitic subjects studied (Table 6–1). It is of interest to note that the mean baseline Ga/TGV ratio of the bronchitic group was in the abnormal range (Ga/TGV ratio value, 0.09 ± 0.03 L./sec./cm. H_2O/L., and it might be argued that significant changes in the Ra of this population would be missed because of the large baseline TGV. However, several asthmatic subjects were observed who

Table 6-1. Plethysmographic responses of test subjects to the inhalation of suggested bogus allergens or irritants

Subjects	No.	Sex M	Sex F	Age*	Ra*† (cm. H$_2$O/L./sec.) B[#]	Ra*† (cm. H$_2$O/L./sec.) PI[¶]	TGV*‡ (L.) B	TGV*‡ (L.) PI	Ga/TGV*§ (L./sec./cm. H$_2$O/L.) B	Ga/TGV*§ (L./sec./cm. H$_2$O/L.) PI
Asthmatic	40	14	26	25.8 ± 7.4	2.22 ± 0.27	3.43 ± 1.35	2.79 ± 0.49	3.00 ± 0.74	0.18 ± .05	0.12 ± .05
Normal	10	4	6	23.7 ± 1.8	1.22 ± 0.36	1.39 ± 0.37	2.86 ± 0.41	2.85 ± 0.41	0.32 ± .11	0.28 ± .09
Restrictive	15	4	11	30.0 ± 9.8	2.77 ± 0.82	3.12 ± 0.89	2.12 ± 0.70	2.04 ± 0.64	0.20 ± .07	0.18 ± .05
Bronchitic	15	10	5	51.8 ± 14.8	3.59 ± 1.44	3.95 ± 1.28	3.91 ± 1.02	4.03 ± 1.05	0.09 ± .03	0.08 ± .03

*Values given are the mean and standard deviation.
†Airway resistance.
‡Thoracic gas volume.
§Conductance—thoracic gas volume ratio.
[#]Baseline measurements.
[¶]Postinhalation measurements.

Table 6-2. Effect of suggestion on airway reactivity in asthmatic subjects

Asthmatic subjects	No.	Ra (cm. H$_2$O/L./sec.) B	Ra (cm. H$_2$O/L./sec.) PI	TGV (L.) B	TGV (L.) PI	Ga/TGV (L./sec./cm. H$_2$O/L.) B	Ga/TGV (L./sec./cm. H$_2$O/L.) PI
Clinical asthma attacks	12	2.29 ± 0.60	4.97 ± 0.87	2.71 ± 0.69	3.10 ± 0.85	0.18 ± 0.03	0.07 ± 0.03
Increased Ra with no symptoms	7	2.26 ± 0.35	3.72 ± 0.41	2.57 ± 0.38	2.83 ± 0.67	0.18 ± 0.05	0.10 ± 0.01
No reactions	21	2.16 ± 0.51	2.44 ± 0.49	2.90 ± 0.73	2.99 ± 0.72	0.18 ± 0.05	0.15 ± 0.05

Abbreviations and measurement values are the same as in Table 6-1.

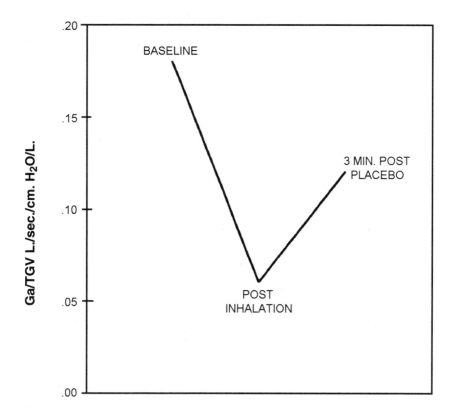

Figure 6–1. Mean Ga/TGV ratio values of 12 asthmatic subjects developing clinical signs and symptoms of bronchospasm in response to the inhalation of a supposed allergen or irritant, and the subsequent response following the administering of a placebo.

had equivalently abnormal baseline Ga/TGV ratio values but who still responded to the experimental situation with a marked fall in Ga/TGV ratio values (e.g., a baseline Ga/TGV ratio value of 0.12, followed by a postinhalation Ga/TGV ratio value of 0.04, observed in one subject).

Discussion

The data demonstrate that an appropriately supplied suggestion is capable of influencing the airway caliber of 47.5% of the asthmatic subjects investigated. Bronchoconstriction or dilatation could be accomplished, depending upon the

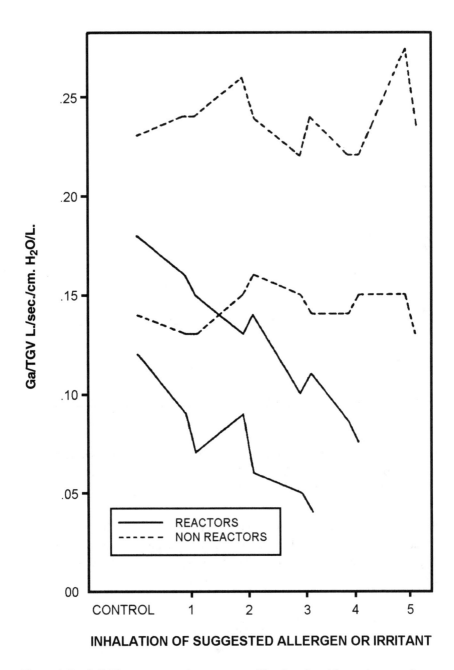

Figure 6–2. Solid lines represent the responses of 2 asthmatic subjects who reacted to the inhalation of suggested allergens with bronchospasm (expressed as a fall in the Ga/TGV ration value). Broken lines represent the responses of 2 asthmatic subjects who did not react to the same test stimulus.

suggestion supplied. This phenomenon was not observed in normal subjects or in subjects with bronchitis or restrictive lung diseases. It cannot be argued that the asthmatics developed their attacks by chance alone under the stresses of the experimental situation, since this would not account for the dramatic reversal of the bronchospasm in those subjects who received a placebo under the same test conditions. The following observation illustrates that the response of the subjects was related specifically to the suggestion. One subject, who was given the suggestion that she was inhaling pollen, developed hay fever as well as bronchospasm. As part of another experiment, she was given the suggestion that the inhalant was dust and the subject then had only an asthma attack without hayfever. On a third occasion, following exposure to supposed "pollen," she once more reacted with hayfever as well as asthma.

Although the independent variable in the present study has been referred to as suggestion, it may be that such a designation is an over simplification. It is possible that certain elements of conditioning may also be operating. If an individual has repeatedly associated the onset of asthma attacks with the presence of a specific agent, it is possible that contiguous stimuli may assume a conditional stimulus value. The present study, however, does not provide sufficient information to permit a distinction to be made about the various types of learning which could be instrumental in bringing about the phenomenon observed in this investigation.

With the demonstration that asthmatics can be divided into two populations—namely, those who react to suggestion with changes in lung mechanics and those who do not, it becomes relevant to inquire about other possible differences between these two populations. For example, are there differences between the two groups in personality, duration of illness, frequency of attacks, or allergic diathesis? These questions cannot be answered on the basis of the available information, and further studies are required before any meaningful comparisons of the two asthmatic populations can be made along these parameters.

The changes in the Ga/TGV ratio observed in the present study occurred primarily because of a fall in airway conductance. The rapidity of both the responses and their reversibility point to a change in smooth-muscle tone as the most likely explanation.[6] In another study, we have demonstrated that atropine is capable of blocking the bronchoconstriction induced by suggestion,[7] indicating that the response of airways to this stimulus is mediated through cholinergic efferent pathways. This hypothesis is in keeping with the observations of Simonsson et al.[8] Those authors have shown that stimulation of subepithelial receptors will trigger reflex airway constriction, which is eliminated by atropine blockade of the efferent limb of the reflex arc. The present study indicates that activation of efferent fibers can occur at a central level without direct stimulation of the afferent side. The exact site of stimulation of the efferent fibers and the mechanism by which they are activated is unknown.

Asthma is a complex disease process, the pathogenesis of which remains unknown. In the light of the present findings, a meaningful assessment of the precipitants of asthma and the treatment of any given asthmatic patient must necessarily include an appraisal of the role played by suggestion. If an individual associates a specific agent with the onset of his asthmatic attacks, there is a likelihood that contact with that substance when the asthmatic is aware of it will induce an asthma attack, regardless of whether that agent at that time is physiologically active. Subsequent provocative tests for diagnostic purposes, if done with the subject's knowledge of the test substance, will probably only enhance the asthmogenic potential of that substance. Similarly, the expectations of the patient will have a marked influence on the efficacy of any given therapeutic regimen.

Research related to the psychophysiology of asthma must necessarily institute suitable controls for the influence of suggestion. In such experiments, it often becomes extremely difficult to provide adequate controls for the large number of complex, interacting psychological variables presumed to be operating. In those instances, it is especially important to be sure that the subject is not responding to subtle cues being communicated by the experimenter. Such cues could operate as a suggestion for a particular response, which would then confound rather than clarify the psychophysiology of asthma.

Summary

The effect of suggestion on the pulmonary mechanics of subjects with bronchial asthma, of subjects with restrictive lung diseases, of emphysematous subjects, and of normal individuals was studied by whole-body plethysmography. Following baseline measurements of Ra, each subject was told that he would be inhaling progressively increasing concentrations of an allergen or irritant which would induce bronchospasm. The substance actually given was nebulized physiologic saline solution. After inhalation of the bogus allergen or irritant, the mean Ra of the entire group of asthmatic subjects rose significantly. This was brought about by a marked rise in the Ra of 19 of the 40 asthmatic subjects. Of those 19 asthmatic subjects who reacted, 12 developed full-blown attacks of asthma with wheezing and dyspnea. All asthma attacks were successfully treated with a saline solution placebo, and 3 min. after the inhalation of the placebo, the Ra had returned to baseline levels. The normal subjects and those subjects with restrictive and nonasthmatic, obstructive lung diseases did not react to the inhalation of suggested bogus irritants or allergens with significant changes in R_a.

References

1. Stein M: Etiology and mechanisms in the development of asthma, in The First Hahnemann Symposium on Psychosomatic Medicine. Lea, Philadelphia, PA, 1962, p 149
2. MacKenzie JN: The production of "rose asthma" by an artificial rose. Amer J Med Sci 91:45, 1886
3. Dekker E, Groen J: Reproducible psychogenic attacks of asthma. J Psychosom Res 1:58, 1956
4. DuBois AB, Botelho SY, Comroe JH Jr: A new method for measuring airway resistance in man using a body plethysmograph: values in normal subjects and in patients with respiratory disease. J Clin Invest 35:327, 1956
5. Briscoe WA, DuBois AB: The relationship between airway resistance, airway conductance and lung volume in subjects of different age and body size. J Clin Invest 37:1279, 1958
6. Widdicombe JG: Regulation of tracheobronchial smooth muscle. Physiol Rev 43:1, 1963
7. McFadden ER Jr, Luparello T, Lyons HA, et al: The mechanisms of action of suggestion in the induction of acute asthma attacks. Psychosom Med 31:134, 1969
8. Simonsson BG, Jacobs FM, Nadel JA: Role of autonomic nervous system and the cough reflex in the increased responsiveness of airways in patients with obstructive airway disease. J Clin Invest 46:1812, 1967

CHAPTER 7

Blood Pressure Changes in Men Undergoing Job Loss
A Preliminary Report

STANISLAV V. KASL, PH.D., AND
SIDNEY COBB, M.D.

Prefatory Remarks

Richard H. Rahe, M.D.

The work of Sidney Cobb and his associate, Stanislav Kasl, was seminal in psychosomatic research in that it greatly helped to move the investigatory laboratory to the work site. Perhaps not since the pioneering studies by Lawrence Hinkle, Jr., had the workplace been seriously considered as a naturalistic source of stressors waiting to be investigated.[1] Whereas Hinkle, and followers, used an epidemiological approach, Cobb and his biochemist colleague, George Brooks,

---

Volume 32, 1970, pp. 19–38.
   From the Institute for Social Research, University of Michigan, Ann Arbor, Mich. 48106.
   The research here reported was supported by grants #CD-00102 and K3-MH-16 from the U.S. Public Health Service and a seed grant from the United Automobile Workers.
   We are indebted to Carolyn Bookspun, Gail Kohn, Winnifred Connelly, Marilyn Jeffs, Vivian Visscher, Jennie Partee, Ruth Van Niman, and Mary Ann Keller for their very careful attention to the taking of BP and pulse rates. The importance of the cooperation of the employees over a span of more than 2 very difficult years was essential to the study and can never be adequately acknowledged.
   Received for publication June 16, 1969; revision received Aug. 7, 1969.

selected biochemical and physiological indicators of stress, utilizing selected subpopulations for study—such as people undergoing job loss.[2]

The physiological consequences of "real life" stress have fascinated many members of this society, including myself.[3] Kasl is to be credited for the exemplary psychosocial and statistical precision that he brought to these studies. What has accrued since, from literally hundreds of similar investigations, is a realization of the astonishing variability of persons' responses to stress. Mean values may show significant differences, but these effects alone obscure substantial variability in subjects' responses. Although a majority of persons may respond with transient increases in adrenergic tone when faced with life-change stress, indicated by small increases in systolic and/or diastolic blood pressure, others will show no pressure changes, and still others will demonstrate a fall in blood pressure. We can now say with some certainty that there is no single stress indicator true for all, or even for most, people. We are now witnessing a rediscovery of these earlier observations in the research arena of psychoneuroimmunology.

References

1. Hinkle LE Jr, Redmont R, Plummer N, et al: An examination of the relation between symptoms, disability, and serious illness, in two homogeneous groups of men and women. Am J Public Health 50:1327–1336, 1960
2. Kasl SV, Cobb S, Brooks GW: Changes in serum uric acid and cholesterol levels in men undergoing job loss. JAMA 206:1500, 1968
3. Rahe RH: Life change, stress responsivity, and captivity research. Psychosom Med 52:373–378, 1990

A longitudinal study was made of blood pressure (BP) changes in married, stably employed men who lose their jobs because of a permanent plant shutdown. Some 150 men, including controls, were seen and followed up to 2 years. Major findings were as follows: (1) The controls showed no significant long-term trends, (2) BP levels during anticipation of job loss and unemployment or probationary re-employment were clearly higher than during later stabilization on new jobs, (3) Men whose BP levels remained high longer: (a) had more severe unemployment, (b) were lower on Ego Resilience, (c) reported longer-lasting subjective stress, and (d) failed to show much improvement in reported well-being, (4) Within the period of anticipation, there was a clear rise in BP which was correlated with subjective ratings of felt stress, and (5) These major BP changes were replicated in preliminary results from a second company.

An examination of some fairly recent reviews of the literature on psychological factors in BP[1,2,3] permits the reader few firm conclusions. While it is true that many studies either find psychological differences between hypertensive patients and normotensive subjects, or show some psychological correlates of BP levels (or reactivity), nevertheless, no overall coherent and consistent picture emerges. Moreover, replication of findings has been difficult, largely because of obvious deficiencies in sampling and because of the frequent use of assessment methods of unknown validity. The rich epidemiological literature is intriguing enough, but drawing inferences from it about the role of specific psychological factors is hazardous because the role of alternate variables—race, genetic endowment, body bulk, nutrition, prevalence of infections, and so on—cannot be ruled out.

Ostfeld and Shekelle[2] believe that the only conclusion which can be safely offered is that "acute psychological stress may initiate sudden and transient elevations of BP in some persons." Unfortunately, it has been difficult to go beyond this general finding and to establish firm links between continuous psychological stress and sustained elevation of BP. What is needed, Ostfeld and Shekelle suggest, is some speculation about:

> the nature of the situations in ordinary life experience that are associated with pressor responses. Looking at them from the point of the person involved, we can distinguish several of their characteristics. 1) The outcome of the event is uncertain. 2) The possibility of bodily or psychological harm exists. 3) Although running or physical resistance may be considered, they are not appropriate behavior. 4) The person involved commonly feels compelled to maintain a vigilant mental attitude until the situation is clarified or ended.

It is the purpose of this report to describe BP changes in men who go through a social stress situation very much like the one outlined above by Ostfeld and

Shekelle: job loss because of a permanent plant shutdown. The men are followed as they go through the stages of employment on the old job, loss of job, unemployment (for some), probationary reemployment, and stable employment on a new job.

Methods

The study is an ongoing longitudinal investigation of the health effects of job loss and the ensuing unemployment and/or job change.[4] The subjects are married men, ages 35–60, who hold a variety of lower skill, blue collar jobs. They have been on their jobs a minimum of 3 years, but are about to lose them because of a permanent plant shutdown. The men are seen by public health nurses at approximately 3–4 month intervals, beginning with the time when they are still on their old jobs but already know about the impending shutdown. The second nurse visit is approximately 1 month after job loss, with other visits coming at 4, 8, 12, and 24 months after the original job loss. During the course of each visit to the man's home, the nurse collects blood and urine specimens, takes blood pressure, pulse rate, height and weight, and uses a structured interview schedule to collect diverse social-psychological and health data. These include: his current employment situation, his economic circumstances, his subjective evaluation of his job and financial situation, questionnaire measures of mental health and affective reactions used in previous studies,[5, 6, 7] and physical health data. After the visit, the nurses rate the respondent on a number of dimensions relating to his mental health and well-being.

Figure 7-1 summarizes the design of the study and the data collection sequence. At the time of Round 1, all of the men are still working; they are about a month and a half away from plant closing and they all know what is about to take place. It is not unreasonable to call this the Anticipation Stage. During Round 2, many men are unemployed and none of those who have found new jobs have yet passed the probationary period of employment. With later Rounds, more and more men have found new jobs and stabilized their employment situation. Some men, however, experience additional job loss or they go through a voluntary job change. The last visit takes place some 2 years after loss of original job.

Because there is a great deal of repeated data being collected, two nurse visits for each Round are necessary; these two visits come 2 weeks apart. The nurse records the BP at the beginning and at the end of each visit. Given the pair of visits within each Round, we thus have 4 BP values on each man for each

Blood Pressure Changes in Men Undergoing Job Loss   121

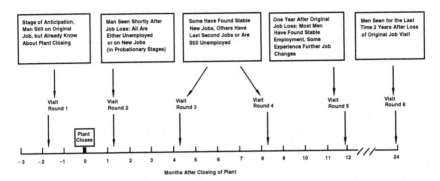

Figure 7-1. Basic design of longitudinal study of men losing jobs and schedule of home visit interviews by Public Health nurses.

Round. A mercury manometer is used with the men sitting up. In recording the BP, all of the nurse interviewers were standardized against the London School of Hygiene testing tape, developed by G. Rose.[8] When necessary, the tape was also used to provide the nurses with additional special training. A subsequent check of accuracy revealed no average systematic bias among our several nurse interviewers.

The design of the study also calls for the use of controls who are continuously employed men in comparable jobs. They are followed for the same length of time and exactly the same assessment procedures are used. The men who lose their jobs and the controls who remain stably employed come from a number of different companies.

Company A: The plant, located in a large metropolitan area, manufactured paint that was primarily used by automobile companies. The men were largely machine operators, assistants in a laboratory, and clerks in shipping and receiving departments. The work was relatively light for most; some did a fair amount of lifting or loading and unloading.

Company B: The plant belongs to a light manufacturing company which makes display fixtures used by wholesale and retail concerns. The factory was located in a community of under 5,000 and was one of two major employers. The men were machine operators, workers on an assembly line, and a few tool and die workers doing relatively light work.

Company D (Controls): The men are in the maintenance department of a large university; they are carpenters and machinists, the latter doing metal welding and installation of new equipment.

Company E (Controls): The plant, located in a metropolitan area, manufactures parts for heavy trucks. The men are machine operators and assembly line workers doing moderately heavy work.

The men from Company C are not included in this analysis.

The men who entered the study were obtained in the following manner. When it was established that a plant would be closing down, we approached the officials of the union local and described briefly to them the intended study. Because we had the full backing from the central UAW union headquarters, we were able to enlist the local officials' cooperation in our efforts. They supplied us with a list of names of men eligible for study (see below for eligibility criteria) and we approached each man individually, asking him to participate. The study was briefly characterized to the men as an effort to understand the health effects of job loss and job change. The number of nurse visits required and the time it would take for each interview were explained to them. The study was described as an important scientific endeavor in an area where lack of relevant data prevents the Union, the Company, and the government from sound policy planning. The backing of the Union was particularly emphasized. In addition, the men were told that if they so wished, we would inform their family physician of any laboratory results which were in any way unusual. The controls were approached in a similar way through our contacts with the UAW and the same appeals for their cooperation were made. They were told about the purposes of the study and it was explained to them that they were needed as continuously employed controls who will not go through any job loss and job change.

Criteria of eligibility for this study were: married male, ages 35–60, with at least 3 years of seniority. Of the 90 men from Company A who fit these criteria, 66, or 73%, agreed to participate. Complete data exist on 56 men which means, for most part, 4 nurse visits 3–4 months apart and some visits 24 months after the original job loss. The men from Company B were picked up considerably later and, consequently, only 3–4 Rounds are generally available on them so far. Of the 70 men eligible for the study, 60, or 86%, agreed to participate. Of the 66 controls from Companies D and E who satisfied the eligibility criteria, 49, or 74%, agreed to participate. Collection of data has been carried out as far as 3 Rounds on 44 men, 39 of whom have complete data for 4 Rounds. Table 7–1 summarizes some of the basic information about the men in the study. It can be seen that on the basic demographic data—age, education, income—the 3 groups of men are roughly comparable. The high seniority of these men shows that these were stably employed men prior to loss of original jobs.

If one looks at Company A men one year after plant closing, one finds that one quarter of them experienced no unemployment, while another quarter went through unemployment exceeding 2 months; the remaining half experienced briefer unemployment periods. Since the plant in Company B closed down more recently, the information on these men is less complete. However, it is clear that the unemployment experience of Company B men has been much more severe;

Table 7–1. Basic data on subject populations in study

Type of company	Typical jobs	Stage of data collection	Number of subjects	Mean age	Mean hourly wage on original job	Mean No. of years of education	Mean No. of years of seniority on original job
Company A: A paint manufacturing plant in a metropolitan area	machine operators, laboratory assistants, shipping clerks	completed	56	46.1	$2.93	10.0	17.7
Company B: A light manufacturing company, making display fixtures; located in a small town	machine operators, assembly line workers	in progress	60	50.0	$2.99	9.4	21.0
Controls: 1) Maintenance department of a large university 2) A plant manufacturing parts for heavy trucks; located in metropolitan area	1) carpenters, machinists 2) machine operators, assembly line workers	partly completed	46	49.4	$3.51	10.7	18.9

one-third of the men were still unemployed some 4–5 months after plant closing.

This report will primarily deal with changes in systolic and diastolic BP (and, to a lesser extent, in pulse rate) as they relate to the employment experience of the men in the study. Inasmuch as data are still being collected about some of the men (given the 24 month follow-up period, the complete data on all of the men in the study will not be in for some time), this report concentrates on the experience of Company A men for the 1 year following plant closing. The less complete data on Company B will be brought in only as a preliminary indication of the extent to which some of the major trends are replicated.

The data below will be presented primarily in the form of difference scores or change scores; i.e., we shall be emphasizing changes within the same person over a period of time. Such change scores do not require the traditional adjustments for age or race (14% of the men in the study are black). However, variables which do themselves fluctuate and are known to affect blood pressure (e.g., body weight) will be examined for their potential confounding of the meaning of the BP change scores.

It is worth noting that the mean BP of the men in the study, taken over all the visit rounds and both on those losing their jobs and the controls, is 131 mm Hg for systolic and 82 mm Hg for diastolic. The corresponding means for men in the same age range and the same average age are 133 and 82, respectively, as reported in the 1960–1962 National Health Survey.[9] We are thus studying BP changes in men whose overall BP levels are equivalent to the national norms.

Results

We may start the presentation of the results by examining the data on the controls. Our interest in the controls is simply to demonstrate that no systematic and reliable changes in BP have taken place. Should any significant changes be demonstrated, then they will have to be taken into consideration in the interpretation of the results on the "experimental" subjects, the men who experience job loss. Table 7–2 summarizes the relevant data. The units of measurement for BP in this and subsequent tables are in millimeters of mercury.

At the bottom of Table 7–2 we see that there is no significant long term trend in the BP levels or pulse rates of the controls. More detailed analyses of changes over time, within visit rounds, and within single visits, failed to reveal any significant differences. The single exception was certain fluctuations in diastolic BP which looked like an interviewing effect. These fluctuations are summarized in the upper half of Table 7–2. Within each Round, the first visit yielded some-

Table 7-2. Summary of blood pressure changes on 44 controls; fluctuations of diastolic blood pressure in *mm Hg* within and between visit rounds

	Within Round 1	Between Rounds	Within Round 2	Between Rounds	Within Round 3	Between Rounds	Within Round 4
Mean drop on diastolic blood pressure between averages of 1st and 2nd visits within Rounds	−2.27		−1.97		−1.67		−0.94
Mean increase on diastolic blood pressure between averages of 2nd visit in one Round and 1st visit of next Round		+1.69		+3.26		+1.84	
Significance of change	<.025	NS	<.05	<.05	NS	NS	NS

Long term changes: Mean over early Rounds vs Mean over later Rounds.
Diastolic blood pressure: Mean rise = 0.90 mm Hg, $p > .30$.
Systolic blood pressure: Mean drop = 0.61 mm Hg, $p > .50$.
Pulse rate: Mean drop = 0.48, beats/min, $p > .50$.

what higher diastolic BP values than the second visit. With later Rounds, this difference became progressively smaller. It is possible that the interview and assessment procedures during the first visit covered topics which were somewhat more disturbing to the men, but that with subsequent visits, the men became more comfortable with the interview topics. It is also possible that, within each Round, the anticipatory uneasiness or anxiety prior to the first visit is greater than prior to the second visit 2 weeks later. In any case, the changes *between* Rounds (i.e., between the second visit of one Round and the first visit of the next Round some 3–4 months later) are in the opposite direction from within the Round changes and we thus get no overall long term trends.

Let us now turn to the findings on the men in Company A. The major change score which was computed involves the difference between 2 time periods: the first 2 Rounds of visits during which the men are under considerable stress (anticipation of job loss and subsequent unemployment or probationary new employment) and the last 2 Rounds of visits, 8 and 12 months after original job loss, during which most men have stabilized on a new job. The means for each time period are each based on up to 8 BP values and the overall change score thus takes into consideration up to 16 separate data points. It should be noted that a few men had experienced additional unemployment at some time during the last two visits; these men have, of course, not stabilized on a new job, and they are excluded from all analyses where the BP levels for these last 2 Rounds of visits are intended to reflect a stabilized employment situation.

The relevant data are presented in Table 7–3. It can be seen that for four-

Table 7–3. Major changes in blood pressure and pulse rate on men in Company A

	Differences between means for early visits (anticipation of job loss and unemployment or probationary reemployment) and means for later visits (stabilization on new job)	Significance of change	Percent of men showing some drop	Correlation of means for early visits with means for later visits
Diastolic blood pressure	Mean drop = 3.06 mm Hg	< .0001	80%	.82
Systolic blood pressure	Mean drop = 5.32 mm Hg	< .0001	80%	.87
Pulse rate	Mean drop = 2.71 beats/min	< .01	67%	.55

fifths of the men, their BP levels were higher during the early visits when they were under considerable stress, than during the later visits when their employment situation had stabilized. The pulse rate data show the same difference but indicate a weaker relationship. The correlations in Table 7-3 reveal that for BP the relative ordering of individuals remains highly stable from 1 time period to the next (of course, each ordering is based on up to 8 BP readings). This is why the BP changes, although rather small in an absolute sense, are nevertheless, highly significant.

The BP changes over time were also analyzed in a somewhat different way: for each individual the slope of the regression line of BP level on time of visit was computed. An examination of these slopes yielded results highly comparable to those just seen in Table 7-3: the same percent of men showed a negative slope and the average steepness of the slope values (different from zero at the same level of significance) agreed with the size of the drop in diastolic and systolic BP seen in Table 7-3.

It was remarked above that the absolute size of the average drops in the BP values is not very impressive from a clinical viewpoint. However, from an epidemiological viewpoint, the average differences are respectable enough. Compare, for example, this amount of change with general cross-sectional population data broken down by age: the mean difference between men in age ranges of 35-44 and 55-64 (i.e., a 20 year difference) is only 2.4 mm Hg on diastolic BP and 11.7 mm Hg on systolic BP.[9]

The average size of the BP drops as seen in Table 7-3 obscures the fair degree of variability in the individual difference scores: some men show rather large drops while 20% in fact show some increase. What are some of the variables which can help us explain this individual variation in these BP change scores? Data relevant to this question are examined next.

When the men were seen 1 year after the original job loss, they were asked a number of retrospective questions about their experience, including the following one: "How long do you think it took you before things got pretty much back to normal?" Five ordered response categories were provided, ranging from "a week or so" to "not yet back to normal even now." In the top of Table 7-4 the responses to this question (condensed to 3 categories) are related to the size of the drop in diastolic BP (scores dichotomized). Two measures of association are used in this table: Goodman and Kruskal[10] gamma, an index specifically developed for data arranged into ordered classes, and Kendall's[11] tau_B with ties. Because of their different treatment of ties, the gamma yields higher values than the tau. However, the test of significance is the same for both and incorporates a correction for continuity.[12]

It is evident that there is a striking negative relationship between the size of drop in diastolic BP and this retrospective evaluation of the job loss experience: those who report a quick return to normal show a large drop in BP, while those who say that a year later things are not yet back to normal show only a small drop, and some even a small rise. The association with the size of drop in systolic BP was weaker and not significant (gamma = −.31, tau = −.15); for pulse rate, the same association also failed to reach significance (gamma = −.30, tau = −.18).

The bottom line in Table 7–4 shows the association of the size of drop in diastolic BP with an objective index of the severity of the unemployment experience, total number of weeks unemployed. The association is in the same direction as with the subjective measure, but is not quite significant. For systolic BP, the same association was just significant (gamma = −.45, tau = −.28, $p < .05$), while for pulse rate the association was virtually zero. The contrast between the association of the objective index of severity and the subjective measure of the job loss experience with the diastolic BP change scores, seen in Table 7–4, merits a comment. (1) One possible explanation is that the objective measure is too narrow a representation of the totality of the objective environment. However, preliminary analysis of other objective variables, such as the respondent's financial situation, failed to reveal any striking association with the BP changes.

Table 7–4. Some variables which account for the size of drop in diastolic blood pressure from early (stressful) visits to later (stabilized re-employment) visits in men in Company A

Size of drop in diastolic BP	Time before respondent's situation stabilized after retrospective evaluation of job loss experience[*]			
	Quickly returned to normal	Moderately slow return to normal	Very slow, not yet stabilized	Total
Large drop	6	13	5	24
Small drop or an increase	0	9	16	25
			Total	49

Other variables	Amount of association and its significance	
	gamma	tau
Ego resilience scale	0.63	0.40, $p < 0.005$
Size of drop in reported irritation	0.67	0.44, $p < 0.001$
Size of increase in reported self-esteem	0.64	0.53, $p < 0.001$
Total number of weeks unemployed	−0.36	−0.21, NS

[*] gamma = −0.78; tau = −0.48, $p < 0.001$.

(2) A second possibility is that the objective measure quite obviously fails to take into consideration the way individuals may differ in reacting to an objectively same or similar stress situation. (The dynamics of such individualized, differential reactions are summarized in Figure 7–2 and are discussed below.) (3) A third possibility is that since for most men the unemployment period took place right after the original plant closing and was not of long duration, the objective index of severity can be expected to be most sensitive to BP changes taking place between plant closing and 3–6 months later, but not as sensitive to changes between plant closing and 8–12 months later. As we shall see below, this possibility does find some empirical support.

The lower half of Table 7–4 reveals other associations of interest. One is with Ego Resilience, a measure developed and validated by Block.[5] It is made up of MMPI items which are in the neutral range of social desirability scale values and should thus be reasonably insensitive to a social desirability response set. The scale is best viewed as a general measure of adjustment or ego strength. It can be seen that high Ego Resilient men tend to have large drops in diastolic BP, while men low on the scale are the ones who show much smaller drops (i.e., they are remaining high).

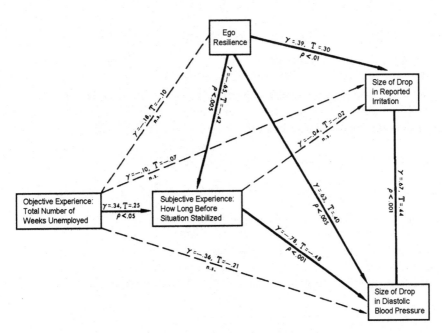

Figure 7–2. Interrelationships among variables presented in Table 7–4: correlates of diastolic blood pressure drop.

On each round, the men answered a lot of questions which have to do with their affective states and psychological well-being. A number of scales were constructed from these items, two of which are Irritation and Self-Esteem. Each scale has 5 items which deal with frequency of feeling irritated or annoyed and with the man's perception and evaluation of himself, respectively. (For additional details of methodology, see Cobb et al.[4]) Difference scores on these scales were then constructed so as to reflect the same change between early and late visits as do the diastolic BP change scores. From Table 7–4 it can be seen that men who experienced a large reduction in Irritation and a large increase in Self-Esteem were also the ones who showed a large drop in diastolic BP. As might be expected, the change scores on these two psychological dimensions were themselves highly correlated (gamma = −.65, tau = −.51).

The associations of changes in systolic BP and in pulse rate with the three psychological measures, Ego Resilience and changes in Reported Irritation, and Self-Esteem, were in the same direction as the associations with diastolic BP changes just discussed. However, in each instance, the association was weaker and did not quite reach statistical significance.

Figure 7–2 summarizes in a schematic form the interrelationships among some of the predictors of the amount of change in diastolic BP from early (stressful) visits to later (stabilized re-employment) visits. Subjective evaluation of the job loss experience clearly mediates the effects of the objective experience on the diastolic BP changes; the index of objective experience by itself shows only a weak association with the BP changes. The association between the indices of objective and subjective experience is significant but clearly not very strong. Here, however, ego resilience emerges as an important conditioning variable: the lower the ego resilience, the longer it took the respondent before he felt his situation had stabilized (gamma = −.65, tau = −.42; in computing this association, the effects of Objective Experience were held constant). Ego Resilience also seems to influence the size of the drop in Reported Irritation, since this drop is explained by neither the Objective nor the Subjective Experience: the lower the ego resilience, the smaller the drop in irritation. Subjective Experience and Drop in Reported Irritation are uncorrelated predictors of diastolic BP change. However, what they do have in common is that they are apparently both affected by Ego Resilience. Clearly, Ego Resilience plays a crucial role and shows both direct and indirect association with the BP changes. In this discussion we are assuming that Ego Resilience can be thought of as a fairly stable personality characteristic.

It should be noted that in Figure 7–2, we could have easily substituted Size of Increase in Reported Self-Esteem for Size of Drop in Reported Irritation. The pattern of interrelationships with other variables, including BP changes, is virtually the same, and the two variables are substantially correlated with each other. This suggests that irritation does not have a unique status in BP dynamics, as might have been inferred from the clinical observations of Alexander[13] and Saul[14] on the role of hostility in hypertension; rather, what we are dealing with in this instance is some more general dimension, perhaps best labelled as affective well-being.

Thus far we have examined BP changes which reflect the most general comparison: the average of early, stressful visits with later, stabilized re-employment visits. We shall now turn to some BP fluctuations which reflect shorter spans of time; specifically, we want to look at the role of anticipation and at the changes which take place shortly after job loss.

Table 7–5 summarizes the data which demonstrate a pure anticipation effect; i.e., BP changes attributable to awareness of impending plant shutdown, but not to actual unemployment or uncertain re-employment. In the upper half of the table we see the BP changes which take place within Round 1. (There are 2 nurse visits, 2 weeks apart, taking place roughly a month prior to scheduled plant closing, and BP is recorded at the beginning and at the end of each visit.) It is clear that diastolic and systolic BP both show a significant rise within this period, while pulse rate shows a nonsignificant drop. Moreover, this BP rise is quite gradual: the BP of the men go up within each visit, and also between visits. The increase seen within Round 1 is in the opposite direction from the modest drop shown by the controls during this same period (see Table 7–2). Thus if the change in the controls indicates an interviewing effect (acclimatization to the interview procedure, or a difference between the content of the first and the

Table 7–5. Changes in blood pressure and pulse rate attributable to anticipation effect alone, on men in Company A

Comparison	Variable	Type of change	Mean amount of change	Significance of change
From initial value during 1st visit to final value during 2nd visit, all within Round 1, anticipation	Diastolic blood pressure	Increase	3.41 mm Hg	$p < .005$
	Systolic blood pressure	Increase	2.34 mm Hg	$p < .05$
	Pulse rate	Decrease	1.85 beats/min	NS
From mean of 2 values for 2nd visit of Round 1 (just before job loss) to mean of up to 8 values for later Rounds (stabilization of new job)	Diastolic blood pressure	Decrease	4.22 mm Hg	$p < .0001$
	Systolic blood pressure	Decrease	6.97 mm Hg	$p < .0001$
	Pulse rate	Decrease	3.33 beats/min	$p < .01$

second interview within each Round) then this interviewing effect cannot explain the observed increase in the men from Company A; on the contrary, it would be attenuating the magnitude of this rise. It is also possible that the difference between the controls and the Company A men is not directly due to any stress of the anticipation of job loss among the latter, but is rather due to the fact that Company A men are increasingly disturbed by an interview which deals, in part, with their current and future life situation. That is, the observed increase in the Company A men may be the result of an interaction between the effects of the interview and of their current life circumstances.

When the men were seen during Round 5, 1 year after original job loss, they were asked a number of retrospective questions about their experience. One technic used here was a kind of a retrospective happiness chart, a graphic presentation of the fluctuations between two poles, "really happy times" and "was really very rough on me," covering retrospectively a period of about 14 months. One score which was computed was the average rating for the period just around the plant closing. Men who rated this period as a relatively happy one showed no increase in diastolic BP within Round 1, Anticipation (mean = 0.09 mm Hg); while the men who rated it as relatively unhappy, showed a large increase (mean = 6.59 mm Hg). The difference between the 2 groups is highly significant ($p < .005$). The strength of this association between the retrospective rating and the rise in the diastolic BP can also be expressed as a gamma of .58 or a Tau of .39. The change in systolic BP failed to show a significant association.

It is also interesting to note that the Ego Resilience scale showed no relationship whatsoever to the rise in either diastolic or systolic blood pressure within Round 1. One is tempted to speculate that ego strength or Ego Resilience may be involved only in the process of recovery from stress and not in the initial anticipatory reaction, the "preparatory" response.

The lower half of Table 7–5 presents data which are parallel to the comparison seen in Table 7–3. The only difference is that instead of the mean for early visits (before and just after job loss) computed for Table 7–3, we only use the mean of 2 BP or pulse rate values for the last visit just before job loss. The differences are slightly higher than those seen in Table 7–3, suggesting that anticipation alone is at least as important a component of the total stress as are the subsequent job loss and unemployment or probationary re-employment experiences. (If one takes only the single BP reading at the end of the visit just before job loss, then the mean differences observed are even larger: 5.24 mm Hg for diastolic and 9.52 mm Hg for systolic.)

It was stated earlier that the overall unemployment experience of the men in Company A was not a very severe one and that much of the unemployment took place within a relatively brief period after plant shutdown. We shall now turn to the BP changes during Round 2, and examine their relationship to this objective index of the severity of the experience, length of unemployment. The change score which was computed is the difference between the means for the first and the second visit within Round 2. Diastolic BP shows a significant drop during this period (mean change = 3.26 mm Hg, $p < .005$), while the drop for systolic BP (2.31 mm Hg) is short in significance. Moreover, the diastolic BP change is related to the objective experience: the less severe the experience, the larger is the drop in diastolic BP (gamma = $-.50$, tau = $-.30$, $p < .025$). The systolic BP change fails to show a similar significant association.

The final analysis of the BP data on men in Company A involved an examination of BP variability in relation to BP means and to the Flexibility-Rigidity Scale of the California Personality Inventory.[15] For each man, all of his BP values (up to 24 separate data points) were used to compute an arithmetic mean and a standard deviation, the index of variability. The relevant data are summarized in Table 7-6 in the lower lefthand part of the correlation matrix. For comparison purposes, the data on the controls are also given, in the upper righthand part of the correlation matrix.

From Table 7-6 it is apparent that a person's BP variability is in part dependent upon his overall BP mean. The dependence is not strong and is greater for systolic variability than for diastolic variability (especially so among the controls). Diastolic and systolic variability are strongly related to each other among the men from Company A ($r = .69$), but only weakly so among the Controls ($r = .26$); the difference between the correlations is significant ($p < .005$).

The correlations with the Flexibility-Rigidity Scale among the men in Company A reveal that the more rigid men tend to be more variable on diastolic and systolic BP ($r = -.32$, $p < .025$ and $r = -.24$, $p = .07$, respectively). The compa-

Table 7-6. Diastolic and systolic blood pressure variability in relation to blood pressure means and flexibility-rigidity, on men in Company A and controls*

		1.	2.	3.	4.	5.
Diastolic blood pressure mean	1.		.11	.71	.38	$-.13$
Diastolic blood pressure variability	2.	.32		.22	.26	$-.20$
Systolic blood pressure mean	3.	.76	.41		.51	$-.31$
Systolic blood pressure variability	4.	.25	.69	.49		$-.11$
CPI Flexibility-rigidity scale†	5.	$-.09$	$-.32$	$-.06$	$-.24$	

*The lower left hand part of the correlation matrix reflects the data on 56 men in Company A; the upper right hand part of the matrix is for 14 Controls.
†High score = flexible; low score = rigid.

rable correlations for the controls are lower, but not significantly so. When the two samples of men are combined, the correlations with Flexibility-Rigidity are $-.27$ ($p < .01$) and $-.19$ ($p = .05$) for diastolic and systolic variability, respectively. It is possible that rigid men, especially those going through such a significant experience as job loss and re-employment, are less likely to be able to maintain a flexible adjustment to their changing circumstances, and thus encounter more temporarily stressful situations. And to the extent that BP may be sensitive to such temporary stresses, to that extent these rigid men would tend to show more BP variability.

Let us finally turn to some preliminary BP findings on the men in Company B. The data are preliminary because: (a) no more than 4 Rounds of visits are available, and (b) the men's unemployment experience was much more severe and only very few men can be said to have stabilized on their new jobs by the fourth Round. Table 7–7 summarizes the diastolic BP changes on the men in relation to their objective experience. The upper half of the table contains the

Table 7–7. Diastolic blood pressure changes on men in Company B

	Mean changes between two early Rounds and two later Rounds		
Men involved	Mean change	Significance of change	Percent of men showing a drop
All 57 men	Mean drop = 0.20 mm Hg	NS	49%
19 men who experienced little or no unemployment	Mean drop = 3.32 mm Hg	$p < .01$	79%
38 men who experienced substantial unemployment	Mean rise = 1.36 mm Hg	NS	34%

Association between unemployment experience and blood pressure change: gamma = .70, tau = .43, $p < .001$.

	Mean changes from anticipation to unemployment or to a new job		
Men involved	Mean change	Significance of change	Percent of men showing a drop
All 58 men	Mean rise = 0.97 mm Hg	NS	50%
17 men who went from anticipation to a new job	Mean drop = 3.34 mm Hg	$p < .07$	76%
41 men who went from anticipation to unemployment	Mean rise = 2.76 mm Hg	$p < .05$	39%

Association between unemployment experience and blood pressure change: gamma = .69, tau = .40, $p < .005$.

change from early to later Rounds, a difference score comparable to the ones examined in Tables 7–2 and 7–3, but covering a somewhat shorter span of time. It is clear that the group as a whole have not yet started to level off. This is to be expected given the more severe, prolonged unemployment. However, a subgroup of 19 men who experienced minimal unemployment does already show a significant decrease, while the other 38 men with substantial unemployment are moving in the opposite direction (a nonsignificant trend). The changes for the 2 groups are clearly significantly different from each other, as seen by the size of the association between BP change and the unemployment experience (gamma = .70, tau = .43).

The lower half of Table 7–7 represents a somewhat more refined analysis of this overall pattern. For the 17 men who were employed from the second Round on, the difference score is between Anticipation and all the subsequent Rounds. For the 41 men who had some unemployment, the difference score is between Anticipation and all those visits during which a man was without a job. Again it is obvious that the 2 groups are moving in the opposite direction and that this difference between change scores is highly significant.

The data on the 41 men were analyzed further: 32 of the 41 men found employment at a later time. For these men, the transition from unemployment to re-employment was characterized by a significant drop in BP (mean = 2.23 mm Hg, $p < .05$). It would seem fair to conclude that the unemployment experience prolongs the stress evident in the Anticipation period and delays the eventual drop in diastolic BP.

The systolic BP data were subjected to the same kind of analysis as just described for diastolic blood pressure. The trends in all cases were in the same direction but, with one exception, failed to reach statistical significance. The exception was a significant association between systolic BP change and the nature of the unemployment experience, Anticipation to new job vs Anticipation to unemployment: gamma = .45, tau = .25, $p < .05$.

These preliminary BP data on the men in Company B are fully consistent with the more detailed findings on men in Company A. Part of this consistency is again the considerably greater sensitivity of the diastolic than the systolic BP changes to the men's changing employment circumstances.

Discussion

This study has examined BP changes in men as they go through an important, stressful experience: job loss, unemployment, and reemployment. It appears to us that certain features of the design of this study make it a particularly suitable one for investigating the dynamics of BP reactivity. Specifically, these features are: (1) The study is longitudinal and it is prospective. (2) All men who fit the eligibility criteria are approached in the plant that is closing down. No self-selection biases are introduced other than those due to refusals. Our refusal rate on these men is about 23%, which compares favorably with one-shot, cross-sectional surveys. (3) Because both physiological and psychological data are collected on the same man, we can carry out a thorough investigation of the covariation of these 2 types of variables over time, that is, as these men go through this important social stress. Along with these strong points of the design there is one major limitation: not beginning the data collection sequence at such an early stage that the men could be first seen before they have any knowledge or suspicion that the plant is closing. For many reasons, this desirable feature of the design proved to be a practical impossibility.

Two lines of comment for discussion are: the possible role of other variables in modifying the generality of the finding or biasing in some way the results, and the general significance of the results.

As has been pointed out earlier, the use of BP change scores obviates the necessity for many of the traditional adjustments, such as for age or race. For example, the 11 Negro men in Company A had a predictably higher overall mean BP. However, the pattern of their changes was in no way different from the remainder of the men. And the magnitude of the change scores was comparable as well, provided one took into consideration the somewhat greater severity of their unemployment experience.

However, the use of change scores does introduce one complication. Change scores, irrespective of the phenomenon under study or the hypothesis in question, tend to be correlated with initial level and with other change scores. Specifically, a higher initial level will be associated with a larger drop (regression effect), and the larger the increase within 1 period the greater will be the decrease during the adjacent next period. These statistical artifacts of change scores become a problem whenever the direction of the effect of the artifact coincides with a hypothesis being tested. Most frequently, this occurs when: (1) we select subjects for their very low or very high initial scores and predict that they will show an increase or a drop, respectively, (2) we select subjects according to their change scores and predict that those with a positive change will show a negative change during the next time period, and vice versa, and (3) we correlate an outside variable with a change score where the outside variable is also correlated with initial level.

A review of the data presented in this paper shows that the first two possibilities do not apply. For example, the change scores presented in Table 7–3 are computed on the *total* group, not just on those subjects whose initial level was high. Similarly, men in Company A show an increase within Round 1 and a decrease within Round 2; but nothing in the artifact of change scores would generate such mean group changes unless the subjects were preselected with regard to a previous change score. However, the third possibility does apply. For example, the associations presented in Table 7–4 could be explained, in part, by an association with initial level. However, this is not the case for two reasons: (1) the association of initial diastolic BP level with the change score is only a weak one ($r = .35$), and (2) the other variables used in Table 7–4 are not significantly associated with initial level. Consequently, computing partial associations where initial levels of diastolic BP are held constant would make no practical difference.

Let us now consider some variables which, whether or not they themselves are subject to change, could be systematically influencing or biasing our results. One such variable is body weight. Change scores in body weight were computed so as to correspond to the major BP change scores used in Table 7–3. Analysis revealed that: (1) There was no significant overall trend, the men losing an average of 0.53 lbs ($p > .45$), and (2) there was an insignificant negative association between changes in body weight and changes in BP. Thus changes in body weight cannot be a variable influencing the pattern of our findings.

Another possibility is that the time of day during which the interview took place could have affected the BP values. Specifically, the possibility exists that while the men who were unemployed were interviewed during the day, the men who were employed, were visited during the evenings. A check of the records revealed that although this tended to be true, some of the working men had evening or night shifts, so that the difference was not significant. The BP data from the National Health Survey[9] were used to get an estimate of the diurnal variation. This variation is small, but there does appear to be some peaking between the hours of 5 and 7 pm. Since the excess of interviews on the unemployed men was during the mornings when the BP levels are below average, and early afternoons when they are about average, one must conclude that time of day is a variable which, if anything, tended to attenuate the obtained relationship between the unemployment experience and BP changes.

Finally, a possibility exists that the nurses introduced a systematic bias; specifically, since they knew the men's employment status, they might have been influenced in some ways by their preconceived ideas about unemployment and its effects. The possibility of such a bias is a real one in the case of direct ratings and evaluations. However, this report has not utilized such nurse ratings. Bias in reading and recording the BP values is a much more remote possibility. Because each interview schedule is filed away upon completion, the nurse seldom knows what the man's previous BP was. And during training, the nurses were sensitized to the general possibility of this kind of a bias. In any case, most of the findings just cannot be explained with reference to this possible bias: the greater sensitivity of diastolic over systolic BP in most of the analyses, the influence of such variables as Ego Resilience scale where the men's scores were not known to the nurses, and the greater sensitivity of the subjective measure over the objective measure of severity of unemployment. And the reader can well imagine the difficulty and additional costs involved in collecting BP values by a person who is otherwise totally unfamiliar with the man's circumstances.

Several comments about the general significance of our results are in order. First of all, findings were presented which linked some changes in BP to certain events in the environment. Our findings are consistent with the observations on soldiers after long combat[16] and survivors of the Texas City disaster,[17] which showed an association between an objective threatening event and elevated BP. BP differences between urban and rural Zulus[18] and among Detroit Negroes living in high and low crime-poverty census tracts[19] have also been attributed, in part, to stresses in the environment. None of the above studies, however, is a controlled longitudinal investigation. Studies of more temporary elevations in BP are more plentiful but less relevant. Nevertheless, it is interesting to note that BP goes up when patients recount unpleasant life experiences or threatening events,[20, 21] or engage in apparently emotionally meaningful interaction with an experimenter.[22]

Beyond linking changes in BP to certain environmental events, the present study was also concerned with variables which influence BP stabilization. Variables which affected the extent of the return to "normal" levels included the subjective perception of the environmental stress and Ego Resilience, a general measure of adjustment. If we accept the assumption that prolonged BP elevation due to stress increases the chances of hypertension (a time-honored hypothesis for which no solid empirical evidence exists), then these variables which influence stabilization might be also seen as influencing the development of hypertension. The supporting evidence from other studies is indirect and tenuous at best. Nevertheless, it is interesting to note that many of the studies reviewed by Scotch and Geiger[3] do suggest a poorer general adjustment among the hypertensives, and perhaps pre-hypertensives as well.[23] (The methodological shortcomings of these studies and the frequent failure to replicate[2] must not be ignored, however.) The data on short-term BP elevations during high stresses suggest that hypertensives may react with a more sustained rise than normotensives.[24–27] Of course, what is needed is a set of prospective, longitudinal studies so that we may begin to substantiate the clinical observations of Reiser and his colleagues[28, 29] concerning the role of stressful life events in the development of hypertension.

The above general comments about the BP changes obtained in our study are clearly more descriptive of diastolic than of systolic BP. Diastolic BP revealed a number of significant differences and associations, while systolic BP, though showing no reversal of trends, did not produce as many reliable differences and associations. The variability of the change scores of the two BP is roughly comparable and the change scores tend to correlate about .50 with each other. It thus appears that diastolic BP, the variable which workers in this area consider the more important and meaningful one of the two, may be more sensitive to the events in an individual's life and his reactions to them. On the other hand, it is possible that the difference merely reflects a greater tendency for the systolic BP to vary with momentary changes in the environment which obscures the longer term trends studied here.

It is our hope that as this study draws to conclusion, we shall be able to plot the course of changes over time of many other physiological and psychological variables. Then we can see how quickly or how slowly they return to normal and how this is influenced by severity of the unemployment experience and how it is modified by psychological reactions and by enduring personality traits. For example, it now appears fairly clear that both BP and serum uric acid[30] show an anticipation effect but that BP may not return to a person's "normal" level as rapidly as serum uric acid does. Cholesterol shows no anticipation effects and appears largely sensitive to the transition from unemployment to employment.[30] Still other variables, such as some of our psychological variables dealing with perception of future and optimism about it, point to an almost permanently damaging effect of the job loss experience.

Summary

The present report describes the results of a longitudinal investigation of BP changes of men who suffer a job loss because of a permanent plant shutdown. The men, who are married and in the age range of 35–60, are followed as they go through the stages of employment on the old job, loss of job, unemployment (for some), probationary reemployment, and stable employment on a new job. Controls, i.e., continuously employed men in comparable jobs, are also studied. This report examines in detail data on 56 men in one company; data on 46 controls and preliminary information on some 60 men from another company are also considered. The major findings were as follows:

1. The controls showed no significant long-term overall trends but some minor fluctuations, an apparent interview effect.
2. BP levels during anticipation of job loss and unemployment or probationary reemployment were clearly higher than during later periods of stabilization on new jobs.
3. Men whose BP levels remained high longer: (a) had a more severe unemployment experience, (b) reported a longer lasting subjective stress, (c) were lower on Ego Resilience, and (d) failed to show much improvement in Self-Esteem or much Reduction in Irritation. These findings held much more strongly for diastolic than for systolic BP.
4. There was a clear rise in BP during the anticipation period. The size of this rise depended upon subjective stress. Anticipation alone produced as much elevation as unemployment or probationary re-employment.
5. BP variability was somewhat higher among men who had higher overall BP means and who were more rigid.
6. Preliminary results from the second company replicated the major associations between BP changes and the person's objective employment situation, so we feel reasonably comfortable about drawing general conclusions from these findings though further replication is clearly indicated.

References

1. McGinn NF, Harburg E, Julius S, McLeod J: Psychological correlates of blood pressure. Psychol Bull 61:209, 1964
2. Ostfeld AM, Shekelle RB: Psychological variables and blood pressure, in The Epidemiology of Hypertension. Edited by Stamler J, Stamler R, Pullman TN. Grune, New York, 1967, pp 321–331
3. Scotch NA, Geiger HJ: The epidemiology of essential hypertension. II: psychologic and sociocultural factors in etiology. J Chronic Dis 16:1183, 1963
4. Cobb S, Brooks GW, Kasl SV, et al: The health of people changing jobs: a description of a longitudinal study. Amer J Public Health 56:1476, 1966
5. Block J: The Challenge of Response Sets. Appleton, New York, 1965
6. Gurin G, Veroff J, Feld S: Americans View Their Mental Health. Basic, New York, 1960
7. Hunt SM, Singer K, Cobb S: Components of depression: identified from a self-rating depression inventory for survey use. Arch Gen Psychiat (Chicago) 16:441, 1967
8. Rose G: Standardization of observers in blood pressure measurement. Lancet 1:673, 1965

9. U.S. Department of Health, Education and Welfare: Blood Pressure of Adults by Age and Sex, United States, 1960–1962 (Ser 11, No 4). National Center for Health Statistics, Washington, DC, 1964
10. Goodman LA, Kruskal WH: Measures of association for cross-classification. J Amer State Assoc 49:732, 1954
11. Kendall MG, Stuart A: The Advanced Theory of Statistics, Vol 2. C Griffin, London, 1961
12. Hays WL: Statistics for Psychologists. Holt, Rinehart, New York, 1963
13. Alexander F: Emotional factors in essential hypertension. Psychosom Med 1:173, 1939
14. Saul LA: Hostility in cases of essential hypertension. Psychosom Med 1:153, 1939
15. Gough H: The California Personality Inventory. Consulting Psychologists Press, Palo Alto, CA, 1957
16. Graham JDP: High blood pressure after battle. Lancet 1:239, 1945
17. Ruskin A, Beard OW, Schaffer RL: Blast hypertension. Amer J Med 4:228, 1948
18. Scotch NA: Sociocultural factors in the epidemiology of Zulu hypertension. Amer J Public Health 53:1205, 1963
19. Harburg E: Stress and Heredity in Negro-White Blood Pressure Differences. Program for Urban Health Research, The University of Michigan, Ann Arbor, MI, 1967
20. Pfeiffer JB Jr, Wolff HG: Studies in renal circulation during periods of life stress and accompanying emotional reactions in subjects with and without essential hypertension: observations on the role of neural activity in the regulation of renal blood flow. Res Publ Ass Res Nerv Ment Dis 29:929, 1950
21. Wolf S, Pfeiffer JB, Ripley HS, et al: Hypertension as a reaction pattern to stress: summary of experimental data on variations in blood pressure and renal blood flow. Ann Intern Med 29:1056, 1948
22. Weiner H, Singer MT, Reiser MR: Cardiovascular responses and their psychological correlates. Psychosom Med 24:477, 1962
23. Harris RE, Sokolow M, Carpenter LG, et al: Response to psychologic stress in persons who are potentially hypertensive. Circulation 7:874, 1953
24. Brod J, Fencl V, Hejl Z, et al: Circulatory changes underlying blood pressure elevation during acute emotional stress in normotensive and hypertensive subjects. Clin Sci 18:269, 1959
25. Malmo RB, Shagass C: Studies of blood pressure in psychiatric patients under stress. Psychosom Med 14:82, 1952
26. Simonson E, Brozek J: Review: Russian research on arterial hypertension. Ann Intern Med 50:129, 1959
27. Wolf S, Cardon PV, Shepard EM, et al: Life Stress and Essential Hypertension. Williams & Wilkins, Baltimore, MD, 1955
28. Reiser MF, Brust AA, Ferris EB: Life situations, emotions, and the course of

patients with arterial hypertension. Psychosom Med 13:133, 1951
29. Reiser MF, Rosenbaum M, Ferris EB: Psychological mechanisms in malignant hypertension. Psychosom Med 13:148, 1951
30. Kasl SV, Cobb S, Brooks GW: Changes in serum uric acid and cholesterol levels in men undergoing job loss. JAMA 206:1500, 1968

CHAPTER 8

Learned Control of Cardiovascular Integration in Man Through Operant Conditioning

GARY E. SCHWARTZ, M.A.,
DAVID SHAPIRO, PH.D., AND
BERNARD TURSKY

Prefatory Remarks

Don R. Lipsitt, M.D.

In 1967, Miller and DiCara[1] published an article that began, "The problem of whether or not visceral responses are subject to instrumental learning (also called operant conditioning or trial-and-error learning) has basic significance for both the theory of psychosomatic symptoms and the theory and neurophysiology of learning." These researchers at Rockefeller University and others spawned a whole new field of research based upon the discovery that autonomic functions once thought to be totally involuntary could indeed be brought under voluntary control. This article is representative of that new field of research, and it has contributed to subsequent advances in the application of psychophysiological studies in humans and in solving clinical problems in psychosomatic medicine referred to as behavioral medicine (including techniques such as biofeedback and other forms of self-regulation). Furthermore, by showing that various autonomic functions could be manipulated singly (differentiated) or in combination (integrated), the value of a systems approach to research on human behavior was greatly enhanced.

Reference

1. Miller NE, DiCara LV: Instrumental learning of heart rate changes in curarized rats: shaping and specificity to discriminative stimulus. J Comp Physiol Psychol 63:7–11, 1967

In previous research, it has been shown that subjects can learn to increase or decrease their systolic blood pressure without corresponding changes in heart rate, or they can learn to increase or decrease their heart rate without corresponding changes in blood pressure. The present paper outlines a method for directly conditioning a combination of two autonomic responses. A system was developed which, at each heart cycle, determines on line whether heart rate and blood pressure are integrated (both increasing or both decreasing) or differentiated (one increasing and one decreasing). To test this method, 5 subjects received a brief light and tone feedback only when their heart rate and blood pressure were simultaneously increasing, and 5 subjects received the feedback only when their heart rate and blood pressure were simultaneously decreasing. Subjects earned rewards consisting of slides and monetary bonuses each time they produced 12 correct heart rate-blood pressure combinations. Significant cardiovascular integration was obtained in a single session. Subjects rewarded for simultaneous increases in heart rate and blood pressure showed small, comparable increases in both, while subjects rewarded for simultaneous decreases showed sizeable decreases in both. Applications of the method in research and treatment are discussed.

Many papers have been published which demonstrate that by providing subjects with feedback of their autonomic activity and rewarding specific changes, it is possible to modify responses in the autonomic nervous system.[1-4] The theoretical and practical significance of this research stems in large part from data showing that learning is specific to the autonomic response that is directly reinforced—i.e., the rewarding of one autonomic response does not seem to produce learning in others.

A series of experiments by Shapiro and associates illustrates the extent of learned autonomic differentiation in man within the cardiovascular system. In one experiment,[5] subjects were given feedback and reward for increasing or decreasing systolic blood pressure while heart rate was simultaneously monitored. Significant blood pressure differences were obtained between increase and decrease subjects without corresponding differences in heart rate. After replicating this result in a second sample of subjects,[6] a similar experiment was performed,[7] except that this time feedback and reward were given for increasing or decreasing heart rate while systolic blood pressure was simultaneously monitored. The results indicated significant heart rate conditioning without corresponding changes in blood pressure.

These data indicate that learned control of blood pressure or heart rate is possible in man, an encouraging finding concerning the application of operant procedures for the treatment of certain forms of hypertension or tachycardia. However, there arises a related question of whether it is possible to control a combination of responses at the same time. For example, if reinforcing blood pressure leads to learned blood pressure control and reinforcing heart rate leads to learned heart rate control, then what procedure is necessary to produce simultaneous learning of *both* blood pressure and heart rate? It would seem that this particular combination of responses should be relatively easy to learn since heart rate is itself one physiologic determinant of systolic blood pressure.[8]

The approach taken in the present paper is that it is possible to condition a combination of autonomic responses by rewarding a subject *only* when he shows the desired pattern. This requires a methodology for measuring *on line* the phasic interrelationships of autonomic activity. Toward this end, instrumentation was developed which, at each heart cycle, determines whether heart rate and blood pressure are integrated—i.e., both going in the same direction, either both increasing or both decreasing, or whether the responses are differentiated—i.e., both going in opposite directions, one increasing and the other simultaneously decreasing, as measured from median levels.

To test the system as well as to attempt the direct conditioning of heart rate-blood pressure integration in man, the following experiment was performed.

Method

Subjects

The subjects were 10 normotensive males between the ages of 21 and 30. All subjects were in good physical health and were paid for participating in the experiment.

Physiologic Measures

Systolic blood pressure, heart rate and respiration were recorded on an Offner Type R Dynagraph. The electrocardiogram was measured using standard plate electrodes and was displayed on one channel of the polygraph. An electronic switch was used to trigger Grason-Stadler (Model 1200) solid state programming equipment at each heart cycle (R spike). The procedure for measuring median systolic blood pressure and median heart rate is based on the method developed in the earlier studies.[5-7] Median systolic pressure is defined as the constant cuff pressure level at which 50% of possible Korotkoff sounds occur. By displaying the Korotkoff sounds on one channel of the polygraph in conjunction with a second electronic switch, it is possible, through appropriate logic modules, to track the number of heart beats accompanied by a Korotkoff sound, and the number of heart beats followed by the absence of a Korotkoff sound. Similarly, median heart rate is defined as the heart rate level (detected by a third electronic switch calibrated in beats per minute) at which 50% of possible fast (above the level) heart beats occurred. This is accomplished by displaying beat-by-beat heart rate on one channel of the polygraph through a cardiotachometer (Lexington Instrument Model 107) and, using appropriate logic modules in conjunction with the third (cardiotachometer) electronic switch, by tracking the number of heart beats (R to R intervals) that are faster than the cardiotachometer level detector. It has been empirically determined that if 36 or more of 50 possible Korotkoff sounds (or fast heart beats) occur, the applied cuff pressure (or cardiotachometer electronic switch) is raised 2 mmHg (or 2 bpm) on the next trial. If 14 or fewer of 50 possible sounds (or fast heart beats) occur, the applied pressure (or the cardiotachometer electronic switch) is lowered by 2 mmHg (or 2 bpm) on the next trial. This procedure provides an accurate means for independently tracking both median systolic pressure and median heart rate at the same time, and for obtaining comparable beat-by-beat information about relative increases or decreases in both responses.*

The tracking of blood pressure-heart rate integration and differentiation at each heart beat is obtained by a program which detects the four possible combinations of these two responses *relative to their median values.* Figure 8–1 shows a representative portion of a polygraph record of the system in operation. Shown are the electrocardiogram, heart rate displayed through a cardiotachometer, the presence or absence of Korotkoff sounds measured at a constant cuff pressure, and two marker channels. The presence or absence of a Korotkoff sound, relative to the constant pressure in the cuff, indicates whether blood pressure is up or down for each heart cycle, while up and down heart rate is relative to the median heart rate. After each heart cycle, one of four possible marks appears on the integration-differentiation (ID) marker. The longest and shortest marks reflect integration—i.e., *up* blood pressure and *up* heart rate produce the longest mark, while *down* blood pressure and *down* heart rate produce the shortest mark. The other two marks reflect differentiation—i.e., *up* blood pressure and *down* heart rate produce the third longest mark, while *down* blood pressure and *up* heart rate produce the second shortest mark. The bottom channel indicates which of the four possible combinations is receiving feedback and reward. In this example, feedback is occurring for *up* blood pressure-*up* heart rate integration.

The extent of beat-by-beat integration, as defined here, becomes the percentage of beats in which both heart rate and blood pressure are simultaneously up or down. Therefore, for a given trial, 100% would reflect complete integration and 0% would reflect complete differentiation. The system is purposefully complicated by the fact that if tonic levels of physiologic activity change, the integration values change accordingly. Consequently, a subject can best succeed at producing rewards in, for example, a *down-down* condition, by lowering both his *median* heart rate and blood pressure, as opposed to changing only the more

---

*See Tursky, Shapiro, and Schwartz:[13] "An Automated Constant Cuff-pressure System for Measuring Average Systolic and Diastolic Blood Pressure in Man" for a complete description of the blood pressure system. Included in their article are data validating the system against blood pressures recorded by surgical catheterization.

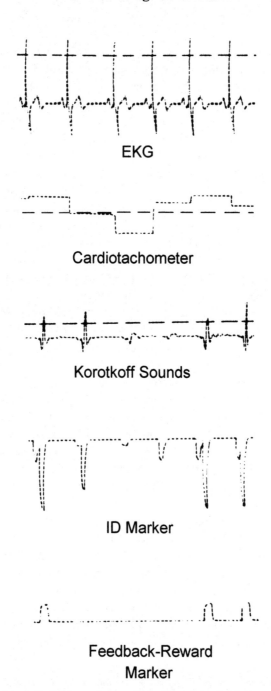

Figure 8–1. Segment of polygraph record of subject rewarded for increasing both his heart rate and systolic blood pressure simultaneously (up-up integration). Horizontal dashed lines indicate level detectors.

phasic characteristics of the two responses. Since the ultimate clinical goal in this research is to affect *tonic* levels of physiologic activity, the ID system proves very satisfactory.

In addition to heart rate and blood pressure, respiration was recorded on the polygraph, using a strain gauge device placed around the subject's chest.

Design and Procedure

On entering the laboratory, subjects were seated in a lounge chair in a sound- and temperature-controlled room, and were connected to the physiologic recording devices. Subjects were told that the purpose of the experiment was to determine if they could learn to control certain physiologic responses that are considered involuntary. They were instructed to refrain from moving and to breathe regularly. Half the subjects received a brief light and tone as feedback each time their blood pressure and heart rate were simultaneously increasing; the other half received the light-tone feedback only when their blood pressure and heart rate were simultaneously decreasing. For every 12 correct responses, a reward in the form of a slide was shown for 3 seconds. In working with normal males, we have found that a potpourri of rewards provides the most interest and incentive. The slides included landscapes, pictures of attractive nude females, and monetary bonuses for succeeding at the task.

All subjects received five adaptation and 40 conditioning trials, each trial being 50 beats in length. Variable rest periods of 20–30 seconds' duration separated each trial. Initial blood pressure levels between groups were made comparable by matching subjects (±4 mmHg) on the adaptation values. The matching procedure also served to eliminate potential experimenter bias effects,[9] since the experimenter did not know what condition the subject would receive until after he read the instructions, left the subject room, and obtained the adaptation data. At the end of conditioning, the experimenter re-entered the subject room and interviewed all subjects concerning what they were doing to control their physiologic activity.

Results and Discussion

The results of this experiment (Figure 8–2) are quite different from the previous research wherein specificity was obtained when a single response was rewarded. As predicted, significant control of *both* blood pressure *and* heart rate was obtained in a single session. Analyses of variance (Biomed 08V computer

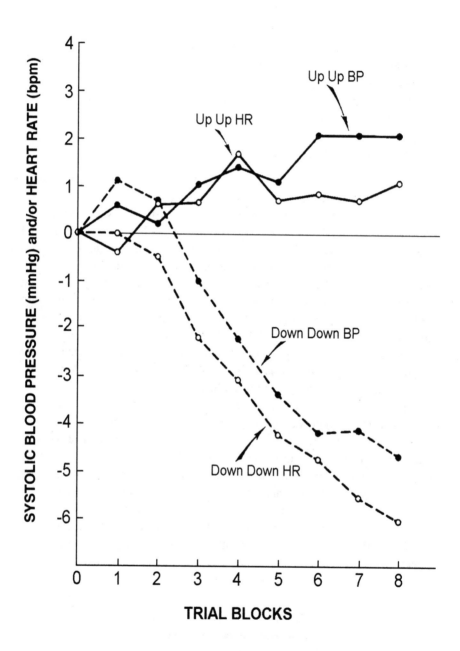

Figure 8–2. Average heart rate (HR) and systolic blood pressure (BP) in subjects rewarded for simultaneously increasing both HR and BP (up-up integration) and for simultaneously decreasing both HR and BP (down-down integration). Each point is mean of 5 subjects, five trials each. Ordinate is both beats/min. and mmHg. All values were adjusted for initial adaptation levels and were set to zero.

analysis) reveal highly significant groups by trial interactions for both blood pressure ($p < 0.001$) and heart rate ($p < 0.001$), demonstrating that the divergence of the blood pressure curves and that of the heart rate curves are reliable. Subjects rewarded for simultaneous increases show small comparable increases in both systems (maximum increase at trial 40 for a single subject of +6 mmHg and +2 bpm), while subjects rewarded for simultaneous decreases show larger decreases in both systems (maximum decrease at trial 40 for a single subject of −12 mmHg and −8 bpm).

Potential respiratory influences on blood pressure and heart rate were considered. As in our previous work, analysis of respiration revealed no systematic differences between groups. Interestingly, there was some tendency for the up-up subjects to report more active mental and task involvement than the down-down subjects. However, these data are too variable to warrant firm conclusions about cognitive correlates of the conditioned autonomic activity.

Analysis of the frequency of the four possible combinations of heart rate and blood pressure revealed that on the average, subjects' blood pressure and heart rate were both simultaneously above or below their respective medians only about 50% of the time (during adaptation, the 10 subjects ranged from 25 to 60%). This fact may explain why when blood pressure or heart rate is singularly rewarded, learning does not occur in the other. In other words, if increased blood pressure is being rewarded, from the heart's point of view, half the time it receives reward when it is increasing and half the time it receives reward when it is decreasing. The hypothesis is put forth that it should be theoretically possible to predict the amount of relationship over time between two autonomic responses by rewarding one and determining the extent to which the other shows simultaneous learning. The reverse hypothesis is that when a single autonomic response is rewarded, the extent to which it is related over time to any other autonomic response is the extent to which those responses will also show learning similar to the response controlling the reward.

The data and theory may have important implications for treatment. If it is clinically desirable to lower the activity of only one response without affecting others, care should be taken to make sure that the other responses are not highly correlated with the symptom in question. If it should be desirable to lower two autonomic responses, it may be necessary to reward the patient directly for the integration of this activity, as in the present experiment. For example, one application of operant autonomic integration may be in the treatment of angina pectoris, where lowering the combination of blood pressure and heart rate can result in reduced cardiac oxygen requirements and therefore in reduced pain.[10, 11] Finally, if two responses are partially correlated, and it is still desirable to lower only one, it may be necessary to reward the patient directly for the differentiation of this activity. The doctoral research of the first author[12] not only demonstrates the direct conditioning of cardiovascular integration on a second sample of subjects, but further demonstrates that the direct operant conditioning of cardiovascular *differentiation* is possible in man.

These data, in conjunction with those in our previous research,[5-7] offer strong evidence for human operant autonomic control. Man can learn to increase both his blood pressure and his heart rate, lower both his blood pressure and his heart rate, or raise and lower his blood pressure or his heart rate. This degree of *learned* autonomic specificity raises important questions as to what controls what in the autonomic nervous system. The present paper offers a method for the study of autonomic integration and differentiation, and outlines a new technic for the control of multiautonomic responses in man.

References

1. Kimmel HD: Instrumental conditioning of autonomically mediated behavior. Psychol Bull 67:337–345, 1967
2. Katkin ES, Murray EN: Instrumental conditioning of autonomically mediated behavior: theoretical and methodological issues. Psychol Bull 70:52–68, 1968
3. Miller NE: Learning of visceral and glandular responses. Science 163:434–445, 1969
4. DiCara LV: Learning in the autonomic nervous system. Scientific American 222:30–39, 1970
5. Shapiro D, Tursky B, Gershon E, et al: Effects of feedback and reinforcement on the control of human systolic blood pressure. Science 163:588–590, 1969
6. Shapiro D, Tursky B, Schwartz GE: Control of blood pressure in man by operant conditioning. Circulation Res 271:27–32, 1970
7. Shapiro D, Tursky B, Schwartz GE: Differentiation of heart rate and blood pressure in man by operant conditioning. Psychosom Med 32:417–423, 1970
8. Berne RM, Levy MN: Cardiovascular Physiology. CV Mosby, St Louis, MO, 1967
9. Rosenthal R: Experimenter Effects in Behavioral Research. Appleton-Century-Crofts, New York, 1966
10. Braunwald E, Epstein SE, Glick G, et al: Relief of angina pectoris by electrical stimulation of the carotid-sinus nerves. New Eng J Med 277:1278–1283, 1967
11. Sonnenblick EH, Ross J, Braunwald E: Oxygen consumption of the heart: newer concepts of its multifactoral determination. Amer J Cardiol 22:328–336, 1968
12. Schwartz GE: Voluntary control of human cardiovascular integration and differentiation through feedback and reward. Science 174:90–93, 1971

13. Tursky B, Shapiro D, Schwartz GE: Automated constant cuff-pressure system for measuring average systolic and diastolic blood pressure in man. Trans Bio Med Engineering 19:271–275, 1972

CHAPTER 9

Effect of Psychosocial Stimulation on the Enzymes Involved in the Biosynthesis and Metabolism of Noradrenaline and Adrenaline

JAMES P. HENRY, M.D.,
PATRICIA M. STEPHENS,
JULIUS AXELROD, PH.D., AND
ROBERT A. MUELLER, M.D.

Prefatory Remarks

Bernard T. Engel, Ph.D.

This article was a collaborative effort between two groups of investigators: James Henry and his colleagues at the University of Southern California and Julius Axelrod and his team at the National Institute of Mental Health. Henry and his co-workers had shown that in mice the social stress of territorial deprivation was associated with a large increase in blood pressure. Axelrod and his colleagues, in a series of Nobel Prize–winning experiments, had described the enzymatic pathways involved in the synthesis of epinephrine. They had further shown that severe pharmacological and physical stresses will induce the production of adrenaline-synthesizing enzymes. These two groups collaborated to show that the environmental stresses present in the social situation could cause a large increase in the production of adrenaline and its associated enzymes. Research such as this helped to set the stage for subsequent work by others who showed that a major mechanism underlying the physiological expression of stress is the activation of corticotropin-releasing factor, which stimulates both sympathetic nerve activity and ACTH release.

Various groups of CBA mice were exposed to differing levels of psychosocial stimulation by mutual confrontation for 6 months after reaching maturity. Their experiences ranged from individual isolation, through standard boxing, to a colony life in an intercommunicating box system containing males and females.

The blood pressures of the socially stimulated groups increased to 170 ± 20 mmHg; those of the boxed and isolated animals remained a normal 126 ± 12 mmHg. Adrenal weights, adrenal noradrenaline and adrenaline, monoamine oxidase, tyrosine hydroxylase (the rate-limiting enzyme in catecholamine synthesis) and phenylethanolamine-N-methyltransferase (PNMT, the enzyme that converts noradrenaline to adrenaline) were all increased in the stimulated groups. A significant decrease in the two latter enzymes was observed in the isolated animals. It is suggested that the increase in catecholamine-forming enzymes resulting from psychosocial stimulation may be neuronally mediated, and that it is not an immediate response as in the case of a sudden discharge of noradrenaline and adrenaline in states of anger, fear or aggression.

Recent studies have demonstrated that a sustained increase in blood pressure can accompany the psychosocial stimulation that develops when the rivals in an animal colony repeatedly confront each other over a prolonged period.[1]

It was assumed that hypertension was due to the many episodes of arousal of the defense alarm response, and the consequent repeated stimulation of the sympathetic nervous system. The work of Brod[2] was cited as an example of the arousal of the defense alarm response in man. He has shown that mental arithmetic in men who are challenged to respond under the duress of a time constraint induces vasodilation in the muscles, vasoconstriction in the viscera, and a rise in blood pressure.[2] Folkow and Rubinstein[3] have demonstrated that these same changes occur in anesthetized rats, when the anterolateral hypothalamus is stimulated. They further showed that when the same region was stimulated chronically, sustained hypertension developed in the conscious rat.[3] Levi[4] and Frankenhaeuser,[5] continue to marshal evidence that rates of catecholamine excretion in human urine are related to such states of arousal, and that noradrenaline is related to "critical and uncomfortable experiences." Recently, von Holst[6] has shown the deleterious effects of persistent sympathetic arousal on breeding and on other parameters in the tree shrew. He reports a fatal outcome if the animals find no surcease from repeated emotional stimulation.[6] In the study of Barnett et al.[7] excessive sympathetic arousal may also be responsible for the death of formerly dominant male rats which fail to survive when placed with a group of strangers. In related work with mice, Bronson and Eleftheriou[8] have shown that a few minutes of fighting each day will lead to an increased adrenal content of cortical hormone. Welch and Welch[9] have demonstrated that 5–10 daily 5-minute bouts of fighting will increase noradrenaline and adrenaline in the brain, as well as in the adrenal glands of isolated animals. These changes persisted for at least 20 hours after the last episode of stimulation.[9] In further work,[10] they showed that mice did not need physical contact, but responded in the same way at the mere sight of violent confrontations involving other mice.[10] Although blood pressure was not measured in the course of these various experiments, there is reason to believe that had this been done, the level would have been found to be elevated.[1]

Since activity of the adrenal medulla is involved with the above phenomena, a study was undertaken to examine whether or not its basic metabolic machinery—the enzymes involved in the biosynthesis and metabolism of the sympathetic neurotransmitter, noradrenaline, and the adrenal medullary hormone, adrenaline, are affected by psychosocial stimulation. Since increases in these enzymes take many hours to develop, the work might point to a mechanism by which long-term pathophysiologic changes could eventuate from transitory episodes of social stimulation. A preliminary communication of this work has already been made.[11]

Methods

The objective was to impose maximum psychosocial stimulation on one series of adult CBA mice, and to contrast the effects with those in a series that had been subjected to as little interaction as possible. The method of using an interconnected box system with a central feeding location was chosen because it provides a system in which floor space per mouse is the same or is greater than that for normally boxed animals; yet, there is repeated confrontation, as the mice traverse the tubes connecting the boxes, and eat and drink at the same central dispenser.[1]

The symbols in the lower part of Figures 9–1 and 9–2 depict the three phases of treatment accorded to 8 groups of animals. (a) The first period was from birth to weaning at 21–28 days for all animals except the isolates which were weaned as early as possible—i.e., at 12–14 days. During this time, the nurslings were either left with their mothers (i.e., Groups 1–4), or were separated from the mother for 2 hours a day by isolation in bottles which were one-third filled with shavings (Groups 5–8). (b) The second period was from weaning at 12–14 days until maturity at 4 months. During this time, Groups 1, 2, 5 and 6 were maintained as siblings, separated according to sex, in standard boxes; Groups 3, 4, 7 and 8 were kept in isolation in 1-pint glass jars as previously described.[1] (c) The third period was from the attainment of full adult life at 4 months until 10 months of age. The animals either remained in boxes as standard siblings (i.e., Groups 1 and 5), or they were isolated in bottles (i.e., Groups 3 and 7). The remaining 4 groups (i.e., 2, 4, 6 and 8) were placed in the interconnected box system with equal numbers of males and females. The maximum number was 34/system. There, they were exposed to intense mutual stimulation.

The eight columns of the three sets of treatments indicate the different combinations that were employed. The control group in the first column experienced standard handling for this laboratory—i.e., the nurslings remained at all times with the mother until weaned at 3–4 weeks of age. The siblings were then separated according to sex, and remained, 6–8/box, in standard $11 \times 7 \times 5$ inch boxes throughout their lives.[1] At the extremes on either side of this standard were the seventh and eighth sets in this design. These experienced the poorest preparation for later social experience, because not only were they maintained alone in bottles for the 14 weeks from weaning to maturity, but they were also separated from the mother for 2 hours a day during the period prior to weaning. Of these two mother-deprived sets, the seventh remained isolated for the entire 6-month adult period, while the eighth experienced the acute reversal, from prolonged

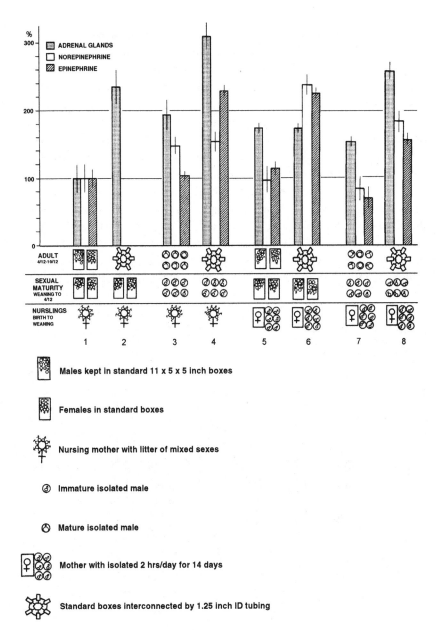

Figure 9–1. Effects of psychosocial stimulation on adrenal gland weight and adrenal norepinephrine and epinephrine content of 8 groups of CBA mice. Figures in bottom three rows symbolize different procedures. Numbers 1–8 are used to identify various experimental groups in text. Controls in Group 1 are normally raised, normally boxed siblings. Asterisks denote differences from these control values in various groups—
*$P < 0.05$; **$P < 0.01$; and ***$P < 0.001$.

isolation to forced socialization in the six-box intercommunicating system.

Once maturity had been attained at 4 months, blood pressures were measured every 2 weeks, with a cuff 6 mm in length and 5 mm in diameter. It has been shown in this laboratory that the systolic pressure of CBA mice, raised and boxed as siblings, reads as 126 ± 12 mmHg, when measured with a cuff of this size.[1, 13] The determination of the pressure thus followed the practices previously described; for the final blood pressure figure in the present study, an arithmetic mean was taken of all values on each animal for the last 2 months of adult life—i.e., from 8 to 10 months of age.

The animal husbandry practices of feeding, watering, etc., were the same as previously described.[1, 13] At autopsy, approximately one-half were killed by placing them in an ether jar, and one-half, by decapitation. Eight males from each group were sampled for the study of biochemical changes in the adrenal glands. In either case, the time—from selection of an animal from a box by a familiar handler (PS), to cleaning and weighing of the gland—averaged less than

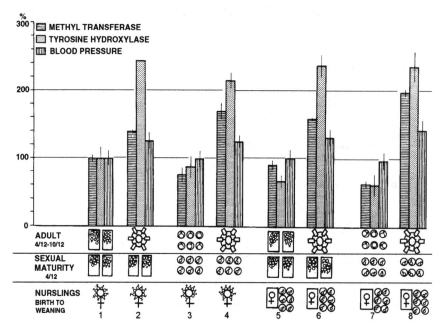

Figure 9–2. Effects of various psychosocial procedures on adrenal content of phenylethanolamine *N*-methyltransference (PNMT) and tyrosine hydroxylase. Final column represents mean of biweekly blood pressure measurements on each of male members of various groups. Meaning of three rows of symbols is indicated on legend to Fig. 9–1. Asterisks denote significant differences from control values as indicated in legend for Fig. 9–1.

3 minutes. The average weight per group of a single adrenal was derived by taking the mean of all the glands in the group—i.e., both right and left glands. After they were weighed, the adrenals were immediately packed in dry ice and shipped air freight to the participating biochemical laboratory. There each gland was homogenized in 1 ml of ice-cold isotonic sucrose with a glass Duall homogenizer, and an aliquot was taken to determine noradrenaline and adrenaline content by the method of von Euler and Lishajko.[15] The remaining homogenate was centrifuged at 27,000 g. Tyrosine hydroxylase,[16] phenylethanolamine N-methyltransferase (PNMT),[17] and catechol-O-methyl transferase (COMT)[18] were assayed in the supernate; and monoamine oxidase (MAO)[19] was determined in the particulate fraction. Tyrosine hydroxylase was chosen because it is the initial and rate-limiting enzyme in the chain forming the catecholamines (Figure 9–3). It is localized in the sympathetic nerves as well as in the adrenal gland. PNMT is found in the adrenal medulla and in some areas of the brain; it converts noradrenaline to adrenaline. MAO and COMT are the enzymes responsible for metabolizing the catecholamines (Figure 9–3).

Results

One group of controls (8 animals) was assigned to the experiment representing Column 1—i.e., they were normally nursed and normally boxed (Figures

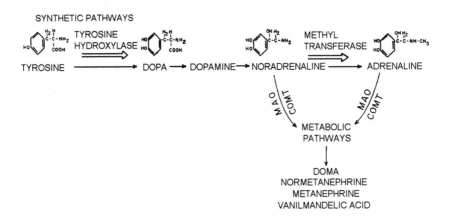

Figure 9–3. Enzymes studied in biosynthesis and metabolism of catecholamines. DOPA = dihydroxy phenylalanine; MAO = monoamine oxidase; COMT = catechol-O-methyltransferase; and DOMA = dihydroxy mandelic acid.

9–1 and 9–2). Their average body weight was 33.0 g and the average weight per adrenal gland was 1.05 mg. Thus, their relative adrenal weight was 3.1 mg/100 g (Table 9–1).

The mean weight per adrenal of stimulus-deprived or isolated male mice was 1.55 mg, and their body weight was 28.3 g, giving a relative weight of 5.5 mg/100 g. For the animals that were strongly stimulated in the intercommunicating box system, body weight was 28.4 g and mean weight per adrenal was 2.5 mg (8.8 mg/100 g). Thus, both the absolute and relative (mg/100 g body weight) adrenal weights of the isolated animals were greater than those of the controls; however, the adrenals of the socially stimulated members of the intercommunicating box system were even greater, being more than double those of the control animals. There was no clear-cut differentiation between any of the Groups 2 through 8. All had significantly larger adrenals than did the controls in Group 1 (Figure 9–1).

The blood pressure of the first group which was normally handled was 129 ± 5 mmHg; this was well within the expected range of 126 ± 12 mmHg. The figure served as a control, and the values for Groups 3, 5 and 7 which were not subjected to intense social stimulation were not significantly different (Figure 9–2). The pressures of the intensely stimulated groups (Groups 2, 4, 6 and 8) all exceeded those of the control by more than one standard deviation. Although they did not differ significantly among each other, Group 8 animals, which were first mother-deprived and then isolated until they were adult, did have the highest mean pressure. Thus, although neither adrenal weights nor blood pressure effectively discriminated between the various socially stimulated groups, the measures did separate the general category of intensely stimulated animals (Groups 2, 4, 6 and 8) from those which were isolated, and from those which were normally boxed (Groups 1, 3, 5 and 7).

Table 9–1. Effect of psychosocial stimulation on adrenal weight

Treatment	Body weight (g)	Mean adrenal weight (mg)	Relative weight (mg/100 g)
Normal	33.0 ± 0.75	1.05 ± 0.12	3.1 ± 0.4
Stimulus deprived	28.3 ± 0.68	$1.55 \pm 0.05^*$	5.5 ± 0.2
Stimulus increased	28.4 ± 0.86	$2.5 \pm 0.15^\dagger$	8.8 ± 0.5

Results are expressed as mean $\pm$ SE per adrenal. One unit of enzyme activity is the P mole product formed per hour.[19] The average weight per group of a single adrenal was taken as the mean of both right and left glands.
*Indicates $P < 0.01$.
†Indicates $P < 0.001$.

The control noradrenaline and adrenaline contents of the glands were 0.42 ± 0.1 μg and 1.42 ± 0.2 μg, respectively. They show significant changes only between those receiving intense social stimulation (Groups 2, 4, 6 and 8) and the controls.

One of the catecholamine-metabolizing enzymes, monoamine oxidase, gave similar results—i.e., the control value was 19 ± 3.0 units; the stimulus-deprived animals showed no differences in enzyme activity, while in the socially stimulated animals (Groups 2, 4, 6 and 8), the monoamine oxidase activity was significantly elevated (36 ± 3.5 units). No changes in the other metabolizing enzyme, catechol-O-methyl transferase, were observed in the socially stimulated, socially deprived, or control groups.

The control level of PNMT was 0.29 ± 0.013 units, where one unit is mμ mole product formed per hour. It was elevated in all categories of social stimulation, and was significantly depressed below the controls in Group 7, in which the animals were mother-deprived and then isolated (Figure 9–2).

The tyrosine hydroxylase parallels the PNMT, the control value being 1.8 ± 0.29 units. The level in stimulus-deprived Group 7 is significantly lower than that in the controls, and is greatly elevated in the stimulus-increased groups (Groups 2, 4, 6 and 8). The data do not permit clear-cut differentiation between the various groups, although in the case of both enzymes, the group with maternal deprivation throughout their lives (Group 7) had the lowest values, and the related Group 8, which was strongly socially stimulated at the end, had the highest.

Discussion

An increase in adrenal weight in animals exposed to intense environmental stimulation has often been described.[9, 20, 21] It is possible that our technic of isolation in small bottles creates an environment which frustrates a programmed drive for physical activity and social interaction; and that in consequence, a mild hypertrophy of the adrenal ensues. However, the underlying mechanism of increase in the size of the organ appears to differ from that in the socially stimulated animals; for, in spite of the hypertrophy, the total content of enzymes remains less than that in the controls.

As in the studies of Welch and Welch,[9] in which mice were exposed to 5 minutes of fighting daily for 10 days, the noradrenaline and adrenaline contents of the adrenal gland were more than doubled in the present work. Welch and Welch point out that even after single brief episodes, the plasma corticosterone remains elevated for hours; they speculated that stimulation of adrenal cortical activity might induce an adaptive increase in adrenal medullary capacity for synthesis and storage.[9]

Increase in rate-limiting tyrosine hydroxylase is important because of its regulatory activity.[22] The question of whether this could be the result of increased discharge of corticoids from the adrenal cortex, or of whether it is due to increased stimulation by the sympathetic nerves remains undecided. However, it has been shown that tyrosine hydroxylase[23] and PNMT[24] require sympathetic nerve activity for their elevation. Further, it was shown that this is transsynaptically induced, requires new protein synthesis, and takes 1–3 days to develop.[25] Finally, if a rat is immobilized by being tied down, there is an increase of tyrosine hydroxylase and PNMT activity that can be partially eliminated by cutting the splanchnic nerves to the adrenal gland.[25a] All this suggests that the increase in enzymes may be neuronally mediated, and indicates that, unlike the discharge of noradrenaline or adrenaline, the enzyme changes take a long time to develop.[12] Thus, despite the brevity of individual confrontation stimuli, the overall effect will be a sustained elevation of the catecholamine biosynthetic enzymes.

There is evidence as to the mechanism underlying the decrease in enzyme levels in isolated animals. Hypophysectomy will lead to a reduction of adrenal PNMT[18] and tyrosine hydroxylase,[26] and this decrease can be prevented by ACTH.[25] On the other hand, adrenal tyrosine hydroxylase activity decreases after the splanchnic nerve supply to the adrenal gland is cut.[25] It remains to be established whether the reduction observed in this paper was due to depletion of the hormone ACTH and/or to reduced sympathetic nerve stimulation, or to other factors.

The blood pressure of the group of animals subjected to increased stimulation was significantly elevated, ranging from 150 to 180 mmHg, with a mean of 168 ± 17 mmHg. Higher values are found in animals and humans, especially in association with renal disease, but not in the early stages of essential hypertension.[27] Blood pressure decreases below normal levels in situations in which there is sharp reduction of stimulation.[24] Smirk[27] has discussed the method of producing such basal levels of blood pressure; recent data on adrenal cortical activity suggest that the same will occur for the 17 OHCS levels, if the individual is made to feel exceptionally secure and in control of his environment.[28] The isolated animal presumably enjoyed such circumstances; and this may be connected with the lowered adrenal medullary enzyme levels. On the other hand, the social situation in the intercommunicating box system leads to a prolonged series of challenging confrontations. It is probable that both the pituitary-ACTH mechanism and the sympathetic nervous system produce long-sustained adrenal responses in these situations which involve intense social stimulation. As von Holst[6] has pointed out, if the stimuli are repeated with sufficient frequency to lead to sustained sympathetic arousal, the results can be fatal.[6]

Handling of the young animals was divided into two periods. The first was from birth to weaning (nurslings), and the second, from weaning to maturity (sexual maturity) (Figures 9–2 and 9–3).

In the first phase, the young nurslings were separated from the mother for 2 hours a day. Isolated young will make ultrasonic squeaks which agitate and attract adults.[29] There is evidence that squeaking may be accompanied by distress, since corticosterone levels rise in 2-day pups isolated for 30 minutes.[30] Thus, the ultrasonic calls may be associated with the neuroendocrine correlates of insecurity in pup as well as in mother. It was our hope that by maintaining the longest possible period of daily individual isolation compatible with continued nursing, a sense of insecurity might be induced, which would be perpetuated during adult life.

The animals were isolated in bottles from 12 to 14 days of age, just after the eyes open, until full maturity at 120 days to prevent them from developing normal patterns of response to stimuli received from other mice.[9] Melzak has used evoked potentials to show that social deprivation impairs the capacity to filter out and select information on the basis of prior experience and information storage.[31] Furthermore, by restricting the mice to very confined and solitary quarters, we hoped to produce animals for whom the social environment in an extended box system differed as much as possible from the circumstances surrounding their developmental period. The purpose of the intercommunicating box system was to provide a space where males and females could intermingle, yet in which the narrow tubes provided a continuous challenge to each animal's position in the dominance-subordinance hierarchy.[1] The central feeding and water station was employed with the object of providing a *behavioral sink* of the type Calhoun has described. This forces contentious animals into confrontation during the search for food.[32] The whole system was intended to induce conflict for territory, yet, at the same time, it permits the nondisruptive brief removal of the mice, box by box, for their regular blood pressure readings.

Both Levine and Denenberg and their associates have made extensive studies[33,34] of the effects of briefly disrupting the relationship between mother and infant rodent during the earliest period of life; recently, they have discussed the implications of their findings at some length. It appears that removing the infants from the mother causes her to behave differently towards them.[35] When exposed as adults to the open field test, such animals are bolder; they also have less plasma corticosteroid elevation when so stimulated, than do animals which are left in an undisturbed mother-pup relationship. However, it remains to be seen what the effects of this type of infantile stimulation may be on adaptability to the social situation in population cages where there is a strong sense of social hierarchy.

Certainly, our formerly isolated animals have difficulty in meeting demands of prolonged and stressful social interaction and role playing; they failed to develop a stable social hierarchy. Thus, Ely[36] has evidence which suggests that in a stable group, the dominant animal has a sustained high blood pressure; this may be much lower or even normal in subordinate males.[36] It appears that in poorly socialized groups, there is so much conflict that dominance can be only briefly held by any one individual, and hypertension is more widespread in the group. It is also true that care for the young is grossly deficient in such groups. By contrast, animals raised from birth in a normally interacting colony proved well adapted to the parental role.

In the present study, PNMT and tyrosine hydroxylase levels were lowest in the mother-deprived animals which continued in isolation, and highest in those mother-deprived isolates exposed to social interaction. This is compatible with our observation of higher blood pressure levels in the colony of isolates which had been mother-deprived. Thus, the overall data would suggest that the early maternal deprivation practiced in these studies may, indeed, have increased the severity of the adult isolate's social inadequacy.

Summary

Eight groups of CBA mice were exposed to various modifications of early experience, including, for some groups, isolation from weaning until adult status was attained. Four groups of adults were then exposed, for 6 months, to an intercommunicating box system which led to repeated confrontations and severe social stimulation.

The anticipated increases in blood pressure, adrenal weight and adrenal noradrenaline and adrenaline were observed in these highly stimulated groups. Monoamine oxidase was also slightly increased. Tyrosine hydroxylase, the rate-limiting enzyme for the biosynthesis of the neurotransmitter, noradrenaline, and phenylethanolamine N-methyltransferase, which catalyzes the conversion of noradrenaline to adrenaline, were both greatly increased in groups experiencing excessive social stimulation.

On the other hand, the stimulus-deprived groups showed a lowering of these two biosynthetic enzymes. Since these enzyme responses take several hours to develop, the data provide evidence of long-sustained adrenal medullary responses to acute episodes of social stimulation.

References

1. Henry JP, Meehan JP, Stephens P: The use of psychosocial stimuli to induce prolonged systolic hypertension in mice. Psychosom Med 29:408–432, 1967
2. Brod J, Fencl V, Hejl A, et al: Circulatory changes underlying blood pressure elevation during acute emotional stress (mental arithmetic) in normotensive and hypertensive subjects. Clin Sci 18:269, 1959
3. Folkow B, Rubinstein EH: Cardiovascular effects of acute and chronic stimulation of the hypothalamic defense area in the rat. Acta Physiol Scand 68:48, 1966
4. Levi L: Emotional stress and sympatho-adrenomedullary and related physiological reactions with particular reference to cardiovascular pathology, in Psychosomatics in Essential Hypertension. Edited by Koster M, Musaph H, Visser P. Karger, Basel, 1970, pp 38–51
5. Frankenhaeuser M: Physiological, behavioral, and subjective reactions to stress. Proceedings of Second International Symposium on Man in Space (Paris 1965). Springer-Verlag, New York, 1967, pp 374–388
6. Von Holst D: Sozialer streis bei tupajas (Tupaia belangeri). Z vergl Physiol 63:1–58, 1969
7. Barnett SA, Eton JC, McCallum HM: Physiological effects of social stress in wild rats, 2: liver glycogen and blood glucose. J Psychosom Res 4:251, 1960
8. Bronson FH, Eleftheriou BE: Behavior pituitary and adrenal correlates of controlled fighting (defeat) in mice. Physiol Zool 38:406, 1965
9. Welch BL, Welch AS: Sustained effects of brief daily stress (fighting) upon brain and adrenal catecholamines and adrenal, spleen and heart weights of mice. Proc Nat Acad Sci USA 64:100, 1969
10. Welch AS, Welch BL: Reduction of norepinephrine in the lower brainstem by psychological stimulus. Proc Nat Acad Sci USA 60:478–481, 1968
11. Axelrod J, Mueller RA, Henry JP, et al: Changes in enzymes involved in the biosynthesis and metabolism of noradrenaline and adrenaline after psychosocial stimulation. Nature (London) 225:1059–1060, 1970
12. Ciarenello RD, Barchas JD: Studies on the elevation of adrenaline forming activity in the rat following prolonged physiologic stress. Psychosom Med (in press)
13. Henry JP, Meehan JP, Stephens P, et al: Arterial pressure in CBA mice as related to age. J Geront 20:239, 1965
14. Zarrow MX, Haltmeyer GC, Denenberg VH, et al: Response of the infantile rat to stress. Endocrinology 79:631–634, 1966

15. Von Euler US, Lishajko F: Improved technique for the fluorometric estimation of catecholamines. Acta Physiol Scand 61:348, 1961
16. Mueller RA, Thoenen H, Axelrod J: Increase in tyrosine hydroxylase activity after reserpine administration. J Pharmacol Exp Ther 169:74, 1969
17. Axelrod J: Purification and properties of phenylethanolamine N-methyltransferase. J Biol Chem 237:1657–1660, 1962
18. Wurtman RJ, Axelrod J: Control of enzymatic synthesis of adrenaline in the adrenal medulla by adrenal cortical steroids. J Biol Chem 241:2301–2305, 1966
19. Wurtman RJ, Axelrod J: A sensitive and specific assay for the estimation of monoamine oxidase. Biochem Pharmacol 12:1439, 1963
20. Christian JJ, Lloyd JA, Davis DD: Role of endocrines in the self-regulation of mammalian populations, in Recent Progress in Hormone Research. Edited by Pincus G. Academic Press, New York, 1965, chap 11
21. Southwick CH, Blund VP: Effect of population density on adrenal glands and reproductive organs of CFW mice. Amer J Physiol 197:111–114, 1959
22. Nagatsu J, Levitt M, Udenfriend S: Tyrosine hydroxylase, the initial step in norepinephrine biosynthesis. J Biol Chem 239:2910–2917, 1964
23. Thoenen H, Mueller RA, Axelrod J: Trans-synaptic induction of adrenal tyrosine hydroxylase. J Pharmacol Exp Ther 169:249, 1969
24. Thoenen H, Mueller RA, Axelrod J: Neuronally dependent induction of adrenal phenylethanolamine N-methyltransferase by hydroxydopamine. Biochem Pharmacol 19:669–673, 1970
25. Mueller RA, Thoenen H, Axelrod J: Inhibition of trans-synaptically increased tyrosine hydroxylase activity by cycloheximide and actinomycin D. Molec Pharmacol 5:463, 1969
25a. Kvetnansky P, Kopin IJ, Weise W: Effect of hypophysectomy on immobilization induced elevation of tyrosine hydroxylase and phenylethanolamine N-methyltransferase in the rat adrenal. Endocrinology 87:1323–1329, 1970
26. Mueller RA, Thoenen H, Axelrod J: Effect of pituitary and ACTH on the maintenance of basal tyrosine hydroxylase activity in the rat adrenal gland. Endocrinology 86:751–755, 1970
27. Smirk FH: High Arterial Pressure. Charles C Thomas, Springfield, IL, 1957, pp 11–15
28. Handlon JH, Wadeson RW, Fishman JR, et al: Psychological factors lowering plasma 17-hydroxycorticosteroid concentrations. Psychosom Med 24:535–542, 1962
29. Noirot E, Pye JD: Sound analysis of the ultrasonic distress calls of mouse pups as a function of their age. Anim Behav 17:340–349, 1969
30. Denenberg VH, Brumaghan JT, Haltmeyer GC, et al: Increased adrenocortical activity in the neonatal rat following handling. Endocrinology 81:1047–1052, 1967
31. Melzack R: The role of early experience in emotional arousal. Ann NY Acad

Sci 159:721–730, 1969
32. Calhoun JB: A behavioral sink, in Roots of Behavior: Genetics Instinct, and Socialization in Animal Behavior. Edited by Bliss EL. Hoeber-Harper, New York, 1962, pp 295–315
33. Newton G, Levine S: Early Experience and Behavior. Charles C Thomas, Springfield, IL, 1968
34. Denenberg VH: Animal studies on developmental determinants of behavioral adaptability, in Experience, Structure and Adaptability. Edited by Harvey DJ. Springer-Verlag, New York, 1966, chap 7, pp 123–147
35. Levine S, Denenberg VH: Early stimulation: effects and mechanisms, in Stimulation in Early Infancy. Edited by Ambrose A. Academic Press, New York, 1969, pp 3–72
36. Ely D: Physiological and Pathological Findings Differentiating "Dominants" and "Subordinates" in Confined Population Systems of CBA Mice. Masters thesis, University of Southern California, 1969

CHAPTER 10

Differences in Perception Between Hypertensive and Normotensive Populations

JOSEPH D. SAPIRA, M.D.,
EILEEN T. SCHEIB, B.A.,
RICHARD MORIARTY, M.D., AND
ALVIN P. SHAPIRO, M.D.

Prefatory Remarks

Joel E. Dimsdale, M.D.

From the earliest days of *Psychosomatic Medicine,* two themes have been repeatedly explored concerning hypertension—hypertensive patients' physiological responses to stressors and their behavioral responses to interpersonal frustration. This classic article by Sapira et al. used a unique stressor to study both of these important themes.

Volume 33, 1971, pp. 239–250.
   From the University of Pittsburgh School of Medicine, Department of Medicine, Psychosomatic and Clinical Pharmacology Sections, Pittsburgh, Pa.
   Supported by Research Grant HE 05711 from the National Heart and Lung Institute.
   The skilled technical assistance of Mrs. Thelma Klaniecki and Mrs. Jean Small is gratefully acknowledged.
   Presented in part at the Annual Meeting of the American Psychosomatic Society, 1970, Washington, DC.
   Received for publication July 3, 1970; revision received Oct. 20, 1970.

Films have long been used as probes for studying psychosomatic processes because they can be so evocative and because they provide a standardized stimulus. This film, however, was something new. Instead of the usual harrowing films of traffic accidents or ritual blood-letting, the authors filmed two vignettes concerning good and bad doctor-patient interactions.

The authors did not find that hypertensive patients had a particularly striking hemodynamic response to the film. However the hypertensive patients seemed oblivious to obvious rudeness on the doctor's part. They seemed, if anything, to focus on any distracting detail OTHER than the rudeness which was the essence of the frustrating film clip.

In this classic article Sapira et al. pose a provocative question: if hypertensives do hyperrespond to stressors, after years of experiencing the unpleasant manifestations of hyperarousal, might they not cope with provocation by trying terribly hard not to perceive it?

A group of hypertensive patients (N = 19) and a control group of normotensive patients (N = 15) were shown two movies depicting two types of doctor-patient interaction. In the first movie, the doctor was rude and disinterested in the patient (the bad doctor). In the second movie, the doctor was relaxed and warm (the good doctor). After viewing the two movies, all patients were interviewed as to their impressions of the two scenes. During the viewing, blood pressure and pulse rate responses in the hypertensive group were small but significantly greater than those in the normotensive group; during the interview, the significantly greater response in the hypertensives was physiologically meaningful. The urinary catecholamine and cortisol excretion rates were no different between the 2 groups. Most striking was the finding that the hypertensive group tended to deny seeing any differences between the doctors depicted in the two movies, while the normotensive group could clearly identify differences in the behavior of the good doctor versus that of the bad doctor.

In a second experiment, the same movies were shown to a hypertensive group and to 3 normotensive groups. The patients were asked to fill out a questionnaire derived from auditing the tape recordings in the first experiment. This questionnaire made it possible to differentiate significantly between the hypertensive and normotensive groups. These data are compatible with the hypothesis that the hypertensive patient may perceptually screen out potentially noxious stimuli as a behavioral response to his hyperreactive pressor system.

Psychophysiologic factors in hypertension have dealt primarily with two aspects of the problem: (a) hyperreactivity of blood pressure to emotional as well as to other types of noxious stimuli has been demonstrated repeatedly; and (b) the personality of the patient with hypertension often has been the subject of investigation; the hypertensive patient has been described as an individual who appears hostile, is unable to express his anger appropriately, and is withdrawn and relates poorly in interaction with others. Some workers have argued that the hypertensive patient internalizes anger with the subsequent activation of physiologic effector mechanisms (e.g., increased norepinephrine secretion, increased neurogenic peripheral vasoconstriction, and/or increased cardiac output) which result in hypertension.[1]

Alternately, however, the apparent hostility of the hypertensive patient might actually represent a psychologic awareness of the body's inherent responsivity manifested as a behavioral pattern whose goal is to permit the individual to avoid situations which may result in noxious stimulation. This behavioral pattern could appear to the observer as withdrawal and hostility.[2] Previous evidence for this hypothesis derives from the work of Weiner, Singer and Reiser,[3,4] who asked hypertensive and normotensive patients to respond to a thematic apperception test card. They found that the hypertensive patients told uninvolved, unemotional stories and had minimal cardiovascular responses, whereas normotensive patients with a variety of other illnesses gave much more elaborate stories and had much more reactivity. Harris et al., using psychodrama, have also obtained data which are compatible with this hypothesis.[5,6]

To substantiate this hypothesis further has been difficult, but the experiment we now wish to describe provides some tentative evidence in its support. It involved recording cardiovascular responses by normotensive and hypertensive subjects during the viewing of a pair of contrasting movies, depicting the interaction between a physician and a patient. In one movie, the physician behaved in a negative and rude fashion to the patient, while in the other, he behaved in a pleasant and warm manner. Originally conceived as a stress situation which might bring out contrasting cardiovascular responses, actually the results were considerably more revealing in terms of the emotional reaction of the subjects, as determined from a poststressor interview.

Methods and Materials

Experiment 1

Nineteen hospitalized patients with mild to moderate essential hypertension, who were not receiving drugs which would interfere with catecholamine or cortisol determinations, and 15 hospitalized, similarly restricted, control patients with a variety of medical problems but *without* hypertension, were individually brought to the laboratory on the day of the test after agreeing to allow us "to record their blood pressure reactions while watching a movie." The 2 groups were well matched with regard to age, sex, race, duration of hospitalization, and familiarity with the experimenter. Four of the hypertensive patients were receiving guanethidine sulfate at the time of the study, and an additional 4 were of the labile type; since the data from these patients were not statistically different from those of the other hypertensive patients, they will not be presented separately.

The protocol is summarized graphically in Figure 10–1. On arrival at the laboratory, each patient voided and the urine was discarded. The patient was

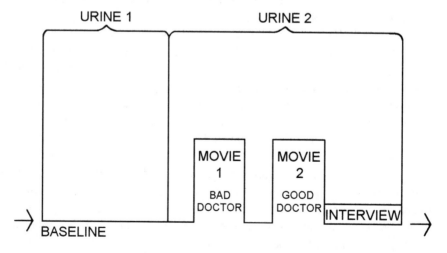

Figure 10–1. Protocol for Experiment 1.

then given two glasses of water to drink, while resting supine for 1 hour. At the end of this hour, a control urine was collected and the patient connected to an automatic blood pressure and pulse rate apparatus as previously described.[7] The investigator then left the room, and the pressures and pulse rates were automatically measured and recorded for 10–15 minutes. By remote control, a *silent* film was then started, consisting of the two movies, each about 5 minutes in duration. The first movie showed a patient visiting a doctor who appeared curt, rude, hurried, disinterested, and annoyed with both the patient and the patient's blood pressure. (This is subsequently referred to as the *bad doctor* movie.) After another rest period, a *good doctor* movie was shown, in which the same patient was seen entering the office of the same doctor. However, in this latter movie, the doctor was relaxed, pleasant, courteous, friendly, and appeared pleased with the patient's blood pressure, and interested in the patient as a person. After the *good doctor* movie was over, the experimenter entered the room with a tape recorder and, for about 5 minutes, interviewed the patient in a quite structured fashion concerning what he or she saw and thought about the two movies. The patient was then disconnected from the recording equipment and the second urine sample was collected.

In this experiment, all patients were interviewed by the same interviewer. In most cases, the interviewer was also the figure playing the role of the *good doctor* and *bad doctor* in the projected movie. However, 5 of the hypertensive patients and 4 of the normotensive patients saw a duplicate film in which a physician, not known to them, played these parts. In both films, the *good doctor* and *bad doctor* movies were approximately equal in the type of camera shots, and the percentage of time spent in various types of doctor-patient interactions—e.g., writing prescriptions, taking blood pressures, talking to the patient, etc.

Pulse rate and blood pressure data were expressed as responses (i.e., the individual's average stimulus value minus that individual's average for the preceding baseline) as previously described.[3] For the blood pressure, the calculated mean arterial blood pressure (diastolic blood pressure plus one-third of the pulse pressure) was used. (Separate analyses of the systolic and diastolic *average* responses and the systolic, diastolic and mean *maximum* responses and the *maximum* pulse rate response failed to yield any additional statistical insights beyond those afforded by the analysis of the average responses of the mean blood pressure and pulse rate; therefore, only the latter will be reported.) Urinary catecholamines and creatinines were determined by previously described methods.[7, 8] Urinary free cortisol was measured by a modification of the method of Mattingly.[9] All urinary catecholamine and free cortisol data were converted to weight per weight of creatinine.

Experiment 2

In Experiment 2, the movies were shown to a group of patients from the outpatient Hypertension Clinic, a group of normotensive arthritic patients attending the Rheumatology Clinic, a group of normotensive patients attending the Dermatology Clinic in the same outpatient facility, and a third normotensive group consisting of laboratory and office personnel who were naive to the psychologic hypothesis being tested. In this experiment, there were no concomitant measurements of blood pressure, pulse rate or urine chemistries, nor were there individual interviews. Instead, questionnaires were administered. For the sake of clarity, the scoring of the questionnaire used for each group will be presented in the Results section.

Statistical analyses were performed by 2×3 analysis of variance or t test for paired values, or, in the case of the questionnaire, by 2×2, 3×2 or 4×2 chi square tests.

Results

Experiment 1

Pulse rate responses are shown in Figure 10–2. Analysis of variance revealed between-group differences for the *good doctor* movie and the interview. For both of these stimuli, the hypertensive patients had a statistically greater pulse rate response than did the normotensive group. Furthermore, there were within-group differences (for both the normotensive and hypertensive) in that the pulse rate responses to the interview were significantly greater than the responses to either of the movies.

The mean arterial blood pressure responses are shown in Figure 10–3. Although the hypertensive group had a significantly greater pressor response than the normotensive group for the *bad doctor* movie, the *good doctor* movie and the interview, physiologically important blood pressure responses were only achieved by the hypertensive group during the interview period. (The magnitude of the interview response is further indicated by the fact that the maximum mean arterial blood pressure response was 20.1 mmHg for the hypertensive group, but only 9.7 mmHg for the normotensive group.) In addition, within-group differences for both the hypertensive and the normotensive groups were noted, in that interview responses were significantly greater than the responses to either of the two movie scenes. Of considerable interest, however, was the absence of a difference in response between the exposure to the

Differences in Perception

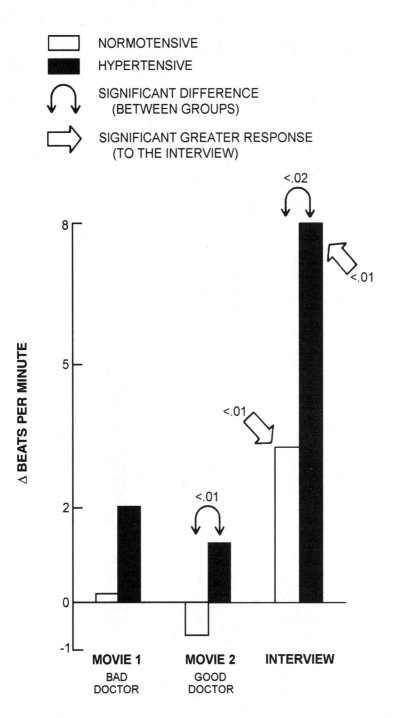

Figure 10–2. Pulse rate responses.

good doctor and the *bad doctor*, particularly in the hypertensive group.

Figure 10–4 shows the urinary catecholamine and steroid responses for the 2 groups. There were no significant differences between the groups for urinary epinephrine, norepinephrine or cortisol. Individual responses are plotted for the

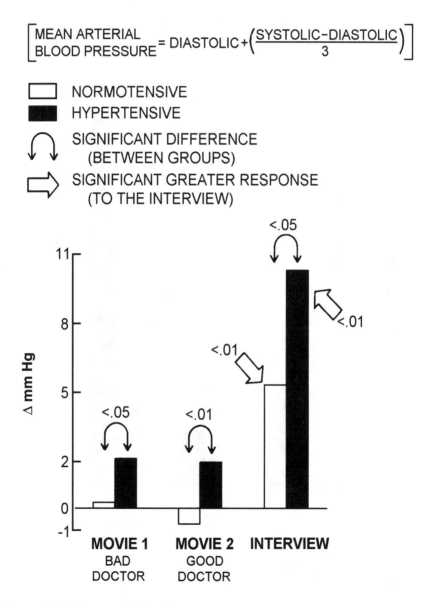

Figure 10–3. Mean arterial blood pressure responses.

Differences in Perception

purpose of indicating the variability of the responses, especially for the cortisol responses.

Figure 10–5 shows the mean arterial blood pressure responses for the hypertensives after this group was split into subpopulations according to whether their interviewer was in the film or not. Those who saw their interviewer in the film had a significantly greater pressor response to the interview, *and only to the interview,* than did the hypertensive patients who saw the neutral physician.

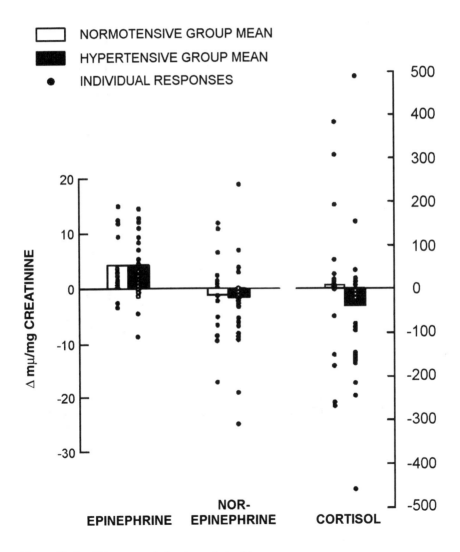

Figure 10–4. Urinary catecholamine and steroid responses.

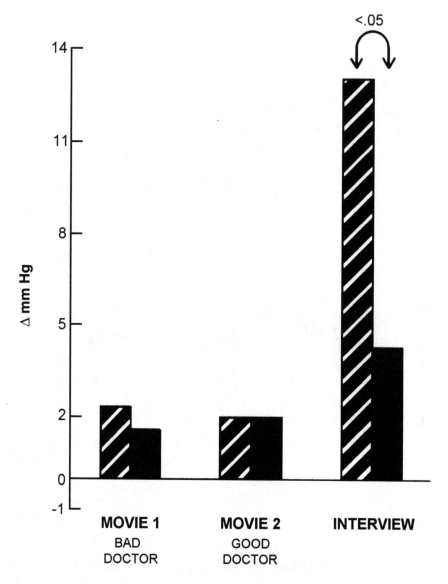

Figure 10-5. Effect of interviewer on mean arterial blood pressure responses of hypertensive group.

Pulse rate responses, urinary catecholamines and urinary free cortisol did not discriminate between the 2 subgroups of hypertensive patients. When the data from the normotensive group were similarly split into the subpopulations, no significant differences between the 2 subgroups were noted for any of the responses.

It had been a working hypothesis of the study that the scenes depicted in the movie strips, particularly the *bad doctor*, would act as pressor stimuli, and accordingly, it was somewhat surprising and disappointing that this was not the case, and that the pressor responses were rather minimal. However, the experimenter who showed the movies and conducted the interviews was impressed by the fact that the hypertensive subjects tended to fail to see obvious doctor-patient interactions in the movies, most particularly represented by a failure to verbalize about the callous behavior of the *bad doctor*. In this respect, the hypertensive subjects appeared to differ from the normotensive patients but obviously, this impression was difficult to quantitate. Accordingly, the tapes were submitted for audit to an observer who was unaware of the diagnoses and who did not know the individual patients. Furthermore, this observer had not been involved in the original planning of the experiment, nor was he in fact attached to the laboratory at the time the data were accumulated, although he was generally familiar with the hypothesis under study.

This "blinded" observer then audited the tape recordings of the interviews from Experiment 1 and from pilot interviews conducted prior to Experiment 1. From his overall impression of each tape, he attempted to assign each interview to a hypertensive or normotensive category. The results of this preliminary experiment are shown in Table 10–1. Of the 15 interviews called hypertensive, in fact, 14 were from hypertensive population; of 13 interviews called normotensive, 11 were from the normotensive population. Although the auditor felt unable to hazard a prediction of group membership for 15 of the interviews ("don't know"), the χ^2 still yielded a P of less than 0.01.

A check list with a scoring system which could be applied to any taped

Table 10–1. Intuition (Series 1)

Category	Population	
	Hospitalized hypertensive	**Hospitalized normotensive**
Hypertensive	14	1
Normotensive	2	11
"Don't-know"	(7)	(8)

$P < 0.01$.

interview then was developed. The check list and scoring system were based on the specific comments—or lack of comments—which each subject made about various specific activities of the doctor and the patient in each interview, and were intended to force the categorization of every taped interview as either normotensive or hypertensive. These taped interviews from the patients in Experiment 1 then were resubmitted to the same observer for scoring. The results are presented in Table 10–2 for 33 interviews. (One tape from the hypertensive group was lost.) A total of 14 taped interviews were called hypertensive, of which all were in fact from the hypertensive population. The 19 taped interviews called normotensive included all 15 normotensive patients and 4 false-negative hypertensive patients. Again $P < 0.01$, by χ^2 analysis.

The following are excerpts from representative transcripts to indicate qualitatively the distinct types of responses.

Normotensive 1

Patient: The first doctor was shaking his finger at the patient and looking in a rather stern manner.

Interviewer: And the second one?

Patient: Well, he had a much more kindly expression in the second movie and seemed more sympathetic . . .

Interviewer: What were some of the things about the doctor's attitude in the first movie in contrast to the second?

Patient: Well, his gestures were such that he seemed to be disapproving. He seemed to be unfriendly towards . . . well, just his general attitude is all I can say . . . the stern manner in which he addressed the patient, frowning and shaking his finger. He was nervously lighting a cigarette and taking short puffs which apparently might indicate that he was annoyed. In the second case he seemed very relaxed in what I could see. He just had a much better attitude toward the patient, that's all.

Table 10–2. Intuition (Series 2)

Category	Population	
	Hospitalized hypertensive	Hospitalized normotensive
Hypertensive	14	0
Normotensive	4	15

$P < 0.01$.

Normotensive 2

Patient: In the first one he seemed nervous or something, frustrated. In the second he would sit back in his chair and relax and talk to his patient.

Interviewer: Why do you think he was like that?

Patient: Well, in the first he picked up the cigarettes . . . he probably was nervous and he didn't seem collected or something. In the second one he seemed more relaxed. He could sit back and feel more relaxed.

Normotensive 3

Interviewer: How would you have felt in those situations?

Patient: With the first doctor like he didn't get a true picture of whether he was sick or not because he had gone to a doctor's office, in the first place it makes him nervous and the first doctor didn't help him relax or be calm to see if you do have high blood pressure. The second one talked to you as if he had all the time in the world to sit there and talk about everything you wanted to talk about. He would let you relax so he would get a true reading. The first one wouldn't have.

Interviewer: How would you have reacted to a doctor like the first one?

Patient: I don't think I would go back to him.

Interviewer: Would you have been annoyed with him?

Patient: Yeah.

Interviewer: And the second doctor, how would you have reacted to him?

Patient: He was a bit OK. I would go back to him. I think he would be the kind that would be interested.

Comment. Perhaps the normotensive group response could be summarized best by that lady who distinguished the first doctor from the second doctor by stating that "the first doctor (bad doctor) acted like one of those smart residents."

On the other hand, the hypertensive patients tended to deny that there were any differences in the behavior of the *good doctor* vis a vis the *bad doctor.* In fact, transcripts of their responses were rather uninteresting because of the paucity of remarks and the frequent pauses in their comments. The following are typical examples of the hypertensive response:

Hypertensive 1

Patient: In both, about the same thing happened. I forced myself to notice some little differences. (pause) Like one of the doctors didn't have a cigarette. (pause) In the second movie. (pause) And the different positions they have the camera in.

Hypertensive 2

Patient: It was telling me to have the blood pressure checked more often. (pause)

Interviewer: Was there any difference between the two scenes?

Patient: In the first he checked both arms, in the second only one arm.

Interviewer: Why do you think that was?

Patient: I don't know.

Interviewer: Were there any other differences?

Patient: No. (pause) The last one gave him a little lecture. (pause)

Interviewer: Was there any other difference between the two doctors?

Patient: One took his glasses off.

Interviewer: Why do you think he did that?

Patient: I don't know.

Hypertensive 3

Comment. The following hypertensive response is unusual in that the patient clearly sees a difference between the first doctor and the second doctor, but is still typical of the hypertensive response in that the patient perceives the *good doctor* as the *bad doctor* and vice versa!

Patient: . . . just noticing the different positions that the camera was in the second time and in the second movie with their hands and talking with their hands, like that. I was trying to think of what the doctor was telling him. (pause) And that's about all.

Interviewer: Was there much difference in the behavior of the doctors, let's say in the first movie and in the second movie?

Patient: In the first movie he kept looking at his watch as though he was trying to rush the patient out and in the second movie he didn't do this but he

Differences in Perception

seemed a bit in a hurry to get him out because he didn't check the blood pressure in both arms and I guess it was a prescription that he gave him and rushed him out.

Interviewer: Well, how did he behave? Did he behave in a different fashion towards the patient in addition to looking at his watch in the first movie as contrasted to the second one?

Patient: My thinking is he seemed a little more nervous and hurried in the second one.

Interviewer: More nervous and hurried in the second one?

Patient: Uh huh.

Interviewer: If you were the patient would it have made any difference to you the way he behaved in one or the other?

Patient: No.

Interviewer: Would you have felt more uncomfortable or any different?

Patient: I think probably in the second movie.

Interviewer: You would have been more uncomfortable in the second movie?

Patient: Yes.

Interviewer: Why?

Patient: Because he didn't keep looking at his watch.

Experiment 2

In an attempt to obtain data more amenable to quantification and because of the difficulties attendant upon editing medical cues out of the tape recordings, a test was developed to permit the movie to be shown to large groups of patients whose responses to a pencil and paper questionnaire could be scored. The questionnaire is shown in Table 10–3. Two things should be noted: (a) every question that is asked about the first doctor is asked about the second doctor; (b) there is no place on the questionnaire for making a response of "don't know" or "can't answer," nor did the accompanying written and oral instructions refer to such a response.

The questionnaire was administered to 24 patients attending the Hypertension Clinic and 25 nonhypertensive patients attending the Dermatology Clinic. *Each* question was then individually analyzed in terms of its discriminant function between the 2 groups. (Intercorrelation matrices and other complicated sta-

Table 10-3. Questionnaire on subject reaction to movies

	YES	NO
1. Were the two scenes the same?	—	—
2. Would you prefer to have the first doctor for your doctor?	—	—
3. Would you prefer to have the second doctor for your doctor?	—	—
4. Did the first doctor listen to the patient?	—	—
5. Did the first doctor talk to the patient?	—	—
6. Did the second doctor listen to the patient?	—	—
7. Did the second doctor talk to the patient?	—	—
8. Was the first doctor interested in the patient?	—	—
9. Was the second doctor interested in the patient?	—	—
10. Should the first doctor have behaved differently?	—	—
11. Should the second doctor have behaved differently?	—	—
12. Was the first doctor worried about the patient's blood pressure?	—	—
13. Was the second doctor worrried about the patient's blood pressure?	—	—
14. Do you think the patient went to the first doctor, even though he was afraid of him?	—	—
15. Do you think the patient went to the second doctor, even though he was afraid of him?	—	—
16. Do you think the patient was becoming angry with the first doctor, but was afraid to let it show?	—	—
17. Do you think the patient was becoming angry with the second doctor, but was afraid to let it show?	—	—
18. Do you know the doctor in the first movie?	—	—
19. Do you know the doctor in the second movie?	—	—

tistical analyses were not evaluated because of the specific intention to develop a simple rating scale.) Oddly enough, the questions had to be scored not for one of two responses, but for one of three responses, since there was a marked tendency on the part of the hypertensive group to *refuse to answer* yes or no. Further, of the 19 questions asked, only four were required to achieve a maximum discrimination between the 2 groups; yet of these four, three questions were specifically concerned with the second doctor (good doctor). The four specific questions and the loading factors are indicated in Table 10–4. A positive number suggests a hypertensive response, and a negative number suggests a normotensive response. Responses of less than a total of 0.10 were designated as normotensive responses.

Using this rating system, we then applied the four questions in a retrospective fashion to the *individual* questionnaires from which the group discriminant loading factors had been obtained. The results are given in Table 10–5. This shows that of the 19 persons called hypertensive by the questionnaire, 16 were in fact hypertensive. Of the 30 patients called normotensive, 22 were normotensive ($P < 0.01$). The same four-item scoring system then was applied *prospectively* to two other nonhypertensive populations as shown in Table 10–6 and of the 29 questionnaires analyzed, only four fitted the hypertensive pattern. A 4×2 chi-square analysis performed on the combined data from the Hypertensive Clinic population and the three nonhypertensive populations yields a

Table 10–4. Four specific questions and loading factors

Loading factors	Yes	No	Refused to answer
1. Were the two scenes the same?	− 0.28	− 0.02	+ 0.36
9. Was the second doctor interested in the patient?	− 0.15	+ 0.25	+ 0.20
11. Should the second doctor have behaved differently?	+ 0.50	− 0.17	+ 0.06
13. Was the second doctor worried about the patient's blood pressure?	− 0.18	− 0.03	+ 0.33

Table 10–5. Four-item questionnaire applied retrospectively

	Population	
Category	Hypertensive clinic	Nonhypertensive dermatology clinic
Hypertensive	16	3
Normotensive	8	22

$P < 0.01$.

Table 10–6. Four-item questionnaire applied prospectively

	Population	
Category	Nonhypertensive-rheumatoid arthritis clinic	Nonhypertensive-section personnel
Hypertensive	4	0
Normotensive	15	10

P is not significant.

P less than 0.01. In passing, it may be noted that the percentage accuracy, when using the questionnaires, never really exceeded that obtained by the initial guessing by the "blind" observer, although the time saving in auditing tapes was considerable.

Discussion

Since this experiment was originally planned as a study of cardiovascular responsiveness to the stress of watching contrasting doctor-patient interactions, the data are subject to a number of criticisms regarding their support of the hypothesis that the hypertensive patient tends to avoid noxious situations. However, several observations seem noteworthy and deserve comment.

First, the hypertensive group had small, but significantly greater, pressor responses to both a movie and to an interview than the normotensive group. Although this might at first seem to be nothing more than the hypertensive patient's well known hyperresponsivity to any type of pressor stimuli,[10] it should be noted that these responses were small, except during the interviews. Perhaps indeed the hypertensive population was attempting to decrease its time at risk for unknown noxious stimuli by reducing the intake of all potentially noxious pressor stimuli, but could not accomplish this when forced to verbalize their observations.

Secondly, it is intriguing to find that the interviewer evoked a greater pressor response from those hypertensive patients who had seen him acting in the role of the *good doctor* and *bad doctor* in the movies (as opposed to those hypertensive patients who saw a neutral physician play the two roles). Although this finding suggests that at some level the hypertensive population did perceive the *bad doctor* as *bad,* it must be emphasized that what is being described as perception is actually an unanalyzed combination of perception, cognition and verbal reporting in a highly structured situation. Nevertheless, the fact remains that this increased pressor response was highly specific in that it was evoked by the interviewer, only in the hypertensive population, only for the interview, and particularly for those patients who had previously seen the movie scenes with the interviewer acting the role of the physician. It is of further interest that this pressor response could distinguish subgroups which were not discriminated by pulse response.

Thirdly, the pressure responses noted do not appear to be related directly to the usual biochemical reactions to a stressor. This statement is made on the basis of the failure of adrenal cortical or medullary hormonal responses to distinguish any of the groups in circumstances where they were clearly distinguished by their cardiovascular reactions. This is in keeping with our previous findings of a lack of relationship between pressor responses and their adrenergic correlates, and the tendency of the pressor response per se to relate to the preexisting state of cardiovascular reactivity, of genetic, and perhaps acquired, origin.[7, 8, 10]

Finally, it appears that the hypertensive group did not report certain observable differences in qualitatively distinct types of doctor-patient relationships. In fact, distortion appeared, as in a few instances where the patient confused the two doctor roles and interpreted the *good doctor* as the *bad* one, or more often, when he considered the second doctor as one "no better than" the first. It was of interest that the questionnaires in the hypertensives could be scored primarily on answers to the questions about the second (*good*) doctor, as if, having denied the existence of a difference, they could not then "admit to their conscious awareness" the concept that there was a *good* doctor, because then there would have to have been a *bad* one—hence, the large number of questionnaires with the only possible alternative, namely, refusal to answer the question.

As indicated, these results may be due to a defect in perception which enables the hypertensive to screen out potentially noxious stimuli as a defense against his cardiovascular hyperreactivity. Within the framework of the present experiment, it is not possible to further clarify this suggestion. Moreover, additional data obviously are needed to confirm these findings, including evaluation of a possible nonspecific reluctance of patients to comment unfavorably about their doctors, study of the reactions of hypertensive subjects to other types of intrapersonal relationships, and the elucidation of the complex components of the perception-cognition-reporting triad which the response to the movies entails. Nevertheless, this technic offers a new approach to a heretofore difficult area to study, and suggests a means to further evaluate and quantitate personality and behavior patterns in certain disease states.

References

1. Shapiro AP: Psychophysiologic mechanisms in hypertensive vascular disease. Ann Intern Med 53:715, 1960
2. Shapiro AP: Psychophysiologic pressor mechanisms and their role in therapy. Modern Treatment. Vol 3. Hoeber Medical Division, Harper and Row, Publishers, New York, 1966, p 108
3. Thaler M, Weiner H, Reiser MF: Exploration of the doctor-patient relationship through projective techniques. Psychosom Med 19:228, 1957

4. Weiner H, Singer MT, Reiser MF: Cardiovascular responses and their psychophysiologic correlates: a study in healthy young adults and patients with peptic ulcer and hypertension. Psychosom Med 24:477, 1962
5. Harris RE, Sokolow M, Carpenter LG, et al: Response to psychological stress in patients who are potentially hypertensive. Circulation 7:874, 1953
6. Kalis B, Harris RE, Sokolow M, et al: Response to psychologic stress in patients with essential hypertension. Amer Heart J 53:572, 1957
7. Sapira JD, Shapiro AP: Studies in man on the relationship of adrenergic correlates to pressor responsivity. Circulation 35:226, 1966
8. Shapiro AP, Nicotero J, Sapira J, et al: Analysis of the variability of blood pressure pulse rate, and catecholamine responsivity in identical and fraternal twins. Psychosom Med 30:506, 1968
9. Mattingly D: A simple fluorimetric method for the estimation of free 11-hydroxycorticoids in human plasma. J Clin Path 15:374, 1962
10. Shapiro AP: An experimental study of comparative responses of blood pressure to different noxious stimuli. J Chron Dis 13:293, 1961

CHAPTER 11

Operant Conditioning of Heart Rate in Patients With Premature Ventricular Contractions

THEODORE WEISS, M.D., AND
BERNARD T. ENGEL, PH.D.

Prefatory Remarks

David Shapiro, Ph.D.

Time is the true test of a classic article in science, and this one passes with the highest marks for clarity of objectives, innovative methods, significant findings, and even-handed conclusions. The study showed that cardiac ventricular function can be brought under operant control in patients with premature ventricular contractions. The beauty of the article is in its details and its many insightful observations. The research was prompted by work in the 1960s showing that human visceral responses can be treated like behaviors and brought

---

Volume 33, 1971, pp. 301–321.
From the Section of Physiological Psychology, Laboratory of Behavioral Sciences, Gerontology Research Center, National Institute of Child Health and Human Development and Baltimore City Hospitals.
The authors would like to thank Drs. Gustav C. Voigt and Kenneth M. Lewis for permitting them to draw patients from the Clinic, and for regular consultation on the patients; Drs. Lewis A. Kolodny and Jay J. Platt for referring Patients 6 and 7, respectively; Mr. Reginald E. Quilter for assisting in the development and maintenance of various instruments used in this study; and Mr. Richard H. Mathias for assisting in the analysis of the ward telemetry data.
Received for publication Aug. 6, 1970; revision received Nov. 23, 1970.

under control by operant conditioning. The study was one of the first attempts to apply these methods to the control of pathological symptoms. Eight patients were studied; each case is described in superb detail. The conditioning procedures were unique, particularly those used to bring variations in an individual's heart rate within present levels ("range contingency"), as was the use of autonomic nervous system drugs to investigate mechanisms behind the changes achieved in heart rate and heart rhythm. The clinical evaluations of the results were comprehensive, including electrocardiographic monitoring of patients in other circumstances, physical examinations, and long-term follow-up. Each case study points out what worked and what did not in the framework of the patient's characteristics and biological and behavioral constraints. The article is a model of applied psychosomatic research.

Operant conditioning of heart rate (HR) was carried out in 8 patients with premature ventricular contractions (PVCs). All of the patients showed some degree of HR control. Five of these patients showed a decrease in PVCs in association with the learning of HR control. Four patients have shown persistence of a low PVC frequency after study, the longest followup being 21 months. Pharmacologic studies suggested that decreased PVC frequency was mediated by diminished sympathetic tone in 1 patient and increased vagal tone in another.

These findings suggest that some aspects of cardiac ventricular function can be brought under voluntary control. Once such control has been acquired, it can mediate clinically significant changes in cardiac function.

For many years, and in a multiplicity of experimental situations, the technics of operant conditioning have been employed to modify and control somatic behavior—i.e., actions involving the use of skeletal muscle.[1] In the last decade, a large volume of additional research has accumulated, indicating that visceral and other involuntary responses also are amenable to operant control.[2,3] Response systems studied have included heart rate,[4-7] blood pressure,[8,9] rate of urine formation,[10] regional blood flow,[11] vasoconstriction,[12] and galvanic skin potential.[13–15]

In addition to reports of operant conditioning of visceral responses in normal man and in animals, there are three studies in which patients with pathologic visceral responses showed improvement after operant training. Engel and Melmon[16] conditioned more regular cardiac rhythms in patients with several kinds of cardiac arrhythmias, and White and Taylor[17] and Lang[18] each conditioned patients to stop or decrease ruminative vomiting.

Several studies have shown the effects of neural impulses on premature ventricular contractions (PVCs).[19] Hypothalamic lesions and stimulation,[20–22] afferent vagal stimulation,[20, 23] efferent cardiac sympathetic nerve impulses,[20, 24] and cardiac sympathectomy[25] all have been shown to produce dramatic changes in PVC frequency. Also, both increases and decreases in PVC frequency have been reported using classic conditioning technics.[26, 27]

Because of these considerations, we undertook a study of patients with PVCs to see if operant conditioning could produce clinically significant control of this arrhythmia.

Materials and Methods

Patients

Selection. Eight patients with PVCs were obtained from Baltimore City Hospitals, and from referrals by private physicians.

Hospitalization procedure. Patients were hospitalized for the duration of the study and given passes each weekend. After admission, they were given a complete physical examination and a standard battery of laboratory tests including a 12 lead EKG and PA and lateral chest X-rays.

Experimental Design

Laboratory. All formal cardiac training took place in the laboratory although each patient was encouraged to practice his technics outside the laboratory as well.

While in the laboratory, the patient lay in a hospital bed in a sound-deadened room. At the foot of the bed was a vertical display of three differently colored light bulbs, an intercom and a meter.

The three lights provided the patient with feedback information about his cardiac function. The top light (green) and the bottom light (red) were cue lights.

The middle light (yellow) was the reinforcer; it was on when the patient was producing the correct heart rate (HR) response. Our system enabled us to feed back this information to the patient on a beat-to-beat basis.

When the fast (green) cue light was on, a relative increase in HR would turn on the reinforcer light. When the slow (red) cue light was on, a relative decrease in HR would turn on the reinforcer light.

The meter accumulated time. Whenever the patient was performing correctly, the meter arm moved, and when he performed incorrectly, it stopped.

One to three 80-minute conditioning sessions were carried out daily. A typical session began with about 10 minutes for the attaching of EKG leads, and of a strain gauge around the lower chest to monitor breathing. Then, the patient lay quietly for 20 minutes more. During the last 10 minutes of this period, a baseline HR was obtained. The feedback lights were off throughout the baseline period. Two to three minutes were allowed for setting the trigger level for heart rate (HR) conditioning. The trigger level was the HR (e.g., in a speeding session) at or above which the reinforcer light would go on. Then the patient had either one 34-minute period during which the feedback lights were on, or two such periods of 17 minutes each, separated by a 10-minute rest period.

Because this was primarily a clinical study, the patient's responses at any stage of the study always dictated the procedure. In general, however, we followed a standard sequence for conditioning. During the initial or control session, the patient simply lay in bed in the laboratory for the prescribed time period. The feedback lights were never turned on. Next, HR speeding was taught for about 10 sessions, followed by HR slowing for about 10 sessions. For about 10 further sessions, a differential contingency was taught, in which the patient alternately had to increase and decrease his HR during periods of 1–4 minutes throughout the session. During these sessions, the green and red cue lights would come on alternately so that the patient would know whether to speed or to slow.

The last training contingency usually was a range situation in which the patient had to maintain his HR between preset upper and lower limits. Only the yellow light would be on when the HR was within this range. When the rate was too fast, the yellow light would go off and the red light would go on, cueing the patient to slow down. When the rate was too slow, the green light would come on, cueing the patient to speed up. Because a premature beat caused the HR to go above range, and the compensatory pause caused the HR to go below range, this contingency also gave the patient prompt feedback every time he had a PVC.

In the range contingency, feedback was phased out gradually. Initially, the feedback was available for 1 minute and unavailable for the next. In later sessions, it was available for 1 minute and unavailable for 3; in the final sessions, it was on for 1 minute and off for 7. By this procedure, the patient was weaned from the light feedback and made to become aware of his PVCs through his own sensations.

Each patient was told in detail about the nature of the experiment, and he was allowed to inspect all his data throughout the study.

Ward. The patient's EKG was monitored three nights per week for 10 minutes out of every hour, using a telemetry apparatus.

Pharmacologic studies. In 3 patients, studies were carried out with the use of some or all of the following autonomically active drugs—isoproterenol, propranolol, atropine, edrophonium, phenylephrine and phentolamine—administered intraveneously. This was done in the laboratory after conditioning had been completed in order to elucidate the mechanism underlying HR and rhythm changes.

Followup. Clinical follow-up was done in the Baltimore City Hospitals Cardiac Clinic by Dr. Weiss, and by the referring physicians. The visits usually included an EKG with a 1–2 minute rhythm strip.

Apparatus

Laboratory. Variations in interbeat intervals were detected by a Beckman-Offner cardiotachometer and converted into electrical signals whose magnitudes were proportional to HR. The cardiotachometer output was also fed into a BRS Electronics Schmitt trigger, which was used to control the patient's feedback. The input to the Schmitt trigger was regulated by a zero suppression circuit on the amplifier to permit adjustment of the trigger point. In order to reduce the hysteresis in the Schmitt triggers, we grounded the emitters. An EKG from a precordial lead was recorded on a Beckman-Offner dynograph, and on magnetic tape using an Ampex SP 300 tape recorder.

Ward. The EKG signal from two chest electrodes was transmitted to a Parks model 220-1 converter and a telemetry receiver in an adjacent room, where the EKG was recorded on a tape recorder for subsequent analysis.

Analytic Procedures

Laboratory. All heart beats were counted automatically, and mean HRs were calculated from these data. PVCs were counted manually, all being counted when they were less frequent (under 10/min); and two to four 1-minute samples per 10 minutes being counted when they were more frequent.

Ward. Mean HR was determined by counting five to six 10-beat samples or five 30-second samples distributed across each 10-minute epoch. All PVCs were counted.

Pharmacologic studies. Heart rate was counted either automatically or manually from a continuous EKG record. All PVCs were counted manually from the same record.

Clinical history and followup. Heart rate and PVC frequency generally were determined from EKGs. Some data were derived from physical examinations.

Results

The results will be presented on a patient-by-patient basis. However, since the findings do suggest some general principles, these will be presented as well. Each of the tables summarizes some of the major findings for each patient; however, specific references to these data will be made in the individual patient presentations.

Patient 1

LR, a 52-year-old Caucasian female, had a history of five myocardial infarctions (MI) in the 13 years prior to study. In association with the last two, 8 months and 5 months prior to study, she had PVCs. Maintenance quinidine therapy was required to suppress them after the last MI. She had been on digoxin for 1 year. Because of persistent diarrhea, the quinidine was discontinued 2 weeks prior to study, and PVCs increased in frequency from about one to two per minute to ten per minute.

Laboratory. Table 11–1 reports the proportion of sessions during which this patient performed successfully as measured by changes in heart rate or (during the range sessions) by percentage of time heart rate was within the correct range. Figure 11–1 shows the absolute heart rates and the frequencies of occurrence of PVCs during the training periods of each session.

During speeding training, the patient was able consistently to increase her HR from baseline in the afternoons but not in the mornings (when she also had few PVCs). In association with these successful performances, her PVCs increased to over 23/min. (Figure 11–2). The patient said that she thought about relaxing to speed her heart. During the slowing sessions, the patient was able consistently to decrease her HR from baseline, and PVCs were consistently less

Table 11-1. Ratios of sessions during which each patient performed successfully to total number of sessions for each contingency

					Range				
				1:1		1:3		1:7	
Patient	Speed	Slow	Differential	CRF	On	Off	On	Off	On	Off
1 (Study 1)	4/9	4/6	7/9	5/6	—	—	—	—	—	—
1 (Study 2)	—	—	—	8/10	3/5	4/5	2/4	3/4	2/4	2/4
2	11/14	5/7	9/9	10/10	2/2	2/2	2/2	2/2	3/3	3/3
3	5/11	9/10	8/10	2/3*	4/4*	4/4*	3/4*	3/4*	5/5*	5/5*
4	6/10	5/10	10/10	5/5	11/11	11/11	7/7	7/7	—	—
5	1/10	9/9	12/14	15/15	—	—	—	—	—	—
6	1/6	5/11	—	13/16	—	—	—	—	—	—
7	2/8	7/10	—	2/4	—	—	—	—	—	—
8	—	16/18	—	15/15	—	—	—	—	—	—

During the range sessions, successful performance was defined as maintenance of HR within the correct range for more than 50% of the time.
*Slow.

frequent—1–4/min (Figure 11-2). She said that she concentrated on breathing maneuvers.

The patient differentiated consistently although she did not increase her HR with respect to her baseline rate during the speeding phases of the sessions. PVC incidence was quite low, under 1/min. At this time, the patient reported that her heart was functioning in a dysrhythmic fashion, when actually it was beating quite regularly. Her cardiograms were shown to her, and the differences between her rhythm strips during the speeding sessions and the present sessions were explained to her in detail. After her misconceptions had been clarified, she subsequently learned to recognize correctly the presence of PVCs.

During the range sessions, the patient consistently maintained her HR within the predetermined, 10-beat range (usually 60–70 beats/min) and PVCs were very infrequent, generally about 0.2/min.

After a 3-week recess, the patient's digoxin was stopped. The only discernible effect was an increase in baseline HR of about 5 beats/min to about 68. Twenty-three further range sessions were carried out. Gradually, the patient's feedback was decreased until it was present only 1 minute out of 8 by the last four sessions. PVCs remained very rare, about 0.1/min. She was discharged off all medications.

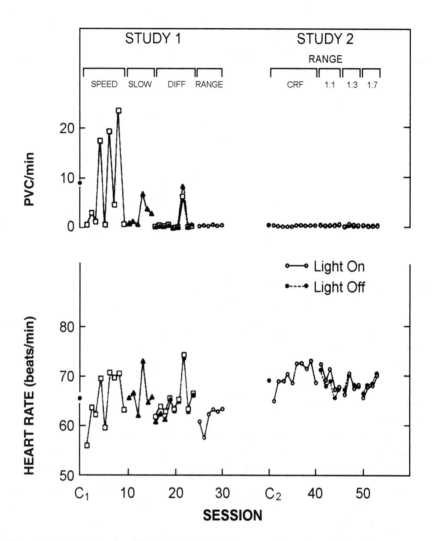

Figure 11–1. Patient 1. PVC and HR levels during training; C1 and C2 are initial sessions during Studies 1 and 2, respectively, when no feedback was provided. Diff, differential conditioning; CRF, continuous feedback; 1:1 feedback on 1 minute, off 1 minute; 1:3 feedback on 1 minute, off 3 minutes, etc; □, speeding; ▲, slowing; ○, range.

Ward. Cardiac activity on the ward (Tables 11–2 and 11–3) paralleled events in the laboratory—ie, her PVC incidence was highest during the period when she was speeding, and lower during the period when she was slowing.

Pharmacologic studies. After the study, we tested the patient with pharmacologic agents. Atropine (1.0 mg) speeded her HR to 98 but did not produce PVCs.

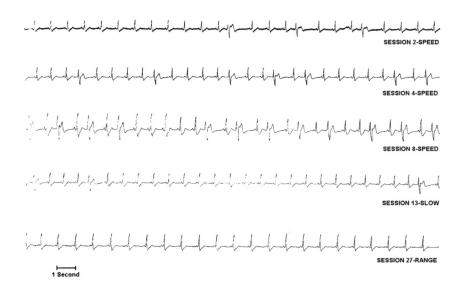

Figure 11–2. Patient 1. EKG rhythm strips during conditioning. These tracings show increase in PVCs during speeding conditioning, and decrease in PVCs during slowing and range conditioning.

Isoproterenol (0.5–1.5 µg/min) speeded her heart rate and produced PVCs when the HR was above 90. The PVC configuration was the same as those she had spontaneously and during conditioning to speed her heart rate. This suggests that decreased sympathetic tone accounts for her diminished PVC incidence.

Followup. Twenty-one months of follow-up data have been obtained. PVCs remained quite low for 4 months, none being seen on five EKGs. Subsequently, they became more variable—commonly about 1/min., but as high as 6/min. The patient continues to be able accurately to identify PVCs. She says she rarely has significant numbers of them at home. When she does, she sits down and rests, and they stop within 20 minutes and do not return.

Patient 2

IW was a 62-year-old Caucasian male with a history of one MI 7 years prior to study. Thereafter, he had intermittent angina on exertion. PVCs were noted first in 1965; they were present on four of six EKGs taken thereafter, at times in a bigeminal rhythm. The average frequency was 14/min on EKG, and 3–5/min clinically. Two months prior to study, his angina worsened. An exercise tolerance test, performed to clarify the relationship between his angina and his PVCs

Table 11–2. Premature ventricular contraction frequencies (PVCs/min) on ward during different phases of study

Patient	Speeding	Slowing	Differential	Range or PVC avoidance
1	10.7	7.6	2.0	0.8
2	1.4	2.3	1.1	0.5
3	34.4	30.0	12.4	—
4	6.6	5.7	5.0	2.1
5	10.2	6.6	4.9	3.8
6	3.1	7.1	—	6.5
7	16.6	4.7	—	9.4
8	—	15.2	—	10.2

Table 11–3. Heart rates (beats/min) on ward during different phases of study

Patient	Speed	Slow	Differential	Range or PVC avoidance
1	66.9	67.5	66.8	67.0
2	51.7	50.9	50.7	50.4
3	82.9	83.4	69.7	—
4	61.0	57.1	56.0	53.2
5	77.3	75.0	71.5	74.0
6	62.5	79.2	—	66.8
7	74.4	76.1	—	72.7
8	—	83.4	—	88.7

produced bigeminy and multifocal PVCs in association with a heart rate of 95–100 beats/min. Modest exercise, raising HR from the usual level of about 55–80 beats/min, was associated with a temporary cessation of PVCs. When the HR slowed below 60, the PVCs returned. A subsequent therapeutic trial on diphenylhydantoin produced no significant change in the PVC frequency or in the patient's angina.

Laboratory. The patient performed successfully in all phases of the study as measured by changes in heart rate (Table 11–1). Figure 11–3 reports his absolute heart rates and PVC incidences during each training session.

In order to speed his heart, the patient said that he thought about "pushing or forcing" his heart to the left, and about its beating rapidly. In several of the

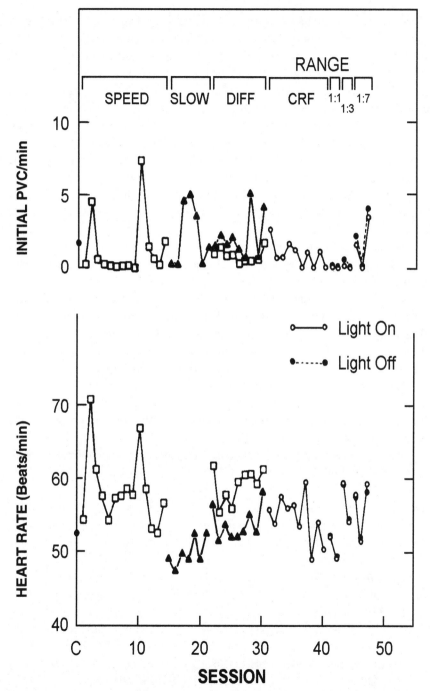

Figure 11–3. Patient 2. PVC and HR levels during training.

speeding sessions, he had long periods of bigeminal rhythm, the PVCs having two configurations. One configuration was like that of the patient's usual PVCs, with the major vector in the same direction as that of the regular QRS. It will be referred to as the *usual type PVC*. The other configuration was seen in the laboratory only in association with HR speeding. Its major vector was in the opposite direction from that of the normal QRS. It will be referred to as the *speeding type PVC*. Apart from the bigeminy, the patient's PVCs were infrequent during speeding, usually less than 1/min. The patient also had several prolonged episodes of bigeminy on the ward recordings of the night after speeding session 11, and on the following night. Both times, these occurred during waking hours when he said he would practice HR control. Many of the bigeminal PVCs on telemetry were of the speeding type. This type of PVC had not been seen on telemetry prior to then.

PVCs were more frequent during slowing, usually 1.5–5/min. They were of the usual type. No bigeminy was seen. He said that he concentrated on the "heart slowing down and stopping."

During the differentiation sessions, PVCs occurred more and more frequently in the slowing periods and less frequently in the speeding periods (Figure 11–4). The PVCs were of the usual type. The patient said that he used the same technics for HR speeding and slowing described above. At comparable heart rates, PVCs were most frequent during HR slowing, least frequent during HR speeding and of intermediate frequency during the baseline periods. These findings suggest that the active processes involved in slowing and speeding the heart were more important in modulating PVC frequency than was the heart rate per se.

During range conditioning sessions, PVCs generally were infrequent, usually less than 1/min.

Ward. Telemetry data showed little variation in HR (Table 11–3). Apart from periods of bigeminy during the waking hours, PVCs were infrequent (Table 11–2). As in the laboratory, they were most frequent during the slowing contingency.

Pharmacologic studies. Studies with autonomically active drugs were done in this patient. Isoproterenol (0.5–1.0 µg/min) led to a HR increase from the resting level of 52 beats/min to 93 beats/min, and to bigeminy and ventricular tachycardia. The PVCs were of the speeding type. The ventricular tachycardia stopped after the isoproterenol infusion was stopped. No anti-arrhythmic agents were required. Atropine (1.0 mg) also speeded the HR to 86 beats/min and increased PVC frequency from 0 to 8/min. These PVCs were of the usual type. Both edrophonium (1–10 mg) and propranolol (0.5 mg every 3 minutes for six times) separately slowed the heart

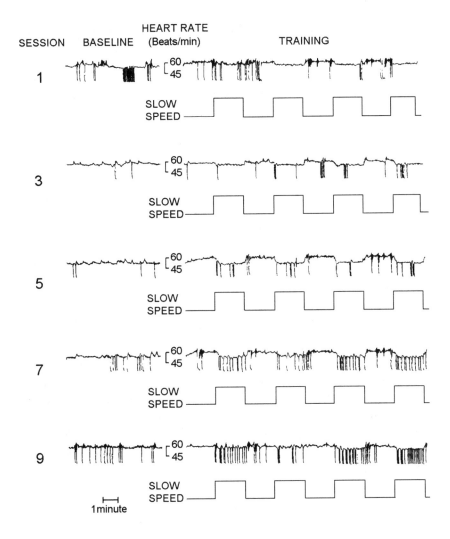

Figure 11–4. Patient 2. Differential HR conditioning. Tracings are cardiotachometer records. PVCs are shown by long vertical lines. As differentiation proceeds, patient speeds and slows appropriately, and PVCs are progressively more concentrated in slowing periods.

to about 48 beats/min, but neither affected the frequency of PVCs. They generally remained below the baseline frequency of 2.5/min. When isoproterenol was readministered (same dosages) after propranolol administration, PVCs increased in frequency to about 10/min although HR did not increase. Their configuration was of the usual type. These results suggest that PVCs of the speeding type were related to increased sympathetic tone. They do not clarify the mechanism underlying the usual type of PVCs.

Followup. The patient has been followed for 10 months since the study. Initially, he continued to have very rare PVCs, averaging 0.4/min on three EKGs. When they were more frequent at home, he said he could decrease them by concentrating on a steady heart beat. His angina continued to worsen, and 4 months after discharge, he had another MI. After recovery from this, the patient's PVCs were somewhat more frequent, averaging 2.2/min in the clinic and, according to him, more at home. He said that it took 15–20 minutes to stop them with HR speeding at home. We therefore readmitted him 9 months after the first study. At that time, PVCs were rare, less than 1/min in the laboratory and on the ward. Because they originated consistently from two foci, quinidine was added to the patient's regimen. This reduced them even further, to one every 4–5 minutes.

Patient 3

MK was an obese 36-year-old Caucasian female with an 8-year history of documented PVCs. They were present on four of six EKGs taken during the 8 years prior to study. The average frequency was 12.8/min. During the last several months before the study, she had had three to four syncopal episodes. An EKG taken by her private physician shortly after one of these revealed unifocal PVCs at a frequency of 21/min. The syncopal episodes had occurred when she was angry or excited. She also reported "a big thumping feeling" in her chest in association with strong emotions and moderate physical exertion such as walking half a mile. To stop this, she said that she sat down and relaxed for half an hour or more.

Laboratory. The patient did not speed consistently from baseline (Table 11–1); however, she did perform successfully in all other phases of the study. During the speeding sessions, PVC frequency was high—up to 40/min (Figure 11–5)—and at times, coupling of PVCs occurred (Figure 11–6). The patient said that she thought about arguments with her children and about running through a dark street during the speeding sessions.

During the slowing sessions, PVC frequency fell to about 20/min (Figure 11–5). The patient said she thought about swinging back and forth in a swing during these sessions.

The patient differentiated well although she speeded from baseline during the speeding blocks in only one session. She slowed during the slowing blocks in all ten sessions. PVCs became much less frequent, usually under 10/min, and at times there were none for periods ranging up to 8 minutes. She said that

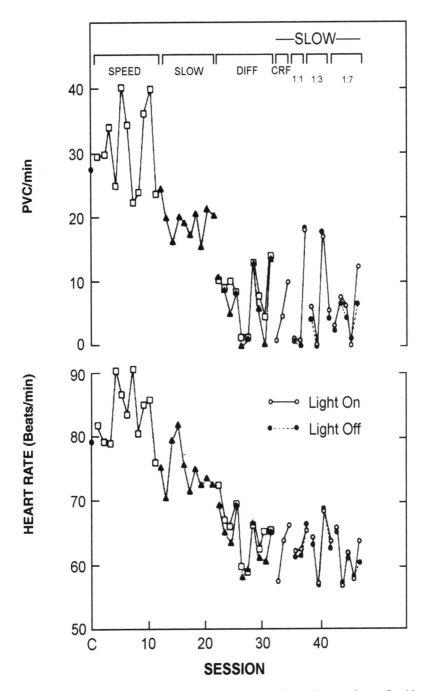

Figure 11–5. Patient 3. PVC and HR levels during training. Slow$_1$ refers to first block of slowing sessions; Slow$_2$ to second block.

she concentrated on the same things described above during the conditioning periods.

Because PVCs were least frequent at the lower HRs, slowing of the HR under 65 beats/min rather than range control was taught next. The patient's HR was under 65 beats/min during twelve of the sixteen sessions. She said that she thought about swinging on a see-saw and about relaxing during these sessions. PVC frequency was usually under 10/min; it was at zero for periods as long as 17 minutes (Figure 11–6).

The patient frequently decreased her PVCs when the training portion of the session began and the feedback lights were turned on (Figure 11–7). Also, the PVCs often returned promptly when the training portion of the session ended and the lights were turned off (Figure 11–7). During the training session in which the light was off part of the time, PVC frequency was as low or lower when the light was off as when it was on (Figure 11–5).

Ward. Cardiac activity on the ward generally paralleled events in the laboratory. Heart rate (Table 11–3) was highest during speeding and slowing, intermediate during the second slowing block (not shown in Tables 11–2 or 11–3), and lowest during the differential conditioning sessions. The PVC pattern was the same as that for HR (Table 11–2). Their lowest average frequency was about 12/min during the differential contingency. At the end of the study, they averaged about 19/min.

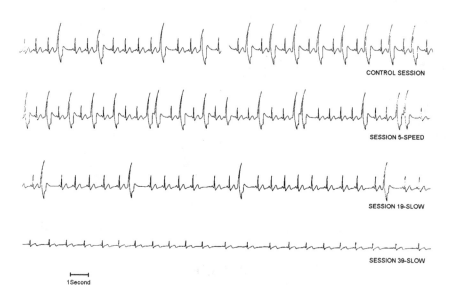

Figure 11–6. Patient 3. EKG rhythm strips during conditioning.

Operant Conditioning of Heart Rate   207

Pharmacologic studies.   Both edrophonium (1–10 mg) and propranolol (0.5 mg every 3 minutes for eight times) separately slowed the heart from about 80 to about 73 beats/min. Neither had any effect on PVC frequency which remained at about 20/min. When administered together (edrophonium, 10 mg at the end of the above administration of propranolol), they slowed the heart from 75 to 60 beats/min and abolished PVCs from a prior level of 20/min. Phenylephrine (7–28 µg/min) in-

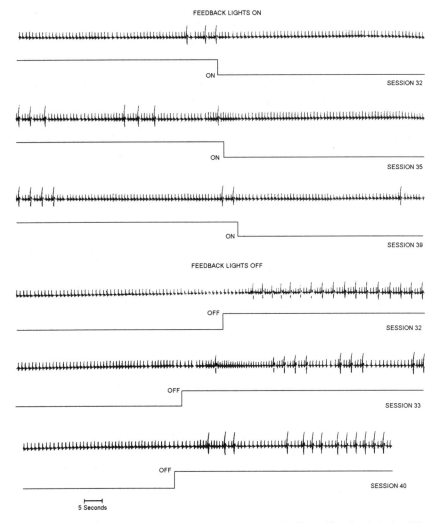

Figure 11–7.   Patient 3.   EKG rhythm strips at onset and offset of feedback during HR slowing. These tracings show that patient was able to stop having PVCs when feedback began, and PVCs returned at end of sessions.

creased the blood pressure from 104/70 to 138/76, slowed the HR from 77 to 54 beats/min, and abolished PVCs from a prior level of 12/min. Isoproterenol (0.5–1.0 µg/min) speeded the HR from 78 to 95 beats/min and stopped PVCs, the prior level being 25/min. Atropine (1.5 mg) speeded the HR from 75 to 97 beats/min and PVCs increased from 19/min to a bigeminal rhythm with 48/min. Phentolamine (5 mg), given at a time when PVC frequency was low (1/min), had no obvious effect on PVCs. It decreased the blood pressure from 108/68 to 90/62, and increased the HR from 75 to 82 beats/min.

These findings suggest that in this patient strong vagal tone inhibits PVCs, regardless of sympathetic input. Weaker vagal tone associated with β-sympathetic inhibition also inhibits PVCs. Vagal blockade leads to frequent PVCs.

Followup. The patient has been followed for 3 months since the study. PVCs have continued to be frequent on EKGs during clinic visits, averaging 17.1/min on three EKGs. However, the patient says that she is able to stop them at home using the HR slowing technic learned in the laboratory. She has not been able to do so in the clinic. She has had no dizziness or syncope since the study.

Patient 4

RL was a 68-year-old Caucasian male with a history of an MI 4 months prior to study. Three months prior to study and after discharge from the hospital, the patient began to have PVCs. These were typically bigeminal or trigeminal, with a frequency of over 20/min, and were unifocal. The PVC occurred well after the preceding T wave, and after exercise, it occurred even later. Also, the PVCs did not increase with exercise; and the patient was unaware of their occurrence. For these reasons, no medications were given to control them.

Laboratory. The patient did not perform reliably during the slowing and speeding training sessions (Figure 11–8 and Table 11–1), and his PVC frequency was highly variable throughout these sessions. He did differentiate consistently, however. Furthermore, he speeded from baseline during the speeding blocks in six of the sessions, and slowed from baseline in seven of them. He said that he moved his shoulders to increase his HR, and lay still and stared at the light to slow his HR. PVC frequency was variable, but was under 10/min in seven of the ten sessions. The PVCs were more frequent in the speeding blocks in seven of the ten sessions.

During the range sessions, the patient said that he generally just watched the light to keep PVCs infrequent. He said that sometimes he also moved his shoulders. PVC frequency was low, under 8/min throughout. During the first five sessions of the range contingency, when the feedback was on during the entire training period, the patient had 2.1 PVCs/min or less (Figure 11–8). As the feed-

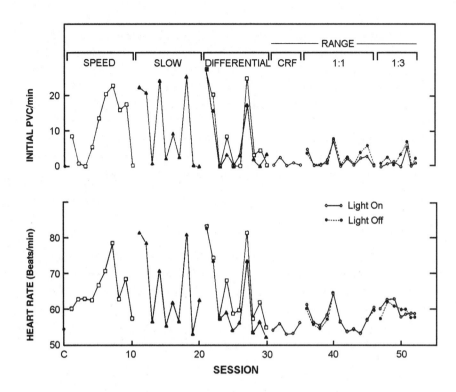

Figure 11-8. Patient 4. PVC and HR levels during training.

back was phased out, PVCs became somewhat more frequent. It is of note that the patient could not tell when he was having PVCs except when the feedback lights were on or when he took his pulse.

Ward. Ward data paralleled the laboratory data. Heart rates (Table 11-3) were highest during speeding and slowing and lowest during the range training. Similarly, PVCs (Table 11-2) were most frequent during speeding and slowing and least frequent during the range contingency.

Pharmacologic studies. No drug studies were performed on this patient.

Followup. Because PVCs were noted to come from two foci (Figure 11-9), the patient was started on quinidine at the time of discharge. PVC frequency has been low on followup visits, averaging 3.2/min on 5 EKGs. Because the patient was unable to detect PVCs except by taking his pulse, he was given twenty-four further training sessions to learn PVC detection. This was done 1 month after the first study. Whereas the patient initially was unable to detect any of his PVCs except by taking his pulse, by the end of the second study, he was able to detect them accurately 35–40% of the time without the light feedback. He said that he felt a sensation of warmth across the precordium when PVCs were occurring. When PVCs were frequent—e.g., 15/min—he also noted diaphoresis.

In one additional followup visit after the second study, there were no PVCs on EKG. During the clinic visit, the patient was able to sense that he was having infrequent PVCs (6/min). He reported that at home he also could sense his PVCs by the precordial warmth—verified by taking his pulse—and by sitting quietly, he could abolish them in half an hour. They stayed away for variable periods of time thereafter, usually for about an hour.

Patient 5

CA was a 73-year-old Caucasian male with a 19-month history of documented PVCs. On thirteen visits to his private physician during the 19 months prior to our study, the patient was described as having no ectopic beats on five occasions, few to moderate ectopic beats ("few," "occasional," "light irregularity of pulse," "irregularity of heart rate") on six occasions, and many ectopic beats on two occasions. The patient said that he could not sense the PVCs.

Laboratory. The patient was unable to speed his heart during the speeding sessions; however, he was consistently successful at slowing his heart (Table 11–1).

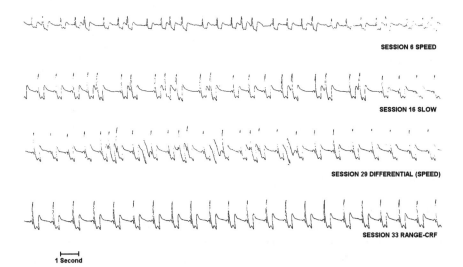

Figure 11–9. Patient 4. EKG rhythm strips during conditioning.

The patient differentiated well (Figure 11–10). He slowed from baseline during all sessions, and he speeded from baseline in five of the sessions, including four of the last seven. In order to speed his heart, the patient said that he thought about bouncing a rubber ball. To slow his heart, the patient said that he counted the amount of time the reinforcement light was on.

PVC frequency was highly variable during the speeding sessions (Figure

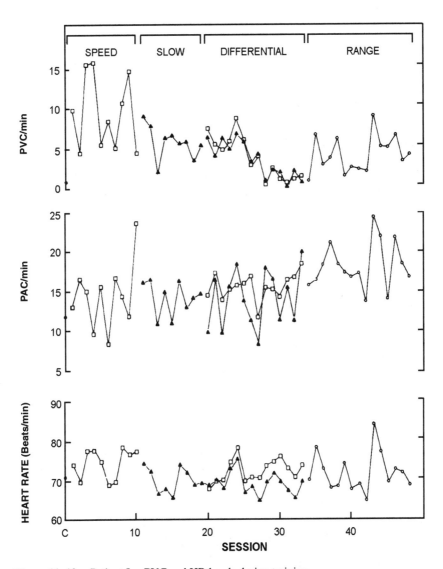

Figure 11–10. Patient 5. PVC and HR levels during training.

11–10). During slowing, PVC frequency declined to about 5/min, and during the differentiation sessions, they fell still further so that there were fewer than three PVCs/min during the last six of these sessions. During the range sessions, PVC frequency remained low, averaging 4/min.

PACs increased slightly during the study, from about 14/min during speeding to about 18/min during the range condition (Figure 11–10). The patient said that he still could not tell when the PVCs occurred.

Ward. There was little fluctuation in HR on the ward (Table 11–3). As in the laboratory, PVCs (Table 11–2) were most frequent during speeding and were fewest during the later range and differential contingencies. PACs on telemetry also paralleled their behavior in the laboratory, being least frequent early (9.5/min during speeding) and more frequent later (17.1/min during the range contingency).

Pharmacologic studies. Drug studies were not done on this patient.

Followup. During 5 months of followup, the patient has been seen three times by his private physician. He was described as having no ectopic beats on two occasions, few to moderate ectopic beats on one occasion, and many ectopic beats on no occasions. An EKG taken 5 months after the study revealed 0.3 PVC/min and 22 PACs/min.

Patients 6, 7 and 8 all failed to learn to control their PVCs. Brief summaries of their cases are included in this report because they highlight important aspects about the limitations of operant training in the control of PVCs.

Patient 6

LS was a 60-year-old Negro male with a 5-year history of cardiac disease, including five hospitalizations for congestive heart failure.

His activities were severely limited by exertional dyspnea and palpitations, and less frequently by angina. He has paroxysmal nocturnal dyspnea about two nights per week. Chest X-ray revealed massive cardiomegaly, with a cardiac/thoracic ratio of 20/27.5. For almost 4 years prior to study, he had had premature atrial and ventricular contractions. Either or both of these were present on eight of nine EKGs during the 4 years prior to study. PVCs averaged 3.7/min and PAC, 1.6/min.

Laboratory. This patient was unable consistently to slow or speed his heart rate; however, he was quite successful at maintaining his rate within a ten-beat range (Table 11–1). His absolute heart rate declined from about 90 beats/min in the early sessions to about 65 beats/min by the end of speeding (slow training was given first in his case). The most likely explanations for this decline in HR are that during his period of hospitalization, he took his medications more regularly, and he reduced his alcohol consumption substantially.

During all training conditions, the frequency of his premature beats was highly variable, ranging from 1/min to 15/min. EKG tracings in the laboratory and on the ward were such that PVCs could not be differentiated from PACs; thus, all are listed together as premature beats.

It should also be noted that the patient drank heavily while on weekend passes so that he was too inebriated to return on Sunday evening as requested, and had to be fetched the next morning.

Followup. In 4 months of clinic followup, the patient continued to have many premature beats. On two EKGs, PVCs averaged 5.9/min and PACs, 9.7/min. His clinical status was unchanged. Thereafter, he was lost to followup. It was learned later that he died at home 10 months after the study.

Patient 7

EC was a 48-year-old Negro male with a history of hypertension for 27 years and cardiomegaly for 5 years, with hospitalization for congestive heart failure 4 years prior to study. After discharge from the hospital, the patient returned to work (manual labor), but he was so limited by dyspnea on exertion, that he was forced to quit. He proved to be little motivated to take a less strenuous job, and despite several professional attempts at rehabilitation, he has not worked since. At the time of study, he was functional Class II-B. The patient had had PVCs for 18 months prior to study, these being consistently present on physical examinations and on EKGs during that time. Their average frequency on three EKGs during that period was 9.0/min. The patient was an active Baptist, attending services twice a week.

Laboratory. The patient did not consistently speed his heart from baseline (Table 11–1); however, he did raise his absolute heart rate throughout the speeding sessions from 61 beats/min at the beginning to 78 beats/min by the end. He said he prayed to speed his heart. Although the patient did consistently slow his heart from baseline during the slowing sessions, his absolute heart rate did not change, remaining at 75 beats/min throughout these sessions. He said he tried to manipulate his breathing, and he prayed to slow his heart.

During the speeding sessions, PVC frequency increased from 6/min to 24/min. During the slowing sessions, PVC frequency was variable, ranging from 10/min to 20/min.

In an effort to enable this patient to gain control over his PVCs, he was given four sessions of training in the range contingency, and nine sessions of training in a PVC avoidance contingency in which a soft tone sounded whenever he had a PVC; his task was to silence the tone. However, PVCs persisted generally between 7 and 20/min, with an average of 12.4/min. HR averaged 76.2. The patient said that he tried mild exercise in bed, as well as praying and changing his breathing to decrease his PVCs.

Ward. Telemetry data (Tables 11–2 and 11–3) indicated that HR did not change throughout the study. However, the incidence of PVCs decreased during the slowing conditioning and then returned to prestudy levels during the range and PVC avoidance training.

Pharmacologic studies. No drug studies were done on this patient.

Followup. During 17 months of followup, he has continued consistently to have PVCs, averaging 6.1/min. His clinical status is unchanged. The patient subsequently revealed that he was afraid that if his PVCs improved, he might lose his disability benefits and have to return to work. It is possible that this concern affected his performance during the study.

Patient 8

JF was a 77-year-old Caucasian male with a history of two probable MIs, the second one being 3 years prior to admission. He was not hospitalized on either occasion, and subsequent EKGs did not reveal definite evidence of an old MI. He also had had diabetes mellitus for 7 years. Shortly after the second probable MI, the patient developed CHF, and was hospitalized. PVCs were noted then for the first time. They did not respond to amelioration of the CHF (digoxin, chlorothiazide and potassium chloride), procaine amide, dilantin, or discontinuing digoxin for several months. They were consistently present thereafter, being seen on all of the nine EKGs taken from that time until the study. They were multifocal in origin, and their average frequency was 12.4/min. The patient said that he could not tell when they occurred.

Laboratory. Although there was evidence of heart rate control (Table 11–1) and a fall in absolute HR from an initial 90 beats/min to 76/min during slowing training, PVC frequency did not decrease. It should be noted that this patient had PVCs of at least four different configurations. Sometimes certain ones were more frequent; sometimes others were. This posed severe difficulties for our HR and PVC detection system. It also made it quite difficult to provide accurate feedback to the patient.

Ward. Telemetry data paralleled events in the laboratory in that HR was lower during the slowing periods (Table 11–3), and PVCs remained frequent (Table 11–2).

Pharmacologic studies. No drug studies were performed on this patient.

Followup. Followup for 8 months revealed no significant changes in the patient's cardiovascular status. PVCs were present on all of four EKGs taken during these visits, with an average frequency of 10.0/min. The patient died suddenly at home 2 weeks after his last clinic visit.

Discussion

This study shows that patients can be taught to control the prevalence of their PVCs. Patients 1–4 showed clear evidence of PVC control in the laboratory, and evidence of transfer of the learned effect to the ward. Patient 1 has sustained her low PVC rate for 21 months, and each of these other 3 patients who have been followed for shorter periods of time reports that he is able to detect and modify his PVCs while at home. Also, Patient 5 has maintained a low PVC frequency for 5 months after the study.

The presence of PVCs is associated with an increased probability of sudden death.[28] Corday et al. have demonstrated experimentally that PVCs can diminish coronary artery blood flow[29] and cerebral blood flow.[30] The fact that Patient 1 has had no further myocardial infarctions in the 21 months of followup, as contrasted with three in the 11 months preceding the study, may be related to her decreased PVC frequency.

In the patients in this study, at least two different mechanisms of PVC control appear to have been involved. The drug studies in Patient 1 suggested that reduced sympathetic tone to the heart was responsible for the decreased incidence of PVCs. As the cardiac sympathetic nerves are known to influence the ventricle strongly,[31,32] this effect probably occurred directly at the ventricular level. In Patient 3, the drug studies suggested that increased vagal tone decreased her PVC frequency. This may have represented a direct vagal effect on the ventricle, as there is anatomic evidence for vagal innervation of the ventricle in mammals,[33,34] and physiologic evidence for vagal effects on the mammalian ventricle.[35,36]

The flexibility of operant conditioning is demonstrated by the fact that PVCs were reduced whether they were mediated primarily by the sympathetic or by the parasympathetic nervous system. This underscores the fact that operant conditioning can be used to alter pathologic conditions mediated by different mechanisms.

Heart rate per se does not determine the presence or absence of PVCs. Similar HRs in Patient 2 were associated with different PVC frequencies depending on the experimental contingency under which they occurred. Also, in Patient 1, HRs between 90 and 100 beats/min induced by isoproterenol were associated with PVCs, whereas similar HRs induced by atropine were not. In Patient 3, the opposite occurred. Atropine-induced HRs above 90 beats/min were associated with PVCs, while similar HRs induced by isoproterenol were not. This also suggests that extensive, short-term, experimental drug studies—of the type carried out in Patient 3—might be useful in clarifying the mechanisms of PVCs in different patients.

The imagery which patients reported while controlling their heart rates has been presented. However, the reports are highly idiosyncratic, and no consistent pattern is apparent.

There seem to be six elements that are important for successful learning of PVC control. These are: (a) peripheral receptors which are stimulated by the PVC; (b) afferents which carry the information to the CNS; (c) CNS processing to enable the patient to recognize the PVC and to provide the motivation and flexibility necessary to enable learning to occur; (d) efferents to an effector organ which can bring about the desired change in the pathologically functioning heart; (e) a heart which is not too diseased to beat more regularly; (f) a homeostatic system in the patient which will tolerate the more normal functioning of the heart.

Patient 4 illustrates the role of the afferent system. He did well at controlling his PVCs when he had continuous feedback in the range portion of Study 1, but did more poorly as the feedback was phased out. After Study 2, he was able to detect his PVCs, and then to reduce their frequency.

Patient 1 illustrates the importance of CNS processing. She had to learn to be comfortable with infrequent PVCs, whereas early in the study, she had been interpreting frequent PVCs as comfortable. This underscores the fact that physicians cannot always rely on the naive patient's interpretation of his physiologic state. The concern which Patient 7 expressed regarding his disability benefits suggests that motivation is also an important, CNS-mediated factor.

The grossly enlarged heart of Patient 6 and the electrically very unstable one of Patient 8 illustrate the importance of the heart itself. These hearts may have been too diseased to beat regularly for prolonged periods of time.

Early intervention may facilitate the learning of PVC control—e.g., during convalescence from an infarction as in Patient 4. (The severity of the arrhythmias which the patients were able to generate in the course of conditioning was striking. Therefore, it would seem advisable not to attempt to condition patients during the acute, postinfarction period.)

This study was not concerned with optimization of technics. It should be possible to accomplish comparable results in much shorter periods of time, as more nearly optimal conditioning technics are employed. For example, studies should be feasible on an outpatient basis; and pretesting with autonomically active drugs such as those used in this study should suggest whether the patient will benefit more from being taught to slow or to speed.

References

1. Skinner BF: The Behavior of Organisms. Appleton-Century-Crofts, New York, 1938
2. Kimmel HD: Instrumental conditioning of autonomically mediated behavior. Psychol Bull 67:337–345, 1967
3. Miller NE: Learning of visceral and glandular responses. Science 163:434–445, 1969
4. Shearn DW: Operant conditioning of heart rate. Science 137:530–531, 1962
5. Hnatiow M, Lang PJ: Learned stabilization of heart rate. Psychophysiol 1:330–336, 1965
6. Engel BT, Hansen SP: Operant conditioning of heart rate slowing. Psychophysiol 3:176–187, 1966
7. Levene HI, Engel BT, Pearson JA: Differential operant conditioning of heart rate. Psychosom Med 30:837–845, 1968
8. DiCara LV, Miller NE: Instrumental learning of systolic blood pressure responses by curarized rats: dissociation of cardiac and vascular changes. Psychosom Med 30:489–494, 1968
9. Shapiro D, Turksy B, Gershon E, et al: Effects of feedback and reinforcement on the control of human systolic blood pressure. Science 163:588–590, 1969
10. Miller NE, DiCara LV: Instrumental learning of urine formation by rats: changes in renal blood flow. Amer J Physiol 215:677–683, 1968
11. DiCara LV, Miller NE: Instrumental learning of vasomotor responses by rats: learning to respond differentially in the two ears. Science 159:1485–1486, 1968
12. Snyder C, Noble M: Operant conditioning of vasoconstriction. J Exp Psychol 77:263–268, 1968
13. Fowler RL, Kimmel HD: Operant conditioning of the GSR. Psychol Rep 7:555–562, 1960
14. Kimmel HD, Baxter R: Avoidance conditioning of the GSR. J Exp Psychol 65:212–213, 1964

15. Shapiro D, Crider A: Operant electrodermal conditioning under multiple schedules of reinforcement. Psychophysiol 4:168–175, 1967
16. Engel BT, Melmon KL: Operant conditioning of heart rate in patients with cardiac arrhythmias. Conditional Reflex 3:130, 1968
17. White JD, Taylor D: Noxious conditioning as a treatment for rumination. Ment Retard 5:30–33, 1967
18. Lang PJ, Melamed BG: Case report: avoidance conditioning therapy of an infant with chronic ruminative vomiting. J Abn Psychol 74:1–8, 1969
19. Scherf D, Schott A: Extrasystoles and Allied Arrhythmias. Grune & Stratton, New York, 1953, pp 253–274
20. Korth C: The production of extrasystoles by means of the central nervous system. Ann Intern Med 11:492–498, 1937
21. Weinberg SJ, Fuster JM: Electrocardiographic changes produced by localized hypothalamic stimulations. Ann Intern Med 53:332–341, 1960
22. Attar HJ, Gutierrex MT, Bellet S, et al: Effect of stimulation of hypothalamus and reticular activating system on production of cardiac arrhythmia. Circ Res 12:14–21, 1963
23. Scherf D, Blumenfeld S, Yildiz M: Experimental study on ventricular extrasystoles provoked by vagal stimulation. Am Heart J 62:670–675, 1961
24. Gillis RA: Cardiac sympathetic nerve activity: changes induced by ouabain and propranolol. Science 166:508–510, 1969
25. Estes EH Jr, Izlar HL Jr: Recurrent ventricular tachycardia: a case successfully treated by bilateral sympathectomy. Am J Med 31:493–497, 1961
26. Peimer IA: Conditioned reflex extrasystole in man. Fiziol Zh SSSR Sechenov 39:286–292, 1953
27. Perez-Cruet J: Conditioning of extrasystoles in humans with respiratory maneuvers as unconditional stimulus. Science 137:1060–1061, 1962
28. Chiang BN, Perlman LV, Ostander LD Jr, et al: Relationship of premature systoles to coronary heart disease and sudden death in the Tecumseh epidemiologic study. Ann Intern Med 70:1159–1166, 1969
29. Corday E, Gold H, DeVera LB, et al: Effect of the cardiac arrhythmias on the coronary circulation. Ann Intern Med 50:535–553, 1959
30. Corday E, Irving DW: Effect of cardiac arrhythmias on the cerebral circulation. Amer J Cardiol 6:803–807, 1960
31. Rushmer RF: Autonomic balance in cardiac control. Amer J Physiol 192:631–634, 1958
32. Sarnoff SJ, Brockman SK, Gilmore JP, et al: Regulation of ventricular contraction: influence of cardiac sympathetic and vagal nerve stimulation on atrial and ventricular dynamics. Circ Res 8:1108–1122, 1960
33. Mitchell GAG: Cardiovascular Innervation. Edinburgh and London, Livingstone, Ltd, 1956
34. Hirsch EF, Kaiser GC, Cooper T: Experimental heart block in the dog, III: distribution of the vagus and sympathetic nerves in the septum. Arch Path

79:441–451, 1965
35. Wildenthal K, Mierzwiak DS, Wyatt HL, et al: Influence of efferent vagal stimulation on left ventricular function in dogs. Amer J Physiol 215:577–581, 1969
36. Daggett WM, Nugent GC, Carr PW, et al: Influence of vagal stimulation on ventricular contractibility, O_2 consumption and coronary flow. Amer J Physiol 212:8–18, 1967

CHAPTER 12

An Integrated Theory of Disease
Ladino-Mestizo Views of Disease in the Chiapas Highlands

HORACIO FABREGA, JR., M.D., AND
PETER K. MANNING, PH.D.

Prefatory Remarks

Jon Streltzer, M.D.

By 1973, psychosomatic medicine had evolved well beyond theories of disease and specificity theories.[1] Fabrega's contributions are an important part of this evolution. In this article, Fabrega and Manning exquisitely reveal how the prevalent approach to patient care that separates mental and physical aspects of illness can cause the alienation of patients from doctors. This article is unusual in that there is no experimental group, no statistics, no quantitative observations, and no case descriptions. Instead, a distinct group of people is the focus of a report that is part ethnography and part philosophy and that highlights and elucidates core issues of psychosomatic medicine: mind-body, sickness-health, illness-disease, and holism versus dualism. This article goes further than recognizing the role of culture in understanding illness—it uses culture as a backdrop

---

Volume 35, 1973, pp. 223–239.
 From Michigan State University, East Lansing, Mich. 48823.
 Support for this study was made possible by NIMH grant #MH 21430-01.
 Received for publication July 10, 1972.

for a theory of illness and demonstrates that the practice of medicine can be viewed from a cultural perspective, with profound implications for understanding of the doctor-patient relationship.

Reference

1. Kimball CP: Conceptual developments in psychosomatic medicine: 1939–1969. Ann Intern Med 73:307–316, 1970

This paper describes the beliefs about illness espoused by Spanish-speaking Mexicans from the Chiapas Highlands. The set of beliefs about illness entails explanations about its causes, mechanisms, manifestations, and consequences and for this reason can be viewed as constituting a theory about disease. The theory of disease described encompasses events and processes that outside observers would classify as mental, bodily, and social. To members of the group, disease and well-being reflect the status of a person's adjustment and functioning in all facets of his life. Disease-related notions, such as pain and physiological functioning, are also explained and reacted to in a holistic fashion, partaking social and mentalistic aspects as well as strictly bodily ones. This integrated theory of disease contrasts sharply with the dualistic view of disease held by practicing physicians of the area. The implications that these matters have for the field of psychosomatic medicine are described and analyzed in the paper. In this regard, currently held Western views about "mental" illness, "physical" illness, social deviance, and human individuality are relevant.

Introduction

This paper discusses selected but critical aspects of beliefs about disease and medical care that prevail among Spanish-speaking peoples of the highland region of the State of Chiapas in southeastern Mexico. The material reviewed represents, on the one hand, a theoretical orientation toward disease that is part of the culture, and also an abstract statement of the way the feelings and conceptions of individual persons of the area are organized and patterned during actual occurrences of illness. It will be seen that the term "disease," which in Western medicine has frequently been used dualistically to indicate alterations of body or mind, in this region is used holistically and includes happenings and processes that observers would view both as sociopsychological and as bodily. Briefly stated, a nondualistic and integrated theory of disease obtains in this region, a theory which includes references to emotions, interpersonal relations, naturalistic processes, and bodily changes. The native theory of disease contrasts sharply with that associated with the modern system of medical care. These differences in orientation toward medical problems are a source of difficulty for persons who seek medical relief in the clinics of the city. We shall see that the conflicts between these two logically independent theories of disease raise questions about the study of disease (viewed generically) in more complex and urban societies, questions that are germane to the theory and practice of psychosomatic medicine. Discussion of these issues will lead to a consideration of the social and medical influences of prevailing views of disease.

Background

Psychosomatic Medicine

It needs to be stressed that theoretical developments associated with the psychosomatic approaches to disease are typical products of Western biomedicine and as such must be seen as outgrowths of a distinct sociohistorical tradition.[1,2] More specifically, one can say that exploration of the mentalistic correlates of biomedical happenings are recent developments in the field of medicine, a field that following the social and theoretical revolutions of the seventeenth and eighteenth centuries has been closely tied to the growth of Western biological science. This is not the place to review the philosophical presupposition of biology nor its unique concepts and modes of explanation.[3] It needs to be emphasized, however, that rigorous scientific attention to mentalistic aspects of biological functioning came relatively late in the history of biology and medicine. One can trace the unfolding of this attention aimed at linking mind and body functioning in early psychoanalytic writings and to many the problems and formulations of "psychosomatic medicine" represent natural and highly creative extensions of psychoanalytic thought.

Physicians influenced by these psychosomatic approaches to disease have rightfully drawn attention to the negative consequences of holding a rigid dualistic position toward disease.[4, 5] The prevailing assumption is that altered processes we may term disease all have both emotional and bodily correlates. A definition of disease that emphasizes a discontinuity between these changes militates against effective treatment.[6] In pointing to the simplicity of the earlier closed and dualistic orientation, investigators have emphasized the theoretical influence of historically bound scientific paradigms such as that associated with developments in microbiology. In the last analysis, however, a society's theory of disease is not only an explanation of how a person (e.g., body, mind, behavior, etc.) is changed during a phase of life we may term illness. An orienting perspective adopted here, and one which we hope to substantiate in the paper, is that a theory of disease is also like a map or blueprint that provides the outline of what members of a culture accept as real. Theories of disease, then, not only explain but also structure the expectations and behaviors of persons during illness itself, thereby directly affecting the nature of the experiences and manifestations of disease. The contemporary unified or systems view of disease expounded by medical theoreticians is in this sense an outgrowth of observations and inferences made by physicians during the course of treating patients who themselves interpreted and reported their problems within the dualistic mold. It is thus possible to see earlier dualistic notions as providing the necessary background against which the unified perspective emerged.

Examining human dispositions and experiences with regard to disease in a group, such as that studied and reported upon here, which is guided by alternative medical orientations offers the student of disease and human behavior an opportunity to study basic characteristics of how man responds to and copes with stress, just as it affords the possibility of uncovering problematic correlates of our own contemporary framework of disease. Like all historically bound paradigms, this framework constitutes our guiding approach to disease and serves to organize if not constrain our questions and observations.[7, 8] What we ask of and look for in patients is determined by our preconceptions of what disease "is." Potentially enriching insights about the nature of disease and human functioning may be anticipated when problems associated with crises, stress, and disordered bodily functioning are probed in a setting such as the one to be described shortly. For here, we can observe the influence of an indigenous Maya approach to disease (which is sociobiologic and nonmental) and its interpenetration with a colonial Spanish culture which largely antedates developments of Western biological science.[9, 10] The material to be described in this paper, in other words, will examine altogether different approaches to illness and disease, approaches that should prove insightful, since comparative analyses of this material may point to characteristics of human functioning that are tied to and concealed within the prevailing Western dualistic mold. In this context, it is notable that workers of the psychosomatic persuasion do not often examine biosocial and psychosocial aspects of disease in non-Western cultural settings.

Cross-Cultural Medical Studies

Although the study of medical problems in nonliterate settings may be seen as a potentially fruitful endeavor from the standpoint of the problems associated with the psychosomatic mode of approach toward disease, a review of the literature of the field of medical ecology and medical anthropology will disclose that investigators all too often ignore this aspect of medical issues.[11] Much of this work, of course, is of an epidemiological sort and the investigators are attempting to delineate the distribution of disease in various social groups. Insofar as the investigator begins his study with a fixed preconception of the disease or diseases he intends to uncover in the field (i.e., a case of disease D_i is realized when indicators I_L-I_Q are found), his framework may be considered closed. He is not likely to look for or notice, much less record, the way in which actual persons experience and orient to the various complex changes and processes that are associated with an actual occurrence of disease. It is often the case that the investigator does not actually see or talk with the person that may later (after suitable samples of his blood or stool specimens are examined) be classified as a "case." Even in the work of recent epidemiologists who are very sensitive to the pernicious effects that a closed-systems approach to disease can have for understanding the nature of disease in human groups, there is manifest little concern for carefully searching for hidden possibly unique correlates of a disease process.[12] The result is, then, that fixed categories vis-à-vis disease are perpetuated, and the way the persons of the group experience, explain, and orient to the disease process is left out of focus. It is precisely in this latter arena—namely in the domain of bodily sensations, emotions, and cognitions—that the student of disease is likely to find material likely to enrich the field of psychosomatic medicine. For it is here where the investigator is likely to learn about the reciprocal influences that sociocultural factors have on bodily happenings.

Culturally oriented anthropologists who study medical issues from the perspective of their traditional discipline represent another group of investigators who are potentially able to contribute to the clarification of problems tied to the nature of human disease. Review of the literature in the field of ethnomedicine (the term used to designate the medically oriented studies of cultural anthropologists), however, will indicate that these types of problems are not given attention.[13] Anthropologists of this persuasion who examine medical problems have simply been content to examine medical issues at the sociocultural level. Illnesses, in other words, have been described mainly in terms of their meanings in the culture (presumed causes, interpretation, etc.) and in terms of the organized reactions that they occasion in the group. Rarely have investigators probed the actual contents of the behaviors and symptoms that indicate socially and psychologically that an individual is ill. When they have, the disease studied has usually been judged to be "psychiatric"—a sociobehavioral alteration presumed to have a functional cause has been studied. The deleterious effects that this has had for anthropology and for medicine generally have already been outlined.[14] Suffice it to say that the bodily correlates of other types of "disease," and by this we mean the physiological symptoms and the way in which these are experienced and evolve through time, have not been described. The guiding assumption appears to be that at most, social, cultural, and psychological categories merely elaborate upon that which is biologically "given." Physicians and biologists conversant with the literature of psychosomatic medicine can anticipate that the effect that culture has on human disease is more pervasive insofar as the relation between psychological factors and biological happenings is direct and continuous.

Research Setting and Methods

The research was conducted in and around San Cristobal de las Casas, a city of some 33,000 people in the highlands of Chiapas in southeastern Mexico. The city is the commercial, social, and religious center for a hinterland which contains about 175,000 Indians of Mayan descent. Within this geographic setting there are three principal ethnic groups: *ladinos,* who are said to be of direct Spanish descent; *mestizos,* or people of mixed Indian and Spanish descent (these two groups speak fluent Spanish, wear Western clothing, and identify with the values and institutions of the Mexican government); and the numerically dominant (outnumbering the other two by 6 or 7 to 1) but socially subordinate group, the heterogeneous *indigena* (i.e., Indian). The characteristics that distinguish the groups are not exclusively genetic or biological, but are rather social and cultural (wealth, power, education, style of dress, etc.).

The data upon which part of the descriptions of the report rest were gathered by means of a technique of ethnographic investigation and description that is current in anthropology.[15] The procedures employed were largely those of systematic elicitation from informants and can be briefly characterized as directed toward discovering native-language questions which regularly and successfully constrain informant responses to a limited set.[16, 17] Questions which are adequate in this sense are termed frames, and the regularly associated answers are called responses. The frame and responses constitute a unit in the description, and such units may be seen related to each other in a variety of ways within the description as a whole. Starting with a shared framework of communication (Spanish was always used as the language), the initial goal is to search for the specific and relevant frames in the domain of interest, namely, illness. These frames are used in the subsequent elicitation process when choices, contrasts, and cognitive boundaries are sought.

The construction of a description of this sort, composed of eliciting frames and responses, and sets thereof, is the immediate goal of the procedure. Such a form of description is a step toward the final goal, the production of an intraculturally valid ethnography, that is, an ethnography in which significant categories and relations are derived from intracultural analysis rather than from externally imposed rubrics. That is, one begins with the assumption that prior knowledge and experience, derived from one's own cultural background or other cultures previously studied, is potentially different from the knowledge and experience of these informants, and the task becomes the discovery of this knowledge that is not one's own, but which people of the culture under study use to identify, evaluate, and act upon in circumstances in which they find themselves. A description which accurately displays what is believed to be the "knowledge" of these informants should allow the anticipation (if not prediction) of events and behavior in circumstances specific to the culture under study in ways that match the expectations of the informants. Appropriateness or inappropriateness of anticipations based on the description is the means of actually testing the description.

In the following research, lay individuals of the regions as well as sick persons, physicians, and folk practitioners were interviewed regarding relevant experiences with medical problems. Persons of both ladino and mestizo background served as subjects. In the substance of the paper, no attempt is made to differentiate between these two social groups, and in line with the conventions adopted by social scientists who study in the Chiapas area, the term ladino is used. This report is part of a larger study designed to evaluate how commonly used symptom terms (e.g., cough, headache, stomach pain) stand in relation to a list of folk illness terms (*colico, susto, detencion,* etc.). Preliminary interviews have been held with a panel of families. During follow-up interviews a representative of the family unit is asked if a member has experienced an illness episode in the previous two weeks. If an episode has been experienced, the respondent is further asked what symptoms were associated with this self-defined problem, what interruptions took place in specified role spheres, and what actions were taken for resolution of the problem. In this research, then, the culturally based rules are inferred from the behavioral consequences associated with known linguistic pairings: symptoms, folk terms, and behaviors.

Ladino and Mestizo Medicine

Underlying Factors in the Etiology of Illness

According to ladinos, an outbreak of illness constitutes evidence that a person's strength, termed by them *consistencia,* has been overrun or depleted. This term refers to various aspects of a person that, importantly, are thought of as conjoined. It includes his inherited constitution. Here, ladinos have in mind not only attributes that are passed on through generations but also factors stemming from the physical, psychological, and moral status of the parents during the time of conception and following through the pregnancy. Features of a person's body and mind both fall within the intention of the term. Bodies that are strong, resilient, constituted of "good food," rest, exercise, and, in the case of men, proper amounts of sexual energy show high *consistencia*. A person's *caracter,* which designates a mentalistic entity, roughly personality, contributes a person's strength or *consistencia*. Together with one's intelligence, education, and previous experiences, personality is believed to contribute to level-headedness. These enable a person to plan and deal effectively with life demands. During times of crisis these traits become more relevant since they allow the person to effectively discharge emotion and tension in a constructive way so that the mind and body are not harmed by excesses of emotion (see below). One last feature of mind is relevant here. A person with a strong *consistencia* is one who does not allow himself to become *sugestionado*. Here, ladinos refer to the ability to withstand suggestions from others as well as preoccupations and worries of any sort. In a setting where persons are always potential targets of envy, anger, spiritistic influences, superstitions, and the general interpersonal machinations of others, a strong person is one who is not overcome by these influences. Thoughts, worries, and preoccupations are seen as potentially harmful to both mind and body.

Centrality of Emotions and Interpersonal Relations

In the causation of illness and disease, ladinos ascribe principal importance to the emotions. Indeed, in ladino theories of disease one can equate the centrality attributed to the emotions with that of "germs" in the Occidental germ theory of disease. The amount ("dosage") and noxiousness ("virulence") of the various *sentidos* (roughly, emotions, feelings) are differentiated, and are believed to affect proneness toward and both the seriousness and actual type of disease that develops. Emotions can actually be ranked as to their pathogenicity, and it is also possible to associate causally illness types with each of the various emotions. Inspection of the list of emotions that are described as pathogenic indicates that pleasantness and unpleasantness are not critical factors. Rather, their amount and persistence in the individual across time appear to be critical. Emotions and feelings are viewed as inevitable, but when present they should be discharged (in action, talk, or thought) or neutralized (as with alcohol) so that the body at no one time or during any one interval carries an excessive load. For emotions, when present in this way, are seen to have deleterious bodily extensions. Related to the pathogenicity of the emotions is the importance that ladinos ascribe to types of interpersonal situations. Arguments, separations, envious coveting, love triangles, intensely satisfying exchanges, etc., all have medical relevance precisely because they give rise to excessive feeling. The personality types or *caracteres* assume relevance here since they reflect an individual's habitual mode of conducting and responding to interpersonal situations.

In contrast to Mayan conceptions,[18, 19] then, in the ladino theory of disease one finds a concept of "person" which refers to a distinct psychological, social, and physical being. Furthermore, all of these related aspects of being are seen as connected and affected in important ways by the emotions. A person's inner "self," for example, is believed to not only respond passively to external situations and occurrences, but also to mediate and monitor actions so as to maintain both consistency with and proper amounts of the emotions. This "self," however, is not only limited to social and psychological factors but has bodily attributes. In the following section, ladino views about the body will be discussed. Suffice it to say here that the body is described as differentiated, the organs are named, their functions described, and their influence on disease recognized and explicitly stated. Diseases and emotions are believed to have specific loci in the organs of the body which are consequently altered and damaged causing the signs and symptoms of disease. The body, instead of being conceived simplistically as a passive repository for evil as in the case of the indigenous medical system, is seen instead as a complex entity composed of separate parts that function together in an integrated manner. Body and mind, then, are conjoined, the core essence of a person, responding to and regulating his various activities.

We may illustrate the relations between these notions by examining outbreaks of illness. The *consistencia* of the person and his personality form a baseline which determine vulnerability. A critical factor is the influence of certain types of interpersonal situations. A frightening occurrence or an embarrassing or shameful incident, for example, are common causes of illness among women, but will rarely affect men who are judged as more resistant along these emotional axes. Arguments and altercations, on the other hand, can affect both sexes. Unless resentments are discharged (by fighting, insulting, or acting out a plan of revenge, etc.), they will subsequently produce physical harm. Hostility is associated with the shortest "incubation period," and furthermore, its effect is judged as rapid and direct. So are excitements, and intensely satisfying or happy situations. Illness can result in days or hours, and although these can be lethal they often are short-lasting episodes. Sadness and envy, on the other hand, produce illness gradually and insidiously; the components or manifestations of the illness, in addition, are general, diffuse, and less dramatic but longer lasting and less easily removed. The type of illness that develops as well as its gravity are a function of the constitution and character of the person and the evolving interpersonal situation. Cleverness and intelligence are traits that modify the severity and duration of emotional states insofar as they enable one to discharge the emotion in a reasonably productive or adaptive way.

Illness conditions can affect groups (families or friends) that are exposed to or participants of interpersonal situations that are inciting. In this sense, the illness may be described as "contagious." Likewise, it follows that friends and relatives occupy important roles in the genesis and development of illness, for they, by intensifying or modifying the reactions of others, are believed to affect the level of emotion and hence its virulence and pathogenicity. By giving advice, offering to perform chores, or otherwise simply supporting those bound up in emotionally trying circumstances, they are said to have strategic influences on illness. It remains to be emphasized that communities or periods of time characterized by social unrest are especially deleterious from a medical standpoint. By contributing to low morale, unhappiness, and worry they can so debilitate the person that they render him vulnerable to frequent and/or serious illness.

Beliefs and Attitudes Toward the Body

Ladino views on illness and disease must be seen as extensions of their beliefs and attitudes about their bodies. A person's body, in many ways viewed as a machine, symbolizes that which is complex, delicate, and above all sacred in the human being. "Our bodies indicate that we carry a portion of God with us. They are the source and focus of our feelings, our energies, and our personalities." Regardless of how much antagonism and resentment may be felt toward someone, it is the case that a ladino maintains awe and respect for his corporeal self. Mystery also attaches to the body, for with the body one is said to be able to apprehend the pain of a loved one, his physical constraints, his disease. "His pain I can feel as my pain" is an assertion that ladinos invoke as proof of the capacity of the body to apprehend and "receive" communications from the bodies of others. Here, in other words, what we may view as sensitivity, empathy, or simply suggestibility, the ladino views as the body's way of actually apprehending and communicating changes in the physical states of others. The fact that sadness, happiness, and other emotions can replace the pain of a disease or the awareness of sensations associated with physiological processes (e.g., weakness, hunger) ladinos take as proof of the continuity or unity of body and mind, for the body's physically compromised state is believed to be actually altered by these experiences. The body can dominate the self in other ways. Attractive and strong bodies are sources of pride and admiration, whereas heavy, unkempt ones bring shame and discredit. Gaining weight is something ladinos claim can be felt, and since it is associated with changes in the blood can be harmful to one's health. Furthermore, extra weight is associated with a changed personality—one becomes less energetic, slower, lazier, more cautious and restrained as a result of gaining weight. To the ladino, another person—a friend or a relative—is not merely a psychological or social type. There is a particular individuality and uniqueness in others which involves their bodily constitution. Social exchanges between close persons are thus also occasions for inquiries about the conditions of one's bodies and health in general. The tiredness of a long journey or the stiffness produced by the strain of a trip allows relatives an opportunity to directly (through massage and heat) or indirectly (by preparation of herbs, the giving of folk preparations, etc.) relate to and intrude within the physical essence of others. In these and other ways, then, ladinos manifest a continual awareness and acceptance of their bodies as extensions of their minds and selves. The centrality, sacredness, and respect for the body is manifested individually and socially. Its mystery and wonder is something they repeatedly experience and make use of in relations with others.

A dramatic illustration of the various influences that are associated with bodily constitution and state is afforded by the condition of pregnancy. First of all, women are afforded a number of social and psychological entitlements and prerogatives as a result of becoming pregnant. Family members are disposed to significantly modify their expectations of and demeanor toward women in this condition, just as they are likely to show a great deal of tolerance for peculiarities of their temperament. Pregnant women are also the locus of unusual powers. Since their bodies contain more heat and are in complex ways altered, they are able to effectuate medical cures denied nonpregnant women. Sprains, joint tenderness, bone pains, or any other reasonably well localized pains believed to be the result of drafts of cold air are particularly susceptible to the ministrations of pregnant women. The heat of the woman and fetus, in other words, can capture and extract the air, thereby relieving if not curing the ailment. This power, however, is not without its liabilities. Women who are pregnant are also dangerous sources of illness. The heat of their bodies can "infect" others, causing either an outbreak of illness or a worsening of one due to other causes. Insofar as women naturally acquire this strength or power during the pregnancy, they are not held responsible for its untoward effects on others.

The Experience of Pain

The unity between mind and body, feeling and biological state and the linkage of these with social processes can be illustrated in the way ladinos speak about and describe pain. The *sensation* of pain does not appear to be differentiated. One does not obtain descriptions of pain experiences such that the quality of this experience as a mentalistic entity is differentiated and seen as separate from the locus, extensions, and presumed source of the pain. "I have a crampy pain in my stomach," or "The pain I am having is continuous" are not assertions likely to be proffered by ladinos. Rather, we obtain remarks such as "I am having the pain of X." Probing the meaning of this statement we obtain "It is the pain of my liver, located here, which was brought on by doing Y after having experienced Z, and the pain is like someone were squeezing me inside, and the vomiting and headache that I am also having are part of the same malady." Physical and social metaphors abound in attempts to elaborate about the pain associated with various conditions which may be seen as focused in discrete anatomical parts. In short, pain, as a distinct sensation or feeling, is not given independent status. What exist, instead, are pains of X, Y, Z, etc., where these are diseases, emotions, anatomical entities, or even situations. Even the word "pain" itself (*dolor*) has limited extension. What we observe frequently are "heaviness," "burningness," "squeezingness," etc., which (although viewed as instances of pain by the observer) are often seen as different sorts of phenomena than "pain" by the ladino—i.e., as separate and distinct units of a disease or situation variously characterized. The uniqueness of these units is not limited to their sources or locations but includes modes of physiological, social, and interpersonal handling. In this broad sense, we may say that what we as physicians think and inquire about as pain, ladinos conceptualize, talk about, and experience as complex wholes, i.e., as chains of behavior, or situations, or as critical episodes. Thus, description of the pain of X will likely include an emotional and/or interpersonally inciting cause; the mechanism and components of the processes that result; a description of the characteristics of the pain viewed as a bodily, psychic, and social entity; the duration of these; and the various ways of controlling and bringing the pain episode to a close.

Additional Factors

Besides reflecting emotional and interpersonal considerations, illness is judged by the ladino to also result from naturalistic factors. Excessive heat; cold drafts of air (especially when an individual is angry or otherwise emotionally excited); insufficient, improperly prepared, or spoiled food; unduly prolonged fastings; excess sexual or other form of physical activity; and last, insufficient or inadequate rest and exercise (or sexual activity) may all be invoked as related factors in the explanation of an occurrence of illness. Naturalistic factors are usually given correlative importance; their causal significance is in association with the issues discussed previously. The ladino theory of disease accommodates most of the usual causes of disease that are expounded in the competing modern system. Thus, genetic factors, pathogenic microorganisms, or physiological dysfunctions may be (and often are) included as contributory explanations. However, careful interviewing discloses that emotional-interpersonal issues underlie these factors and are considered basic.

Acts of malevolence attributed to witches are frequently said to be the sources of illness, though persons differ as to how frequently they resort to this type of explanation. The degree of acculturation seems to be a factor, since more Westernized and urbanized ladinos invoke this cause less frequently. Acculturation is neither a necessary nor sufficient condition for belief in witchcraft, however. A person's level of morality and looks of distrust and suspiciousness are related, though asserting this is partly a tautology. In this cultural setting the form assumed by distrust is precisely that of accusations and suspicions of witchcraft. Sources of alleged witchcraft are fellow ladinos and especially the *indigena*. Most ladinos view him as the ultimate irrational and malevolent agent that holds a potential influence on their well-being. Meaningless or otherwise unexplainable outbreaks of serious disease eventually are attributed to their "senseless" actions.

The Mechanism of Disease

The manner in which the ladino explains the relations between the multiplex factors that are implicated in an occurrence of illness can be described as homeostatic. An optimal range of function and structural integrity underlies health. Each of the classes of factors discussed earlier represents sources of disturbances that can upset this range. The various factors can combine with or oppose the others, so that notions of balance and equilibrium are also implicated in health and illness.

The linkages between the various classes of factors that underlie and affect health are mediated by the person's blood and by his nervous energy (or activity). The latter two elements are viewed almost as isomorphic. Emotional excitements, physical essences reflecting the state and strength of the body, and deleterious exogenous influences that affect health all directly affect the blood and in fact are judged as part of the blood. Native practitioners, consequently, by pulsing the sick person, learn from the blood the nature of the disease and its cause. The blood, then, literally is seen as carrying the emotions throughout the body and in this way affects the structure and function of the organs.

An Integrated Theory of Disease

The preceding considerations should indicate that in contrast to the views held by the Maya of this region,[18,19] for ladinos the entity disease (or illness) is a relatively complex entity. Among Maya, disease is conceptualized abstractly, and the influences of body, social relations, and supernatural factors are not separated but merely condensed and fused. The social and legal consequences of illness are salient. Among the ladinos, on the other hand, a number of factors (seen as related) are identified and almost invariably held to be implicated in an occurrence of disease. These rest on rather elaborate, if not complex, notions about human functioning. The causes of disease, in short, touch on aspects of personality, social relations, and strictly biological functioning, all of which are seen as linked almost in a homeostatic and feedback manner. The self or personality and the body emerge as complicated entities. Furthermore, we observe that disease—as a time-bound state denoting compromised human functioning—is likewise highly differentiated. Ladinos distinguish between disease types on the basis of rate of onset, duration, and severity as well as symptom components. It may be the case that these aspects of disease are associated causally with personality, interpersonal relations, biophysical constitution, and prevailing situation. It nevertheless follows that a more refined entity is envisioned by ladinos when they speak about disease. This is also reflected in their description of the manifestations of disease, for they elaborate not only on the kinds of physiological behaviors (symptoms) that can take place but also on the many different types and levels of constraints imposed by disease. What persons do and do not do during an illness state is as much a function of the causal factors that are invoked as of the type of disease that has developed.

The ladino theory of disease can be labeled "integrated" because a number of alternative domains frequently viewed in an analytic sense by others as separate and nonoverlapping are treated by them as conjoined and continuous. Among these domains we may include mind vs. body, social vs. psychological, and genetic vs. environmental. Attention was drawn to the unified way in which ladinos view their bodies and their *caracteres*. Just as these two domains overlap and fuse, so also do the naturalistic and supernaturalistic. It will be recalled that physical factors as well as spiritistic or diabolical influences are given importance in disease causation. These two classes of happenings likewise appear to be fused. Various "natural" occurrences, for example, are viewed by the ladino as evidence of the mysterious and occult. A broken glass, window, or plate symbolizes a communication that something evil and tragic will occur soon. The broken fragments are consequently placed in water in order to neutralize their effects. Portions of garlic are kept attached to doors, undergarments may be worn inside out, and holy water sprinkled across windows and doors to keep spiritistic emanations from intruding. A barking dog at night, a flying vulture, or a screeching owl are not only animals but also the transformed essences (*naguales*) of the devil himself or of persons who have a compact with the devil. Dreams are critical openings into the supernatural and the mysterious; their content portends, causes, or reflects bodily changes of a harmful and threatening sort. In these and innumerable other ways, then, the natural and supernatural "orders" are connected by the ladino and are treated by him as phenomena that are conjoined. In an analogous fashion, ladinos combine the points of view that are entailed in the "nature vs. nurture" conflict. Environmental and genetic factors are given equal and related roles in disease causation, with these two classes of occurrences affecting and modifying the other in a Lamarckian manner. In the area of health and disease, children profit in a genetic and physicalistic sense from the habits and experiences of their parents.

The integrated view of disease that prevails among ladinos is manifest in still another manner. In a previous study the striking characteristics that ladinos from the town of Tenejapa ascribed to what we would term psychotic disturbances were outlined.[20] The causes of this type of illness are not judged as different from those of other types of illness. Furthermore, although ladinos may view the psychotically disturbed person as altered and changed in important ways during the time that he is ill (and this would include organismic changes), no stigma or other form of social discreditation (or differentiation) attaches to the person following recovery. Mental illness, in short, is not the occasion for morally censuring an individual—it is judged as an illness similar to others. The differential valuations that elsewhere are placed on afflictions of the mind as opposed to the body are thus not observed in ladino communities. Related to this, we observe that many behavioral alterations that an outside observer may describe as psychiatric—depressive or paranoid reactions, antisocial outbursts, character disorders, etc.—are frequently also judged by ladinos as indications of illness, though the nature of this illness is not differentiated in any special way.

The illnesses, in other words, would not be described by them as purely emotional, although these psychological (as well as social) aspects would be acknowledged. Illnesses of this type may even be called excessive envy or greed or sadness due to painful separations, etc., with the situational and interpersonal roots included as indications of the illness state. Importantly, however, discussions with ladinos disclose that they consider the afflicted person or persons as also *physically* changed and ill—i.e., specific organs as well as the blood is described as altered and diseased. We observe, then, that among ladinos of the Chiapas region psychiatric illness, in the way that we think of this entity, has no unique and separate status. Attitudes and dispositions about its causes and attributes are continuous with those of other illnesses, and in addition, the belief that it reflects dysfunction of only one type of system (mind vs. body) is eschewed.

Disease, Mind-Body Conceptions, Medical Care, and Social Change

The fact that illness in the highlands is seen as a state having many diverse but interconnected facets has logical implications for the treatment of illness. Many of these have been covered in the literature but they bear a brief repetition here.[21, 22] For one thing, requesting treatment from a practitioner is the occasion for the sharing of a host of personal concerns which, as we have tried to indicate, are viewed as components of the illness. Data about how the body is functioning is simply one type of information that is exchanged. Furthermore, personal relations with the practitioner become critical; his humanity, trustworthiness, and alleged powers in various domains which outsiders may view as separate if not irrelevant to disease, are critical. Special technical competence, in other words, is but one of many attributes that a practitioner must possess. Ladinos believe that one who knows about the mysteries of the body must know about the mysteries of the soul, of the spirits, of the proper forms of conducting social relations, and of the future itself. This follows from the "sacredness" that surrounds the body, from the fundamental role that it has in reflecting and mediating self-consciousness and a social reality which includes the supernatural, and from the identity that these sociobiologic issues have with what we would term "medical issues." Thus, the transaction between the practitioner and his patient is the focus of social, psychological, and moral as well as bodily matters. Insofar as illness refers to and reflects both personal and interpersonal issues, the self-presentation of each participant is critical[23]: morality, illness, and self,

An Integrated Theory of Disease 237

in other words, are fused and all three are continuous with how one behaves. During medical treatment practitioner and patient both become parties to a crucial situation that has roots in and effects on highly private and socially meaningful issues. The transaction, thus, must establish consensus vis-à-vis blame, shame, malevolence, and propriety. In this context, trust and distrust become critical. This is the case because a medical evaluation entails the examination of motives, the evaluation of character, and the opportunity to judge the espousal of norms; diagnosis is in part equivalent to socially and morally typing another; and treatment brings the opportunity to share in and help resolve another's crisis of living by modifying his conduct.

A person's view of theory of disease naturally determines what he will do in order to get well. If the theory is broadly shared by members of the culture, as it is in the highlands, it will also determine the kind of treatment that he receives from a folk practitioner. In the case of ladinos, we note that the native theory directly implicates domains that medical theorists currently believe importantly affect the cause, components, persistence, and resolution of disease.[24, 25] Stated succinctly, if it is desirable to handle and treat disease in terms of the various separate but linked systems that are believed to be implicated in any one instance or occurrence, then ladinos (because of their native theory of disease) to some extent accomplish this among themselves. Thus, not only do they view disease as having a holistic basis, they also treat it in this fashion. Assuming the validity of the view of disease expounded by medical theorists and presuming that ladinos can point to sources of psychosocial tension and interference in a reasonably accurate manner, we can infer that ladinos to some extent deal effectively with disease. What they lack, of course, is effective ways of directly modifying physiologic and chemical changes that are also associated with disease. It is the ability of modern medicine to affect this domain that draws many ladinos to seek care from physicians. This visit to a physician, however, often has interesting if not ironic consequences.

When a ladino visits a physician he experiences an orientation to his problem that is markedly different from his own. A "modern" view that fractionates the native holistic and integrated view of disease is encountered. For there he is probed in a very precise and intensive way about his body (its appearance, function, and sensations) but not about his feelings, moods, dispositions, and social relations. Little confidence and trust can be placed in procedures and strategies that stem from a framework and orientation that is judged as highly formal and mechanistic, especially when these procedures are coordinated by an impersonal individual who appears uninterested in the varied personal and social goings-on which are believed to cause alterations in bodily states and in fact give these their significance. For the ladino patient, one result of having his medical problems reduced in this fashion and of receiving interpretations about bodily matters that are not only discordant but frequently viewed as insufficient and simplistic is skepticism, alienation, and a lack of compliance with medical regimens. A search for a more "understanding" practitioner follows, and not infrequently, a deterioration of a problem for which there is an "available" cure. Countless instances can be recorded of persons who have withdrawn from "modern" treatment when no immediate cure was forthcoming, with consequent deterioration in health status.

Our research indicates that ladinos themselves and their native practitioners have available various modes for effectively dealing with alterations in most of the system components that we (abstractly) may judge as implicated in an occurrence of disease. Their mode of care lacks refinement in one of these components, namely the strictly biological. It is in this narrow segment of the spectrum of disease where physicians can be most effective. However, these lack "competence" or credibility in the other system components or portions of the spectrum of disease that ladinos judge as logically contained in and indicated by an occurrence of disease. Physicians are thus often not visited, or their advice ignored precisely because of their narrow approach to disease. The result, thus, is lack of coordination and disarticulation between treatment modalities and a consequent worsening or nonimprovement of the "disease."

Many factors can be invoked as reasons why folk systems of medical care are supplanted by Western biomedical conceptions and practices. We can classify these roughly into two types: (a) patent limitations of the folk system (objectified as high infant mortalities, high disease prevalence, etc.) and (b) evidence (visible and inferential) that Western "modern science" can profoundly change, alter, and control nature (not just illness matters). However, the spread of modern medicine cannot be seen as a process that simply erodes and takes the place of native views and practices, but rather as a pervasive undermining (with consequent disarticulation of) established modes of thinking, feeling, and behaving. In the highlands, conceptions about disease, indeed experiences of and with disease, are isomorphic with those that articulate one's personal identity and also give meaning to social relations. What is more, all of these form the fabric of what we may term "medical care." It is not surprising, then, that the intrusion of Western medicine to such a setting brings with it more than decreased infant mortality and rates of infectious diseases; it brings with it the destruction of the previously mentioned unity that is seen in social relations, body, and self. Insofar as it operates through specialized occupational and suboccupational groups (nurses, internists, psychiatrists, surgeons, etc.), medicine tends to segmentalize the person in various ways. Each of these groups has a perspective that is organized by separate premises, obligations, and explanations, all of which are in conflict with native understandings. Problems are somewhat arbitrarily divided into "mental" vs. "physical," "social" vs. "medical," natural vs. "superstitious," thereby producing disarticulations. In other words, what to ladinos is a single crisis having broad ramifications is in this new system or view a heterogeneous collection of "problems" each of which has a separate cause and locus. In this process of differentiation and specialization, Western medicine not only fragments and undermines the native cultural system thereby creating conflict, but it brings with it the rigid dualistic notions that many physicians see as being central to the disaffections patients often feel with medical care in urbanized societies.

Comment

From a historical perspective, the ladino-mestizo medical care system and the beliefs on which it is based represent a culmination of a developmental process issuing originally from Iberian culture which was transformed and synthesized by contact with indigenous Mayan cultures.[9, 10, 26, 27] The most notable aspect of the highlands is its conservative atmosphere, a consequence of the power and durability of native values and traditions. The ideas current in the highlands can be traced to Spanish conceptions of health and illness. One of the principal paradigms organizing these conceptions is the Greek humoral theory, associated with Hippocrates. Related views are prevalent throughout Hispanic cultures. Originally introduced to Latin America in the sixteenth and seventeenth centuries and taught in medical schools established by the Spanish in Mexico and Peru, the ideas were spread by missionaries and subsequently diffused throughout Mexico and Central and South America. The four humors (i.e., blood, phlegm, yellow bile, and black bile) are normally in a state of equilibrium in the person's body. Natural adjustments are made to everyday events and changes in physical demands, but health is signified by a warm, moist body maintaining a balance among the four basic elements. In contrast, illness is believed to result from humoral imbalance said to be caused by an excess of one of the four, and reflected metaphorically in an excessively hot, cold, moist, or dry body. There is a strong culturally sanctioned emphasis upon the restoration of balance. Foods, drinks, herbs, and medicinal substances, themselves also classified into hot or cold categories, may be used to maintain health or to return the body to a previous healthful state. A further extension of the balance notion intrinsic to this version of the humoral theory is that of the emotions themselves, which are seen as a reflection of the degree of balance obtained in social relations and "inside" a given person. Previous investigators have not adequately explicated the extensiveness and universality of the conception of balance and holism in Latin cultures. Often they have taken a basically Cartesian dualism abroad. In these types of analyses it is assumed that body and mind, because they may have an independent logical status, are also viewed as empirically separated, with changes confined to a separate domain.

In assuming the biomedical framework of disease which rests on quite rigid dualistic assumptions, researchers often see "cultures" or "values" as contributing to the cause of disease or to its expression. In the study of the cultural patterning of presenting symptoms, for example, specific diseases are used as a control, or independent fact, with "expression" of symptoms (e.g., pain) a dependent variable associated with membership in Irish, Anglo-Saxon, or Italian ethnic-descent groups. Anglo-Saxons and Irish report fever, more sharply focused and located symptoms, and less intense pain.[28, 29] We can interpret this set of findings in a fashion consistent with inferences drawn from the findings of the study reported here. Anglo-Saxons, coming from a tradition that both spawned and supported the leading medical advances in past centuries, may have learned to see their bodies within a more impersonal dualistic framework, identifying illness as a body or physical experience. The "discrepant" behaviors of Latins and Italians when they are sick may in part reflect current and past differences in the way concepts about disease are understood and acted upon in Hispanic and Mediterranean cultures. The latter groups may not share the Anglo-Saxon attachment to a sharp body/mind distinction, and in this sense, the expression of pain or discomfort may not simply be a result of emotional or temperamental factors as these are affected by a universal biological entity (i.e., "disease"), but rather the expression of fundamentally different orientations of what disease represents. Interpretations of illness "behavior" in modern settings, by both social scientists and physicians, may thus be traced to implicit biomedical assumptions combined with simplistic if not naive identification of a cultural tradition.

Modern psychosomatic medicine and the unified view of disease, seen in the light of these historic and logical considerations, may represent an attempt to reconstruct in a highly refined manner a view of illness that (a) was previously dominant at a particular point in time in selected cultures (principally those that are glossed by the terms "Latin," "Mediterranean," or "expressive"), and (b) is presently held in variable degrees by subcultural groups, e.g., Italian-Americans, Mexican-Americans, Puerto Ricans, etc. Furthermore, as mentioned earlier, this modern view of disease must be seen as a response to the earlier dualistic one which itself was a product of historical circumstances. Taken together, the dualistic and integrated views of disease dramatize the point that facts taken logically as evidence of disease in one framework are nondisease or epistemologically nonexistent in the other. In other words, attention is drawn to the social and historical bases of what disease "is."[8, 14] This point has interesting implications. If one assumes that the natural biological tendency of man is to view and respond to crises and stress in some integrated or at least undifferentiated way, then one can posit that rigid conceptions about what these crises are may affect how one in fact behaves and responds during them. Theories about or views of these "crises" (i.e., disease), then, literally contribute to the very essence of what is indicated by them. One is thus drawn to the position that the "natural history of disease" is not invariant and fixed but rather a consequence of changes in the functioning of connected systems, *each of which is affected by symbolizations about the meaning of and bases for these changes.*

There are social implications that can be drawn from the material presented in this paper. Currently, there is much confusion and ambiguity in contemporary American society about where medical matters begin and end, and also about the nature of the boundary between the medical and the social. No clear solutions to these dilemmas are forthcoming, though factors underlying the dilemmas may perhaps be better understood in the light of the material reviewed. Thus, in many ways, features of the contemporary problems of health and illness, of deviance and of welfare, of social control and crime, may be seen as residues of the fractionization of the more holistic and integrated system associated with the simple folk societies such as those of the Chiapas highlands. Here we refer to confusion about whether an individual is volitional, whether he is responsible for his behavior, whether or not he is to be discredited for his actions, or whether he is to be seen as a pawn of bodily or mental forces over which he has no control. To the extent that portions of one's behavior can be ascribed to autonomous units that are fostered by rigid dualistic notions, to that extent individuals are able to claim lack of responsibility for something which in a compelling way is a feature of the self. However, in a setting where notions that self and body cannot be dissolved, and both are in fact intimately and inextricably linked in social relations, behaviors we may gloss or label as mental illness, crime, deviance, and alcoholism (to name a few) are not separated and distinctly marked. In these settings, such behaviors are not isolated and viewed as unwilled and determined in some impersonal way nor are they problematic and a source of ambiguity and confusion to the individual or to the social system. Instead the behaviors are interpreted and given significance within the integrated and comprehensive view of self-body and social relations that prevails. In other words, the consequences and causes of "mental illness" or "deviance" or whatever else we may wish to label these behaviors can seemingly never be separated from an equation involving both *external* relations (friendships, kinship ties, associations) and the *condition of the body and the self* as perceived and defined. These behaviors are thus viewed as an inseparable part of the individual and his family and group, and are matters of their doing and for which they are responsible. They may be viewed as complex, lethal, and unfortunate but rarely as ambiguous, unwilled, or confusing. It may be then that contemporary dilemmas about medicine and society, and ambiguities about ways of dealing with them, result in part from the fractionization that is a feature of the modern view, a fractionization that is associated with the creation of separate domains each of which has causes that are somehow beyond the individual's locus of control.

References

1. Ackerknecht EH: A Short History of Psychiatry. Hafner Publishing Co, New York, 1971
2. Lipowski ZJ: Review of consultation psychiatry and psychosomatic medicine, I: general principles. Psychosom Med 29:153–171, 1967
3. Simon MA: Matter of Life: Philosophical Problems of Biology. Yale University Press, New Haven, CT, 1971
4. Engel GL: A unified concept of health and disease. Perspect Biol Med 3:459–485, 1960
5. Wolff HF: A concept of disease in man. Psychosom Med 24:25–30, 1962
6. Hinkle LE: Ecological observations of the relation of physical illness, mental illness, and the social environment. Psychosom Med 23:289–297, 1961
7. Kuhn TS: The Structure of Scientific Revolutions. University of Chicago Press, Chicago, IL, 1970
8. Fabrega H: Concepts of disease: logical features and social implications. Perspect Biol Med 15:583–616, 1972
9. Foster GA: Culture and Conquest: America's Spanish Heritage. New York, Wenner-Gren Foundation, 1960 (Viking Fund Publications in Anthropology, 27)
10. Beltran GA: Medicina y Magia. Mexico, Instituto Nacional Indigenista, 1963
11. Fabrega H: Biennial Review of Anthropology. Edited by Siegel BJ. Stanford University Press, Stanford, CA, 1971, ch 3, pp 167–229
12. Cassel J, Patrick R, Jenkins D: Epidemiological analysis of the health implications of culture change: a conceptual model. Ann NY Acad Sci 84:938, 1960
13. Fabrega H: The study of medical problems in preliterate settings. Yale J Biol Med 43:385–407, 1971
14. Fabrega H: The study of disease in relation to culture. Behav Sci 17:183–203, 1972

15. Tyler SA: Cognitive Anthropology. Holt, Rinehart & Winston, New York, 1969
16. Metzger D, Williams G: Some procedures and results in the study of native categories: Tzeltal "Firewood." Amer Anthrop 68:389–407, 1966
17. Fabrega H, Metzger D, Williams G: Psychiatric implications of health and illness in a Maya Indian group: a preliminary statement. Soc Sci Med 3:609–626, 1970
18. Fabrega H: Dynamics of medical practice in a folk community. Milbank Mem Fund Q 48:391–412, 1970
19. Fabrega H: Some features of Zinacantecan medical knowledge. Ethnology 9:25–43, 1971
20. Fabrega H, Metzger D: Psychiatric illness in a small ladino community. Psychiatry 31:339–351, 1968
21. Kiev A: Magic, Faith, and Healing. The Free Press of Glencoe, New York, 1964
22. Frank JD: Persuasion and Healing. Schocken Books, New York, 1963
23. Goffman E: The Presentation of Self in Everyday Life. Doubleday, Garden City, NY, 1959
24. Engel GL: Sudden death and the "medical model" in psychiatry. Can Psychiatr Assoc J 15:527–538, 1970
25. Lipowski ZJ: Psychosocial aspects of disease. Ann Intern Med 71:1197–1206, 1969
26. Foster GM: Relationships between Spanish and Spanish-American folk medicine. J Amer Folklore 66:201–218, 1953
27. Harwood A: The hot-cold theory of disease. JAMA 216:1153–1158, 1971
28. Zborowski M: People in Pain. Jossey-Bass, San Francisco, CA, 1969
29. Zola IK: Culture and symptoms: an analysis of patients' presenting complaints. Amer Sociol Rev 31:615–630, 1966

CHAPTER 13

Socio-Ecological Stress, Suppressed Hostility, Skin Color, and Black-White Male Blood Pressure
Detroit

ERNEST HARBURG, PH.D.,
JOHN C. ERFURT, B.A.,
LOUISE S. HAUENSTEIN, PH.D.,
CATHERINE CHAPE, M.A.,
WILLIAM J. SCHULL, PH.D., AND
M. A. SCHORK, PH.D.

Prefatory Remarks

Kathleen C. Light, Ph.D.

A new generation has been born and grown to adulthood since the 1967 Detroit riots were a source of national attention and concern. When Detroit smoldered in 1967, other communities of our nation awoke and looked at themselves, trying to see if the same tensions and angers were lying below the surfaces of their everyday routine, suppressed but potentially explosive. When Los Angeles exploded in much the same way in the 1990s, a similar nationwide period of awakening and self-scrutiny began.

Harburg and his associates began their bold effort to study the social issues of sudden violent action by disadvantaged people in poor neighborhoods during this climate of heightened public awareness. Their goal was to use a simple and easily verified physiological measure—blood pressure—to provide objective evidence of the greater burden of life stresses experienced by these people, because of their lesser socioeconomic resources, because of the neighborhoods in which they had to live, and because of their skin color. Furthermore, Harburg and his colleagues attempted to weave together the threads of the literature on the clinical psychology and health implications of suppressed hostility with their understanding of the practicalities of survival as a poor black male in an inner-city neighborhood, where fears of arousing the attention of criminals or of the police were equally great.

This work was so broad in its scope that it has influenced widely disparate areas of research in the years since its publication. Included in these areas are epidemiological research on social-environmental factors associated with elevated blood pressure in blacks and whites alike,[1,2] and research on racial/ethnic differences in cardiovascular stress reactivity.[3] The study's impact was also substantial in regard to the linkage of anger and hostility to increased risk of hypertension and coronary heart disease. It is especially compelling that, although the type A behavior pattern has undoubtedly been the focus of greater scientific attention, many investigators employing type A assessments in their research have recently reported that the hostility component of the type A pattern appears to show the strongest association to cardiovascular health outcomes.[4,5]

To name this work by Harburg and associates as a classic is to confirm the obvious, which is that these scientists chose an important issue to study, examined this issue with appropriate rigor, and then wrote about their findings with clarity and insight. The enduring message of this article derives from these strengths, but particularly from the fact that the social and economic factors that inspired this work to begin in the late 1960s are still with us. Dealing with these factors, both scientifically and politically, remains current in the 1990s and will almost certainly do so into the 21st century.

References

1. Cruickshank JL, Beevers DG: Epidemiology of hypertension: blood pressure in blacks and whites. Clin Sci 62:1–21, 1982
2. Johnson EH: Behavioral factors associated with hypertension in black Americans, in Behavioral Factors in Hypertension: Handbook of Hypertension, Vol 9. Edited by Julius S, Bassett DR. New York, Elsevier, 1987, pp 181–197
3. Anderson NB, McNeilly M, Myers H: Toward understanding race difference in autonomic reactivity: a proposed contextual model, in Individual Differences in Cardiovascular Response to Stress. Edited by Turner JR, Sherwood A, Light KC. New York, Plenum, 1992, pp 125–146
4. Dembroski TM, MacDougall TM, Costa PT, et al: Components of hostility as predictors of sudden death and myocardial infarction in the multiple risk factor intervention trial. Psychosom Med 51:514–522, 1989
5. Houston BK, Chesney MA, Black GW, et al: Behavioral clusters and coronary heart disease risk. Psychosom Med 54:447–461, 1992

Four areas in Detroit were selected by factor analysis of all census tracts as varying widely in socio-ecological stressor conditions. High Stress areas were marked by rates of low socio-economic status, high crime, high density, high residential mobility, and high rates of marital breakup; Low Stress areas showed the converse conditions. All areas were racially segregated. The sample in each area provided about 125 married males, living with spouse, aged 25–60, with relatives in the city. Blood pressure levels were highest among Black High Stress males and showed no difference among Black Low Stress and White areas. Suppressed Hostility (keeping anger in when attacked and feeling guilt if one's anger is displayed when attacked) was related to high blood pressure levels and percent hypertensive for Black High Stress and White Low Stress males; Black Low Stress men with high pressures were associated with anger in but denying guilt. White High Stress high reading were most associated with guilt after anger. For Blacks, skin color was related positively to blood pressure and High Stress males had darker skin color than Black middle class males. Black High Stress men with dark skin color and suppressed hostility had the highest average blood pressure of all four race-area groups.

Introduction

The data in this paper are taken from a project entitled "Stress and Heredity in Black-White Blood Pressure Differences."[1] The purpose of the project is to test environmental and genetic aspects of the well known fact that American Negroes have higher blood pressure levels, and higher morbidity and mortality from hypertension, hypertensive heart disease, and stroke than their White compatriots.[2,3] The causes of most instances of high blood pressure are unknown; however evidence for the idea that inhibited, contained, or restricted anger is associated with higher blood pressure has been cited often.[4,5] This report presents new evidence collected on Black and White married males residing in High and Low Stress areas in Detroit. The hypothesis is that coping responses which indicate Suppressed Hostility are related to high blood pressure.

The major concept of Suppressed Hostility used in this paper is taken from Newcomb, who argues that the process of keeping feelings or ideas "repressed" in the Freudian sense is (a) learned in its origins through social interaction, and (b) has social consequences which are manifest in behavior and communication.[6] The indicators of suppression therefore are amenable to observations during social situations which induce emotional and behavioral response. The term "suppressed" in Newcomb's view indicates that the person may be aware, in varying degrees, of hiding hostile feelings in social situations of high arousal, such as when attack is viewed as noxious.

Noxious stimuli usually elicit hostility.[7] It is necessary however that such stimuli be appraised as noxious in order to arouse hostility. A series of studies indicate that when the aggressive behavior of others is perceived as "justified," there is less anger and hostility response than when the aggression is viewed as "arbitrary."[8,9] This appraisal applies to one's own behavior as well as to the behavior of others. If one's own delivery of noxious stimuli is felt to be justified, then the accompanying hostility is felt to be morally correct either at the time or later. Conversely, if display of hostility is judged to be improper, then feelings of guilt arise, which act to inhibit expression of hostility. For some persons, their training to inhibit hostility may be so strong, they feel guilt *later* even if their displayed hostility at the time of arbitrary attack is felt to be justified. This is especially so when the attacker is high in legitimate authority and control of resources, e.g., policeman, boss, parent.

By Suppressed Hostility, therefore, we refer to a coping process of inhibiting negative attitudes in situations where the person is the target of appraised noxious stimuli (attack) from a source of power. Operationally, suppressing hostility to such an attack involves (a) not overtly displaying hostility to the attacker, and (b) feeling that such display should arouse guilt.

That chronic suppression of hostility is related to higher levels of blood pressure has been observed fairly consistently, using interview alone[10] or with other clinical methods on persons with hypertensive levels[11] and by experimental modes on normotensives.[12, 13] More recently a series of studies clearly indicate that standardized forms of attack can elicit significant rises in blood pressure[14] for Whites and Blacks.[15] In the present study, our concern is with home blood pressure level at a point in time and with its sociopsychological correlates. While the literature on patients suggests that Suppressed Hostility is associated with higher blood pressure levels, either chronically or as a reactive state, it is not clear what kinds of coping patterns are related to the normotensive levels of "normal" adults in daily life attack situations.

There have been many historical and social analyses which assert that, due to the cultural traditions of slavery and subsequent social oppression of Negro Americans,[16] Black males in American society are forced repeatedly into social positions and situations where they are attacked yet must restrain their expressions of hostility.[17, 18] These analyses hold that in urban areas, such situations are chronic for the lower income, working class Black males residing in high crime areas where the police tend to be perceived as sources of arbitrary aggression; this in turn arouses anger and hostility which would be punished if displayed. Similar conditions and perceptions probably also prevail for White males in low income, high crime areas. For both workers and middle class Blacks, not only the policeman, but the White homeowner who refuses to sell on racial grounds can be appraised as insulting and noxious, thereby inducing hostility which might worsen the situation if displayed. Again, refusal to sell a desired house can also be directed at Whites, for their nationality or religion, even though this occurs less frequently. In sum, for members of certain social statuses, which can be defined by race, sex, and residence, the role relationships of "Citizen and Police," and "House Buyer and Seller," may increase stressor conditions and the use of certain coping responses, such as Suppressed Hostility.

The major objectives of this present inquiry then are 1. to describe the social distribution of types of coping patterns, e.g., Suppressed Hostility, by race-residence groups in an urban area among married males, and 2. to relate such patterns to their health consequences, i.e., blood pressure levels. Specifically, the major hypotheses are as follows: 1. Suppressed Hostility will vary between High and Low Stress residents, 2. between Blacks and Whites, and 3. will be related to higher levels of blood pressure.

Method

Selection of High and Low Stress Areas

The first objective was to select residence areas in Detroit which varied in extremes of High Stressor and Low Stressor conditions relative to the city.[19] Rates were computed for each of 382 census tracts in Detroit on 1965 data for variables reflecting the concepts of economic deprivation, residential instability, family instability, crime, and density. It is assumed that such combined rates, at their endpoints, indicate social environments which vary objectively in chronic exposure to stressor events. The rates per census tract were factor analyzed and the 382 tracts were each assigned factor scores[20] for the two emergent factors: Socioeconomic Status (SES) and Instability. Data, not shown, indicate that the final selection of four primary study areas (Black High and Low Stress, White High and Low Stress) *were in the extreme quartiles* of factor scores. Table 13–1 shows actual rates of the study tracts after selection on the basis of factor scores.

Table 13–1. Rates for primary stress areas, Detroit, 1965[a]

Characteristics Total Dwelling Units:	Black		White	
	High Stress N = 4118	Low Stress 1910	High Stress 4410	Low Stress 1811
A. Socioeconomic Variables				
1. Median income	$4,627	$8,670	$5,417	$8,030
2. Median education (years)	9.6 yrs	13.2 yrs	9.0 yrs	11.7 yrs
3. % Unemployed	4%	0%	0%	0%
4. % Home ownership	19%	92%	40%	90%
5. % Professional/managerial	9%	49%	7%	19%
B. Instability Variables				
1. Adult crime rate (per 10,000)	89.0	55.9	60.0	9.9
2. Juvenile crime rate (per 10,000)	17.2	6.4	13.5	1.3
3. Marital stability[b]	1:2.9	.00	1:12	.00
4. % in residence 5 years or more	27%	51%	48%	86%

[a] These data are from a 4% sample of the City of Detroit by the Transportation and Land Use Study, except for crime data supplied by the City of Detroit Police Department.
[b] This is a ratio of the number of separations and divorces to the number of marriages.

The rates show predicted sharp differences between High and Low Stress across median income, median education, crime rates, and marital breakup. This same pattern is revealed in other rates (not shown), e.g., school truancy, "drop-outs," welfare registration, Aid to Dependent Children, and so forth.

Selection of the Sample

One major purpose of the larger Project was to estimate the relative contributions of stress and heredity blood pressure levels. The Stress Area Sample then in this report consists of persons: 1. residing in one of the four stress areas; 2. of a given race, Black or White; 3. aged between 25 and 60 years; 4. married and living with spouse; and 5. having relatives (siblings and first cousins) in the Metropolitan area. The sampling and interviewing was carried out in two stages. First, in *Stage I,* a door-to-door *census* was taken in each of the four Stress Areas to classify potential sample members. The census refusal rate was about 2–3% in each area. Next, each person classified as having the five sample traits already described (potential sample member) was visited by a trained interviewer. This *verification* interview checked the criteria traits of the person and data on the relatives. If verified, we requested the person's cooperation in the study, and arranged an interview by a nurse. In *Stage II,* trained nurses of the same race as the respondent were then randomly assigned to interview the randomly selected persons residing in High and Low Stress areas, changing the area each week for each nurse. The refusal rate for nurses was similar across all areas and averaged about 4%.

The final sample of married males having the desired traits within each of the four race-stress area groups, and the design of the analysis, is shown below.

Measure of Blood Pressure

All nurse-interviewers were carefully screened through a minimum of 20 hr of training in both survey technique and a standard blood pressure technique[21]

	Black Males		White Males	
	High Stress $N=118$	Low Stress 134	High Stress 120	Low Stress 120
Mean age (yrs.)	40	39	40	43
Mean weight (lbs.)	176	181	176	181

for the nine-month data collection (October, 1968–June 1969). A reading was taken at the start of the interview, another about five to ten minutes later, and a third about ten minutes later during the first half hour of medical history and before the sociopsychological items. A standard new mercury sphygmomanometer (Baumanometer) was used, with Velcro cuff at heart level, and all parts were checked each day for effectiveness.[22] Nurse performance was quality controlled at various time-points during the data collection by double stethoscope readings with the supervisor. Readings in the home were taken on the left arm, with the respondent seated and arm resting on a table. First, a palpatory pressure was read to relax the person and to allow the nurse to estimate the initial systolic reading. Next, an auscultatory reading was taken; systolic was recorded at the first sound, and diastolic at the cessation of sound, or fifth Korotkoff point. A Latin-Square design was executed before field work by 15 nurses on 15 subjects in a classroom setting to test for both (a) nurse, and (b) instrument differences. No significant differences were found for either main effect for either systolic or diastolic pressures. However, digit-preference differences were present, with the usual preference for "0." Our design required that blood pressure readings be calculated as the mean of the first three readings. This statistically minimized digit preference differences in subsequent analyses and reduced the errors of instability from a single, casual reading.

Analyses are performed with two dependent variables, Mean Diastolic and 4 Category Diastolic: *Mean Diastolic*—mean of the first three diastolic readings (fifth phase) taken in the first half hour of interview, about 10 minutes apart; *4 Category Diastolic*—groupings having clinical import, (a) ≤83 mm; (b) 84–89 mm; (c) 90–94 mm; and (d) 95+ mm. These are coded as Low Normal, Normal, Borderline, and Hypertensive. The category "95+ mm" Diastolic is labeled "Hypertensive" and regardless of which indicator (level or category) is used, they are both indicators of higher risk of mortality from coronary and cerebral attacks.[3, 23] The analysis is based on diastolic pressure because it is highly correlated with systolic and prior experimental studies indicate greater diastolic reactivity to attack.[12, 13, 15, 24, 25]

Measurement of Skin Color

In a Pilot Survey (1966–67) and in this Major Study, skin color was rated on a four-point scale by the nurse-interviewers. The four points were for Blacks/Whites: 1. "Very Light/Fair (white)," 2. "Somewhat Light (tan)/Somewhat Fair," 3. "Somewhat Dark (brown)/Somewhat Dark," and 4. "Very Dark (brown or black)/Dark." The nurses were instructed to choose a person whom they knew who had the rank-order of skin color specified by the scale, and use this person's image as a standard for comparing with the respondent. They were told to take the area on the forehead between the eyes as the target skin area. In each field study, Pilot and Major, the four points showed a symmetrical distribution. As to validity, in each field study a Genetic Distance Scale was significantly related to height, a trait with known high heritability. This same Genetic Scale was related to ratings of skin color for Blacks in both the Pilot and Major Study.[26, 27]

Measure of Coping Patterns and Suppressed Hostility

These items are developed from earlier work[28, 29] and were structured as follows: *Attack by Policeman*—"Now imagine that you were doing something outside and a policeman got angry or blew up at you for something that wasn't your fault. How would you feel?" and, *Attack by Houseowner*—"Now imagine that you were searching to find another place to live in, and finally found one for sale or rent which you liked, but the owner told you that he would not sell or rent to you because of your religion or national origin or race. How would you feel about that?" The response categories for both items were as follows: "1. I'd get angry or mad and show it, 2. I'd get annoyed and show it, 3. I'd get annoyed, but would keep it in, 4. I'd get angry or mad, but would keep it in, 5. I wouldn't feel angry or annoyed." After each item a measure of moral feeling was also asked: "Now suppose you got angry or mad at the (owner) and *showed* (him/her) you felt this way. How would you feel about it *later* if you did this?" and the responses were: "1. I'd feel very guilty or sorry, 2. I'd feel somewhat guilty or sorry, 3. I'd feel a little guilty or sorry, and 4. I wouldn't feel at all guilty or sorry."

Following Funkenstein, King, and Drolette[12] the categories were next recoded into dichotomies: for the Attack items, "Anger Out" (codes 1 plus 2) and "Anger In" (codes 3, 4, 5); and the Guilt items "Guilt" (codes 1, 2, 3) and "No Guilt" (code 4). We then constructed nominal variables to describe coping patterns which are labeled "Anger-Guilt" (to Policeman or Houseowner) with this four-category code: 1. Anger Out/No Guilt, 2. Anger Out/Guilt, 3. Anger In/No Guilt, and 4. Anger In/Guilt. The first code is the operational definition for "Expressed Hostility;" the last code is for "Suppressed Hostility." Each code category is *not* an additive Index score; it refers to a subset which contains all the persons who gave the indicated two responses to the given situation. The use of Funkenstein et al.'s terms of "Anger In" and "Anger Out" is solely for ease of labeling; we did not measure the biological responses of anger.

Results

Stress Area Characteristics

Certain characteristics of the four Stress Area Samples which pertain specifically to Detroit should be described. The *White Low Stress* sample is a few years older on the average than the other area samples, is three-fourths Catholic, resides in an all-White area, 84% were raised in the Detroit area, and they average about 10 years in their residence. These traits are shared with a wider Northeastern area where this tract is located. (Detroit is about 35% Catholic.) Other data, not shown, indicate strong anti-Black biases in this populace. Almost conversely, the *Black Low Stress* sample is younger, is 91% Protestant, resides in an area which in 1960 was all White and in 1970 was almost all Black; 80% have lived there less than 5 years. Furthermore, 72% of the wives are working, either full or part-time, and 21% of them as professionals or managers. It must be added that this tract area in 1965 was not only at the top 1% of all Black tracts on our Socioeconomic Status factor scores, but was also in the top 5% for *all* 382 tracts in Detroit. This group is an historically new Black middle class—new social migrants to their "socioecological niche." The *White High Stress* sample is half Protestant, half Catholic, mostly workers, one-third from the South, one-fourth in apartment houses (about 65% of Detroiters reside in single-family dwelling units). Both White areas were 99+% White in 1960 *and* in 1970, even though the Black population of Detroit rose from 28% to 44% in this decade. For the *Black High Stress* sample, as expected, this area shows the lowest median income, Occupational Prestige Score, and home ownership, and shows the highest percent operatives and laborers, and percent family head unemployed (even in 1968). The usual discrepancy of higher education and lower income relative to the White working class is also present. Residential mobility appears as high as the White High Stress—over two-fifths have changed residences within five years. There are other data which allow us to assume that much of this movement is either within the area or from equivalent areas in Detroit,[30] especially for the Blacks moving from the path of "urban renewal." Finally, it should be noted that the Black High Stress area is contiguous to the "12th Street" tract in which the "Detroit Rebellion" erupted in 1967, and where the Pilot Study was done in 1966–67.[31]

In another report on this survey[32] evidence is presented indicating that residents of High and Low Stress areas do differ significantly in perceptions of their areas in the predicted directions. For example, (for both males and females) about 77% of the Black High Stress persons and over 50% of the White High

Stress persons desired to move to a different neighborhood, compared with about one-fourth of persons in the Low Stress tracts. High Stress persons reported 2 ½ times more likelihood of being "beaten or robbed when out at night," 6 times more hearing of "fights with weapons" last year and 3 times more hearing of a "person assaulted or beaten," than did their Low Stress counterparts. Blacks reported 4 to 5 times more likelihood of arbitrary anger from Police than Whites. The Black High Stress area lies within the area sampled in the "after-riot" and "one-year later" studies by the Detroit Free Press; each survey showed that about 65% of the residents felt that Detroit "police brutality" was a major reason for the 1967 outburst.[33] The next major reasons were (in 1968) overcrowded living conditions (55%), poor housing (54%), and lack of jobs (45%). Finally, in the present study, chances of Houseowners refusing to sell because of the respondent's religion, national origin, or race was "somewhat, fairly or very likely" among 65% of the Blacks in both stress areas, 13% of the White High Stress and 4% of the White Low Stress areas.

Stress Area and Blood Pressure

Next, in regard to blood pressure differences, results of the present survey show that in all comparisons between blood pressure levels in High and Low Stress areas, for males and females, Black and White, the systolic and diastolic averages (adjusted for age, overweight, and other variables) were higher for residents of the High Stress areas.[32] Further, the Black High Stress males had significantly higher blood pressure levels than Black Low Stress males, who in turn showed equivalent readings for three of four comparisons with White males. Black High Stress males also had the highest blood pressure levels (and White Low Stress females had the lowest) of all eight race-sex-residence groups. It should be noted that for males, higher blood pressure levels were related to "being raised in Detroit" rather than being migrant; this relationship was significant for Blacks. The rest of this paper concerns the relationship of Suppressed Hostility to blood pressure for Black and White, High and Low Stress males, with emphasis on Black High Stress males.

Anger, Guilt, and Blood Pressure

Before examining the coping patterns of Expressed and Suppressed Hostility, we should first describe the main effects of its component responses—Anger and Guilt—and blood pressure by attack roles. Table 13–2 examines the relationship of mean diastolic blood pressure to each of the separate attack roles and response variables among the four social groups. For the Black High Stress men, blood pressure levels are higher for Anger In and for Guilt responses to

Table 13-2. Response to attacker role and mean diastolic (mm) and percent hypertensive (95+) by race and stress area

Attacker role and reaction	Black								White							
	High Stress				Low Stress				High Stress				Low Stress			
	(N=118)	$\bar{X}$	SD	% 95+	(N=118)	$\bar{X}$	SD	% 95+	(N=118)	$\bar{X}$	SD	% 95+	(N=118)	$\bar{X}$	SD	% 95+
A. Policeman																
Anger Out	85	84.4	10.5	16	100	82.6	10.5	12	85	80.7	9.3	11	87	81.8	11.5	13
Anger In	33	88.6	13.4	27	34	82.7	9.9	15	35	81.6	12.6	17	33	82.2	11.1	15
t =		1.82[b]				0.07				0.43				0.18		
No Guilt	87	84.1	10.2	17	97	83.5	11.2	15	63	78.7	9.9	10	66	81.8	11.4	12
Guilt	31	89.6	13.9	26	37	80.3	7.5	5	57	83.5	10.3	16	54	81.9	11.3	15
t =		2.32[a]				1.62[c]				2.61[a]				0.05		
B. Houseowner																
Anger Out	69	85.2	10.1	17	86	81.2	8.6	8	66	79.4	8.8	8	88	80.9	10.8	13
Anger In	49	86.1	13.3	22	48	85.3	12.5	21	54	83.0	11.7	19	32	84.7	12.5	16
t =		0.43				2.22[a]				1.94[b]				1.64[b]		
No Guilt	87	84.7	10.3	17	105	83.2	11.0	15	80	79.5	10.1	9	92	81.3	11.1	11
Guilt	31	87.8	14.3	26	29	80.5	7.2	3	40	84.1	10.2	20	28	83.9	11.9	21
t =		1.29[c]				1.26				2.33[a]				1.08		

[a] $p < 0.02$ (1-tail)
[b] $p < 0.05$ (1-tail)
[c] $p < 0.10$ (1-tail)

both attack roles, as are the percent Hypertensive (95+ mm.). These differences however only approach statistical significance for the Police role. For the Black Low Stress men, singular results appear in that those reporting hypothetical No Guilt show higher levels of blood pressure and of 95+ readings; however their Anger In responses continue to show high readings. For Whites, men in both High and Low Stress living areas follow the same trends as do the Black High Stress men, that is, higher levels for Anger In and for Guilt.

For both attack roles, significant responses within groups can be seen most clearly for Black High Stress males toward the Policeman, and for White High Stress males toward the Houseowner who discriminates. Across all four groups, Guilt to the Police and Anger In to the Houseowner appear most significant. As a summary statistical test, a count of the number of times the percent Hypertensive (95+ mm) appears higher in the predicted direction shows this ranking occurs in 14 of the 16 tests ($p < 0.002$), with the remaining two responses consistent in the No Guilt direction for the Black middle class. (This probability was calculated from the formula

$$p(r \text{ successes}/N, p) = \binom{N}{r} p^r q^{N-r}$$

The values used were

$$p(14/16, p = 0.50) = \binom{16}{14} 0.50^{14}\, 0.50^2$$

The null hypothesis is that a greater proportion of hypertensives were no more likely to occur in Anger In or Guilt groups than in Anger Out or No Guilt groups.*

Coping Patterns of Anger and Guilt: Distributions

Having observed that the Anger and Guilt components are, in general, related to blood pressure, we can now examine their logical combinations, or coping patterns. The first question concerns simple distributions of Anger-Guilt coping patterns as they occur in the four race-area groups. Table 13–3 shows that variations exist in patterns between and within groups depending on the attack role. Within each race group, responses to Police attack show slight Stress Area differences. Across groups, however, Blacks report more Anger Out-No Guilt pattern (Expressed Hostility), while White males express more Anger Out-Guilt. This latter pattern may reflect a stronger norm among Whites than Blacks that

---

*See Hays WL: Statistics for Psychologists. New York, Holt, Rinehart & Winston, 1963.

Table 13–3. Coping patterns by attacker role, race, and stress area

Pattern variable: Attacker role and coping pattern	Black				White			
	High Stress		Low Stress		High Stress		Low Stress	
	%	(N)	%	(N)	%	(N)	%	(N)
A. Policeman								
(1) Anger Out-No Guilt	58	(69)	56	(76)	41	(49)	42	(50)
(2) Anger Out-Guilt	14	(16)	18	(24)	30	(36)	31	(37)
(3) Anger In-No Guilt	15	(18)	16	(21)	12	(14)	13	(16)
(4) Anger In-Guilt	13	(15)	10	(13)	17	(21)	14	(17)
Total	100%	(118)	100%	(134)	100%	(120)	100%	(120)
Chi-Square:	N.S.				N.S.			
	Black vs. White: $p < 0.05$ (all comparisons)							
B. Houseowner								
(1) Anger Out-No Guilt	50	(60)	56	(75)	42	(51)	60	(72)
(2) Anger Out-Guilt	8	(9)	8	(11)	13	(15)	13	(16)
(3) Anger In-No Guilt	23	(27)	23	(30)	24	(29)	17	(20)
(4) Anger In-Guilt	19	(22)	13	(18)	21	(25)	10	(12)
Total	100%	(118)	100%	(134)	100%	(120)	100%	(120)
Chi-Square:	N.S.				9.84; $p < 0.02$			
	Black vs. White: N.S. (all comparisons)							

Policemen (in 1968) should be treated with respect at all costs. Toward the Houseowner's discrimination, however, both Black and White Low Stress men are similar. Again, White High Stress men show the least Expressed Hostility of the four groups. For both attack roles, there is a tendency for the High Stress area males to report more use of Anger In and Suppressed Hostility than their counterparts in the Low Stress areas. It is also important to note that for the entire sample, 40–60% of the men reported the Expressed Hostility pattern toward both attack roles, and that only about 10–20% responded with Suppressed Hostility. We will return later to the question of consistency of responses across role-situations.

Coping Patterns and Blood Pressure

Now we can examine the major question: what are the blood pressure readings for those persons showing Suppressed Hostility as they compare with persons showing other Anger-Guilt patterns, and especially that of Expressed Hostility?

Figure 13–1 allows a visual examination of the data presented in Table 13–4. Three patterns are revealed: First, for Black High Stress and for White middle class men, higher blood pressure readings occur for persons reporting Suppressed Hostility; second, Black middle class men with coping responses of Anger In-No Guilt show higher blood pressure levels; and third, for White working class, Guilt seems more related to blood pressure levels than does Anger. Again a summary test shows that in six of the eight comparisons, men with the Suppressed Hostility pattern have a higher percentage of hypertensives than do the groups with Expressed Hostility ($p < 0.11$).** Again the exception is the Black Low Stress group.

Suppressed Hostility (its components or as a pattern variable) can be conceived as both a role-situational response and a consistent personal response across role situations. Criteria are lacking as to how many and what types of role situations must be tested before degree of personal consistency can be defined. Our data indicate that for Black High Stress males ($N = 118$), the average diastolic level for a subset of men who report Anger In to *both* Police and Houseowner attack roles ($N = 22$ or 19%) and another subset reporting Guilt after hostility in *both* situations ($N = 17$ or 14%) is, in each case, 91.1 mm, or Borderline Hypertensive. This level is significantly different ($p < 0.05$, 1-tail) in comparison to those who show Anger Out to *both* attack roles, 85.5 mm, ($N = 58$ or 49%), or in a separate test, No Guilt to *both* attack roles, 84.2 mm ($N = 73$ or 62%). Similar results apply to White Low Stress men for Anger In to *both* attack roles ($p < 0.02$; 1-tail) and lie in the predicted direction but are not significant for Guilt to both attacks. For White High Stress men, results are significant only for Guilt after hostility to *both* attacks ($p < 0.02$; 1-tail).

Coping Responses, Skin Color, and Blood Pressure

Prior results had shown that a measure of skin color was related to blood pressure levels for Blacks in a statistically significant, moderate, and linear manner,[34, 32] especially clear for Black males. In the present survey, skin color was also related to Stress Area, such that High Stress Black males (and females) had ratings of significantly darker skins than Low Stress Blacks (gamma, +0.23; chi-square: 9.37; $p < 0.05$). Degree of skin color in American society is another strong status indicator (besides race, income level, and occupation) which is associated with sociopsychological stressor conditions, i.e., the darker the skin, the more chance for discrimination and prejudice. The question was asked,

---

**The exact test formula is: $p\ (6/8,\ p = 0.50) = \binom{8}{6} 0.50^6\ 0.50^2$; Hays, op.

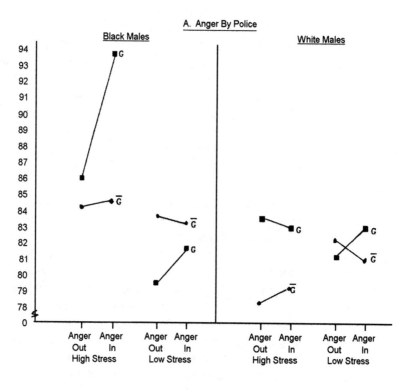
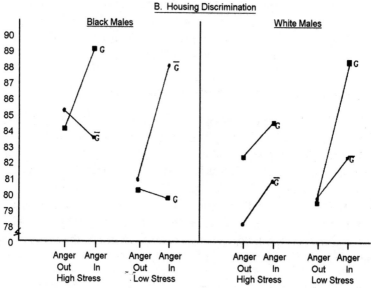

Figure 13–1. Coping patterns and mean diastolic blood pressure (mm) by attack role, race and stress area; ■—■ G(Some Guilt), ●—● G̅(No Guilt).

Table 13-4. Coping patterns and mean diastolic (mm) and percent hypertensive (95+) by attacker role, race, and stress area

Pattern variable:	Black								White							
	High Stress				Low Stress				High Stress				Low Stress			
Attacker role and coping pattern	(N=118)	$\bar{X}$	SD	% 95+	(N=118)	$\bar{X}$	SD	% 95+	(N=118)	$\bar{X}$	SD	% 95+	(N=118)	$\bar{X}$	SD	% 95+
A. Policeman																
(1) Anger Out-No Guilt	69	84.0	10.1	16	76	83.6	11.5	16	49	78.6	8.6	8	50	82.1	11.9	12
(2) Anger Out-Guilt	16	85.8	12.3	21	24	79.5	5.8	7	36	83.7	9.6	14	37	81.4	11.0	13
(3) Anger In-No Guilt	18	84.4	10.8	19	21	83.3	10.1	7	14	79.3	13.9	14	16	81.1	10.3	13
(4) Anger In-Guilt	15	93.7	14.8	33	13	81.8	10.0	15	21	83.2	11.7	19	17	83.2	12.1	18
$F =$		3.13[b]				1.02				2.27				<1		
t(1 vs 4) =		3.03[a]				0.56				1.75[b]				0.36		
B. Houseowner																
(1) Anger Out-No Guilt	60	85.3	9.6	17	75	81.2	9.1	9	51	78.4	8.3	4	72	80.9	10.9	13
(2) Anger Out-Guilt	9	84.3	13.2	19	11	80.8	5.1	22	15	82.6	10.2	18	16	80.7	10.5	8
(3) Anger In-No Guilt	27	83.5	11.8	27	30	88.2	13.7	22	29	81.3	12.7	18	20	82.6	12.1	8
(4) Anger In-Guilt	22	89.2	14.7	27	18	80.3	8.4	6	25	84.9	10.3	20	12	88.3	12.8	33
$F =$		1.08				4.09[a]				2.49				1.54		
t(1 vs 4) =		1.38[c]				0.36				2.63[a]				2.09[a]		

[a] $p < 0.02$ (1-tail)
[b] $p < 0.05$ (1-tail)
[c] $p < 0.10$ (1-tail)

therefore, whether the status combination for Black males, of High Stress residence area, darker skin, and certain emotional responses to attack, might isolate a subset of persons with higher blood pressure levels than revealed by combinations of variables already presented. For this analysis, the four-point variable of skin color was dichotomized to yield a two-point "Light" and "Dark" scale to provide sufficient numbers in each cell.

From data in Table 13–5 it seems clear that darker skin color is related to higher blood pressure levels; that the patterns of Dark-Guilt and Dark-Anger In result in the highest level in each four-pattern comparison across both attacker roles; and that these persons show significantly higher levels than do Dark-No Guilt or Dark-Anger Out persons. However, the percent Hypertensive in this high pressure pattern does not differ from percents already reported for prior-reported emotional responses, namely 25%–33%. When high blood pressure is defined to include Borderline (90+ mm), then the increases in percent do appear.

Table 13–6 presents the resultant patterns formed by combining skin color, Anger, and Guilt responses. We were not trying to account for all the patterns, especially for patterns numbered 2 and 3 with small N's. The predictions are indicated by the four t-test comparisons. First, for both Police and Houseowner, blood pressure levels were higher for dark-skinned males who suppressed hostility than for lighter skinned males who expressed hostility (t-test, 1 vs 8). Second, contrary to prediction, among light-skinned Blacks, for both attacker roles, there is no difference between Expressed and Suppressed Hostility (t-test, 1 vs 4); however, among dark-skinned males, these differences were as expected (t-test, 5 vs 8). Third, men with dark skin and Suppressed Hostility had higher levels than did those with light skin and Suppressed Hostility (t-test, 4 vs 8). Fourth, blood pressure levels of dark-skinned men with Anger In was higher for those who also felt Guilt than for those who did not (t-test, 7 vs 8). Taking the criteria of 95+ mm and 90+ mm (high blood pressure) the direction of results is similar to that for mean levels.

Effects of Age and Overweight

As a final analysis (data not shown), because both age and percent overweight are known correlates of blood pressure, we assessed the effects of these two variables on the relationship of the Anger-Guilt variables and blood pressure. For Low Stress males, both Black and White, adjustments for age and overweight indicate that the significant relationships of the components Anger and Guilt, related separately to blood pressure in Table 13–4, were not affected by overweight, but were affected by age adjustments, i.e., for Low Stress men only, the relations apply more to older than to younger men. When Tables 13–5 and 13-6 were retested using blood pressure adjusted (by regression) for age and overweight, the results were unchanged.

Discussion

The trend of data indicates that the components of Suppressed Hostility—not displaying hostility when arbitrarily attacked, and feeling guilty about dis-

Table 13-5. Skin color, attack response and mean diastolic (mm) and percent diastolic category by attacker role for black high stress males

Pattern variable: Attacker role, respondent's skin color and response	(N = 118)	$\bar{X}$	SD	% 95+ mm	% 90+ mm
A. Policeman					
(1) Light-No Guilt	31	82.9	9.7	19%	29%
(2) Light-Guilt	11	82.9	11.5	27	27
(3) Dark-No Guilt	56	84.8	10.5	16	34
(4) Dark-Guilt	20	93.3	14.0	25	60
	$F = 4.15^a$				
	$t(1 \text{ vs } 4) = 3.28^a$ $t(3 \text{ vs } 4) = 2.94^a$				
(1) Light-Anger Out	31	83.2	10.7	23%	32%
(2) Light-Anger In	11	81.9	8.5	18	18
(3) Dark-Anger Out	54	85.0	10.4	13	35
(4) Dark-Anger In	22	92.0	14.3	32	55
	$F = 3.30^b$				
	$t(1 \text{ vs } 4) = 2.81^a$ $t(3 \text{ vs } 4) = 2.46^a$				
B. Houseowner					
(1) Light-No Guilt	30	82.9	9.2	20%	30%
(2) Light-Guilt	12	82.8	12.5	25	25
(3) Dark-No Guilt	57	85.7	10.8	16	35
(4) Dark-Guilt	19	91.0	14.7	26	58
	$F = 2.23$				
	$t(1 \text{ vs } 4) = 2.43^a$ $t(3 \text{ vs } 4) = 1.75^b$				
(1) Light-Anger Out	25	84.2	10.3	24%	36%
(2) Light-Anger In	17	80.9	9.7	18	18
(3) Dark-Anger Out	44	85.7	10.0	14	39
(4) Dark-Anger In	32	88.8	14.3	25	44
	$F = 1.94$				
	$t(1 \text{ vs } 4) = 1.52^c$ $t(3 \text{ vs } 4) = 1.18$				

[a] $p < 0.02$ (1-tail)
[b] $p < 0.05$ (1-tail)
[c] $p < 0.10$ (1-tail)

play—are both related to higher blood pressure levels, and that Suppressed Hostility, the combination of Anger In and Guilt is more associated with higher blood pressure levels and percent hypertensive than other combinations, across married males, 25–60, with relatives in the city, residing in extremes of urban residential areas. These trends hold in general for both systolic and diastolic pressures. Black High Stress males not only had the highest blood pressure

Table 13–6. Skin color, anger-guilt patterns and mean diastolic (mm), % diastolic category (95+ mm and 90+ mm) by attacker role for high stress black males

Pattern variable: Skin Color-Anger-Guilt	($N = 118$)	$\overline{X}$	SD	% 95+ mm	% 90+ mm
A. Policeman					
(1) Light-Out-None	25	83.5	10.0	20%	32%
(2) Light-Out-Guilt	6	82.0	14.5	33	33
(3) Light-In-None	6	80.2	9.0	17	17
(4) Light-In-Guilt	5	84.0	8.2	20	20
(5) Dark-Out-None	44	84.3	10.3	14	32
(6) Dark-Out-Guilt	10	88.0	11.0	10	50
(7) Dark-In-None	12	86.5	11.3	25	42
(8) Dark-In-Guilt	10	98.5	15.2	40	70
$F = 2.58^b$					
1. $t(1-8) = 3.65^a$					
2. $t(1-4) = 0.09$; $t(5-8) = 3.69^a$					
3. $t(4-8) = 2.41^a$					
4. $t(7-8) = 2.55^a$					
B. Houseowner					
(1) Light-Out-None	21	84.3	9.6	24%	38%
(2) Light-Out-Guilt	4	83.5	15.7	25	25
(3) Light-In-None	9	79.6	7.9	11	11
(4) Light-In-Guilt	8	82.5	11.7	25	25
(5) Dark-Out-None	39	85.8	9.8	10	33
(6) Dark-Out-Guilt	5	85.0	12.7	20	60
(7) Dark-In-None	18	85.5	13.0	22	33
(8) Dark-In-Guilt	14	93.1	15.2	29	57
$F = 1.38$					
1. $t(1-8) = 2.23^a$					
2. $t(1-4) = 0.39$; $t(5-8) = 2.06^a$					
3. $t(4-8) = 2.10^a$					
4. $t(7-8) = 1.87^a$					

[a] $p < 0.02$ (1-tail)
[b] $p < 0.05$ (1-tail)
[c] $p < 0.10$ (1-tail)

levels of all groups, but those with Suppressed Hostility averaged above diastolic levels at which increased insurance "debits" are applied[35] and lie in the Borderline hypertension category, both indicating higher risks of earlier mortality.[36] This relationship was also seen for White males. Interpretation of these results raises a number of issues, some of which can only be raised but not tested by this study.

The first issue deals with the effects of residing in High and Low Stress areas or "socioecological niches" and use of coping patterns. High Stress men reported more use of Anger In than Low Stress men. A weak trend suggests that married middle aged men in High Stress areas report Suppressed Hostility more than similar men in Low Stress areas. We assumed that residents of High Stress areas would report that the possibility of arbitrary police anger and housing discrimination against themselves was higher than would be reported by persons in higher income, lower crime areas. Data, not shown, reveal that these differences and other indications of negative perceptions of their residential environs did exist, in the expected direction,[37] between Black and White High and Low Stress areas. Slightly more use of Suppressed Hostility toward hypothetical attack by Police or Houseowner in High Stress areas, therefore, may be due to adult situational factors inducing fear of punishment, and/or to early family training. It should be noted that an additive Index of Anger In (trichotomized after adding nine Anger Out/In situations) correlates with Diastolic Categories more for High Stress men ($N = 238$, gamma = 0.28; chi-square = 14.2; $p < 0.05$) than for Low Stress males ($N = 254$, gamma = 0.16; chi-square = 5.3; N.S.). Results already shown indicate that both Black and White areas contribute to this finding. Special note for further analysis must be made concerning the association for White High Stress males between Guilt and blood pressure levels. For these men, Guilt to *both* attack roles was significantly related to diastolic blood pressure levels and to Diastolic Categories (gamma = 0.44; chi-square = 21.8; $p < 0.01$).

The internal processes of Suppressed Hostility deserve further analysis to sharpen future research. Psychologically, suppression of hostility from self-awareness and display of hostility to others can be separate processes. In the former, persons can not report their awareness of hostile attitudes accompanying physiological "anger" even when arbitrarily attacked; in the latter case, regardless of awareness, such hostility is *not* displayed. We assume, following Newcomb,[6] that the person who lacks awareness must reveal this error of self-perception through overt communication and behavioral "faults" in the situation or by recall later. Chronic faults probably create heightened psychological tension for the organism through uncontrolled feedback from others. In the matter of displaying hostility or not, such omission or commission may or may not be "appropriate" to the situation, depending on various status roles and consideration of norms. When the attack or threat of attack is "massive," however, such as in *actual* Policeman and Houseowner situations, we assume a person would usually be aroused. There would then be many forms of "inappropriate" responses which would have consequences then or later for the person—for example, inappropriate hostility,[38] yielding,[39] a build-up of resentment,[28] and training in the mechanism of denial.[40]

Concerning the behavior of denial, data from the present Project reveal that higher pressures were associated with Black Low Stress males who reported "no guilt" after hypothetical display of anger to both attacker roles. We interpret this No Guilt response as a form of denial. As members of middle class society, and as leaders in the current Black Movement, these men probably did not want to report, as did many of the White middle class counterparts, that they would feel guilt over protesting an attack by Policeman or Houseowner. In the Pilot Study, Black High Stress persons who reported consistently positive evaluations of their neighborhood, early family life, present marital life, and so forth—evaluations that were opposite to those of the majority of their neighbors—also had higher blood pressure levels[1]; however, the results in the present data are mixed.

Next, viewing our results from a psychophysiological approach, data from other mammals and from humans are utilized in a theory of hypertension suggested by Henry and Cassel.[41] In this view, critical early life stressor situations are conditioned to "defense-alarm reactions" which are described as all-out mobilization of the organism's internal resources. In the stressor-exposed adult, however, repeated arousals of this alarm reaction through the organism's perception of repeated threat might lead to vascular disturbances. Other authors suggest that such vascular dysfunction might result when, "in civilized man 'defense-alarm' reactions are produced, the somatomotor component is usually more or less effectively suppressed; in other words, the originally well-coordinated somatomotor, viscerometor, and hormonal discharge pattern becomes dissociated."[42] The resultant effect over time is to place increased blood pressure load on heart and vessel. There is also the intriguing hypothesis that once elevated blood pressure levels are attained, this may react in turn to inhibit the "rage" response.[43]

The phrase "civilized man" in the above quotation could be specified to include strong early-life and adult-life conditioning to induce Suppressed Hostility responses in certain people within certain family types.[44] Such family training for males is probably: 1. more from "respectable poor" and "upward mobile" and "upper class" families, who are 2. high in religiosity, 3. high in emphasizing "harmony" in interpersonal relations, 4. high in guilt induction, 5. high in respect for upper status prestigeful, community members, and 6. the more dominant parent uses "arbitrary authority"[28, 29]—all acting to induce a coping pattern of Suppressed Hostility. If Suppressed Hostility were induced largely through familial or adult sociopsychological processes, then experimental measures of reactivity to stressors in laboratory conditions should[24, 25, 45] take into account the type of early family authority system as well as coping patterns available in the situation.

Finally, what can be learned from the results showing that darker skin color is related to blood pressure, and that darker skin and Suppressed Hostility responses appear to "interact" for High Stress Black males and relate to higher blood pressure levels? First, one must speculate about the possible physiological relations of skin color and high blood pressure, if all avenues of inquiry are to be pursued toward understanding of hypertension.[46] Next, from a sociopsychological view, strong evidence shows that being Black in the United States is associated with lower levels of occupational prestige, education, and income (e.g., Ref. 47). Correlational analysis of our data further suggests a negative association of socioeconomic status and skin color, i.e., the darker the skin, the lower the occupational level, education, and income. This holds for Black males and Black females, and interestingly, for Whites also.[32] Darker skin is also related more to residence in this study's High Stress area than in the Low Stress area. (We must also report, however, that a relationship of darker skin color with individual perception of discrimination is not found in our data.) Rated skin color, therefore, as opposed to self-rating or subjective color, can be viewed as another ascribed status which, because of its peculiar American historical context, is another stressor condition for Blacks. While this conclusion is perhaps obvious in regard to social class and residence, and in job discrimination, the further *direct* relation of skin color to blood pressure demands further inquiry within Black (*and* White) populations. In closing, we can add a note that, in this survey, while a genetic effect was positive for skin color, there is to date very little genetic effect concerning blood pressure.[27]

Summary

1. Black High Stress males showed significantly higher blood pressure levels than other race-stress area male groups.
2. Blacks showed higher percent of Anger Out-No Guilt to Police attack (about 58%) than Whites (about 41%) but there were no differences in Expressed Hostility to Houseowner discrimination. For the latter situation, White High Stress males showed lower Expressed Hostility (42%) than the other race-area groups (about 55%). High Stress males did report more

Anger In to attack than did Low Stress men.
3. Tested separately, the responses of Anger In and Guilt to both attack roles, Police and Homeowner, were related to higher blood pressure levels and to higher percent Hypertensive. However, Black Low Stress men showed a reverse pattern, namely, higher readings were related to a response of No Guilt toward both attack roles.
4. Suppressed Hostility was related to Hypertensive blood pressure category (95+ mm) for High Stress Black and White males for both attack situations. White, middle class men also showed this pattern, but most clearly in response to housing discrimination. Again, higher pressures for Black Low Stress males were exhibited for the Anger In-No Guilt coping style, while White High Stress levels were most associated with level of Guilt after anger.
5. For Blacks, darker skin color was related to higher blood pressure. For Black High Stress men, the combination of rated darker skin with Anger In or Guilt after anger showed significantly higher levels for each comparison within attack role and skin color response patterns. Prediction of percent having high blood pressure (90+ mm) was highest for High Stress darker skinned men with Suppressed Hostility.

A project as large as this must necessarily draw on the knowledge and skills of many agencies and persons. Acknowledgment of support to all is not possible; therefore, the following list is a partial one.

Initial support in the form of seed money from the Office of Research Administration of The University of Michigan was critical in allowing this project to start. Our special thanks to Dr. Rudolph Schmerl, Dr. Samuel Fox's encouragement, funds from the Center for Chronic Disease Control, U.S. Public Health Service, and Mr. Robert Thorner's administrative skills within this Center, made the pilot survey viable.

Local resources of The University of Michigan in Ann Arbor have also been utilized in various ways with an equally high degree of cooperation. Informal consultation with a core group of authorities in ecology, biostatistics, hypertension, survey methods, sampling, and human genetics has been established for the duration of the Project. The computer facilities of The University of Michigan, the Institute for Social Research, and Wayne State University, including program consultation, have been used extensively.

Active consultants to this Project include: Dr. Jeremiah Stamler, Dr. Sibley W. Hoobler, and Dr. Theodore M. Newcomb. Other persons informally consulted were: Dr. Frederick Epstein, Dr. Otis D. Duncan, Dr. J. E. Keith Smith, and Dr. John Scott. They each have contributed much to this Project. Our special thanks to Dr. Stevo Julius, Dr. Robert Smith, Dr. Adrian Ostfeld, and Dr. John Cassel.

Cooperation from local agencies in Detroit has been superb. The Visiting Nurses Association and the City Department of Health were most helpful in recruitment, and in solving minor problems. The City of Detroit, Department of Police, has furnished through its statistical units, all the crime and delinquency records requested, in an efficient and most pleasant manner. The Mayor's Committee for Community Renewal Program has been most helpful in every request for data, maps, etc., made by Project personnel. Wayne State University campus facilities and graduate students' aid were arranged by the Department of Sociology and Anthropology, which also allowed use of a field office in the department, and appointed the Project Director an Adjunct Professor. Wayne State University provided facilities for training purposes, and facilitated administrative matters. Other agencies aiding the Project were the City of Detroit Planning Commission and the Metropolitan Services Agency. Many persons in Detroit have been consulted on a variety of problems, and all have freely given of their time and ideas.

The public health nurses who actually collected the data through snow, rain and High Stress areas did an excellent job, guided by two superb nurse-supervisors: Mrs. Mildred Harvin (Pilot Study) and Mrs. Revera Munce (Major Study).

Our Detroit Advisory Committee must be thanked for their time, helpful criticisms and support: Dr. Mel Ravitz, Dr. Francis Kornegay, Dr. John Caldwell, Miss Sylvia Peabody, Dr. Leonard Moss, Dr. Ross Stagner, Dr. Robert Smock, Mr. Homer Hall, and Dr. Milton Palmer.

Appreciation must also be expressed to Mr. William Ash, the mathematician-programmer who served this project well at its inception, and to Mr. Eugene Beauregard for initial direction of field work in the Pilot Study.

Finally, we must express our appreciation for additional grants of support from the Michigan Heart Association and the National Association of Mental Health, Inc., at critical periods of work.

References

1. Harburg E, Schull WJ, Erfurt JC, et al: A family set method for estimating heredity and stress, I: a pilot survey of blood pressure among Negroes in high and low stress areas, Detroit, 1966–67. J Chron Dis 23:69–81, 1970
2. Stamler J: Lectures in Preventive Cardiology. New York, Grune & Stratton, 1967
3. Stamler J, Stamler R, Pullman TN: The Epidemiology of Hypertension. New

York, Grune & Stratton, 1967
4. Davies MH: Is high blood pressure a psychosomatic disorder? a critical review of the evidence. J Chron Dis 24:239–258, 1971
5. McGinn NF, Harburg E, Julius S, et al: A review of research on psychological correlates of blood pressure. Psych Bull 61:209–219, 1964
6. Newcomb TM: Social Psychology. New York, The Dryden Press, 1950, pp 372–374
7. Buss AH: The Psychology of Aggression. New York, Wiley and Sons, 1961
8. Pastore N: The role of arbitrariness in the frustration-aggression hypothesis. J Abnorm Soc Psychol 47:728–731, 1952
9. Rothaus P, Worchel P: The inhibition of aggression under nonarbitrary frustration. J Pers 28:108–117, 1960
10. Ayman D: The personality type of patients with arteriolar essential hypertension. Amer J Med Sci 186:213–223, 1933
11. Wolf S, Wolff HG: A summary of experimental evidence relating life stress to the pathogenesis of essential hypertension in man, in Hypertension. Edited by Bell ET. University of Minnesota Press, Minneapolis, MN, 1951
12. Funkenstein DH, King SH, Drolette M: Mastery of Stress. Harvard University Press, Cambridge, MA, 1957
13. Ax AF: The physiological differentiation between fear and anger in humans. Psychosom Med 15:433–442, 1953
14. Hokanson JE: Vascular and psychogalvanic effects of experimentally aroused anger. J Pers 29:30–39, 1961
15. Gentry WD: Bi-racial aggression: effect of verbal attack and sex-of-victim. Paper presented to Southeastern Psychological Association, Miami, 1971
16. Elkins SM: Slavery: A Problem in American Institutional and Intellectual Life. University of Chicago Press, Chicago, IL, 1959
17. Clark KB: Dark Ghetto. New York, Harper Torch, 1965
18. Grier WH, Cobbs PM: Black Rage. New York, Bantam Books, 1969
19. Erfurt J, Harburg E, Rice R: A method for selection of census tract areas differing in ecological stress (multilith report), 1970
20. Harmon HH: Modern Factor Analysis. University of Chicago Press, Chicago, IL, 1960
21. Kirkendall WM, Burton AC, Epstein FH, et al: Recommendations for human blood pressure determination by syphygmomanometers. Circulation 36:980–988, 1967; see also Weinstein BJ, Epstein FH, et al: Comparability of criteria and methods in the epidemiology of cardiovascular disease. Circulation 30:643–653, 1964
22. Wilcox J: Observer factors in the measurement of blood pressure. Nursing Research 10:4–17, 1961
23. Kannel WB, Gordon T, Schwartz MJ: Systolic versus diastolic blood pressure and risk of coronary heart disease: the Framingham Study. Amer J Cardiol 27:335–346, 1971

24. Gambaro S, Rabin AI: Diastolic blood pressure responses following direct and displaced aggression after anger arousal in high- and low-guilt subjects. J Pers Soc Psy 12:87–94, 1969
25. Schill TR: Aggression and blood pressure responses of high- and low-guilt subjects following frustration. J Consult Clin Psy 38:461, 1972
26. Schull WJ, Harburg E, Erfurt J, et al: A family set method for estimating heredity and stress, II: preliminary results of the genetic methodology in a pilot survey of Negro blood pressure, Detroit, 1966–67. J Chron Dis 23:83–92, 1970
27. Schull WJ: A family set method for estimating heredity and stress, III: heredity and blood pressure. Paper delivered at Society for Epidemiological Research Meeting, Houston, TX, May 5, 1972
28. Harburg E: Covert hostility: its social origins and relationship with overt compliance. University of Michigan, doctoral dissertation, 1962
29. Harburg E, Kasl SV, Tabor J, Cobb S: The intrafamilial transmission of rheumatoid arthritis, IV: recalled parent-child relations by rheumatoid arthritics and controls. J Chron Dis 22:223–238, 1969
30. McAllister RJ, Kaiser EJ, Butler EW: Residential mobility of blacks and whites: a national longitudinal survey. AJS 77:445–456, 1971
31. Report of the National Advisory Commission on Civil Disorders. Bantam Books, New York, 1968
32. Harburg E, Erfurt JC, Chape C, et al: Socio-ecological stress, smoking, skin color and black-white blood pressure: Detroit. Paper delivered at Michigan Cardiovascular Research Forum, Detroit, Michigan, October 15, 1971
33. Detroit Urban League: A Survey of Attitudes of Detroit Negroes After the Riot of 1967; and Return to 12th Street: A Follow-Up Survey of Attitudes of Detroit Negroes, October, 1968. Coordinated with the Detroit Free Press
34. Boyle E Jr: Biological patterns in hypertension by race, sex, body weight, and skin color. JAMA 213:1637–1643, 1970
35. Personal communication re blood pressure level from Metropolitan Life Ins. Co., 1971; see also Lew EA: Blood pressure and mortality—life insurance experience, in The Epidemiology of Hypertension. Edited by Stamler, et al, op. cit. pp 392–396
36. Julius S, Schork MA: Borderline hypertension—a critical review. J Chron Dis 23:723–754, 1971
37. Kasl SV, Harburg E: Perceptions of the neighborhood and the desire to move out. Amer Inst of Planners J 38:318–324, 1972
38. Kalis BL, Harris RE, Sokolow M, et al: Response to psychological stress in patients with essential hypertension. Amer Heart J 53:572, 1957
39. Harburg E, Julius S, McGinn NF, et al: Personality traits and behavioral patterns associated with systolic blood pressure levels in college males. J Chron Dis 17:405–414, 1964
40. Croog SH, Shapiro DS, Levine S: Denial among male heart patients. Psych

Med 33:385–395, 1971
41. Henry JP, Cassel JC: Psychosocial factors in essential hypertension: recent epidemiologic and animal experimental evidence. Amer J Epidem 90:171–200, 1969
42. Charval J, Dell P, Folkow B: Mental factors and cardiovascular diseases. Cardiologia 44:124–141, 1964 (see p 130)
43. Baccelli G, Guazzi M, Librette A, et al: Pressoceptive and chemoceptive aortic reflexes in decorticate and in decerebrate cats. Am J Physiol 298:708–714, 1965
44. McLeod JM, Harburg E, Price KO: Socialization, liking and yielding of opinions in imbalanced situations. Sociometry 29:197–212, 1966
45. Shapiro D, Crider A: Psychophysiological approaches in social psychology, in Handbook of Social Psychology, Vol III, Second Edition. Edited by Lindzey G, Aronson E. Reading, MA, 1969, pp 1–49
46. Robins AH: Skin melanin concentrations in the affective disorders: possible relationships to the catecholamine hypothesis. Psych Med 2:391–396, 1972
47. U.S. Department of Labor: Social and Economic Status of Negroes in the United States—1970. Washington, DC, U.S. Government Printing Office, (Ser P-23, No 38) 1970

CHAPTER 14

Depression in Infant Monkeys
Physiological Correlates

MARTIN REITE, M.D.,
I. CHARLES KAUFMAN, M.D.,
J. DONALD PAULEY, PH.D., AND
A. J. STYNES, M.S.

Prefatory Remarks

Christopher L. Coe, Ph.D.

Research with nonhuman primates has had a significant impact on a number of topics in psychosomatic medicine, but probably one of the largest contributions has been in the area of childhood psychopathology and depression. Seminal studies, such as this article by Reite et al., provided strong empirical support for the belief that animals could be used to model human depression. This particular experiment was a technological tour de force in its day; the investigators utilized implantable biotelemetry to record simultaneously heart rate, body temperature, and EEG in a noninvasive manner. They were able to show that the agitation and depressive phases of the infant's separation response were associated with distinctive physiological profiles. Moreover, the onset of the depressive phase could be anticipated by a night of disrupted sleep and hypothermia. The findings raised the question of whether this type of reactive depression reflected a compensatory and energy-saving conservation-withdrawal stage or was instead a maladaptive reaction indicative of emotional overload and physiological dysfunction. This interpretative issue remains unresolved to this day.

Introduction

The depressive component of the agitation-depression reaction frequently seen in monkey infants separated from their mothers is considered one of the best animal models of human depression.[1,2] While most interesting behaviorally, a more complete understanding of the nature of the reaction has been severely hampered by the lack of data on the physiological status of the separated infant. This report for the first time presents certain physiological data including heart rate (HR), body temperature (BT), and sleep patterns during 36 hours of maternal separation in four pigtail (*M. nemestrina*) infants.

Methods

Our infants were born in the Department of Psychiatry Primate Laboratory, where they were raised by their mothers in a social group pen containing an adult male and 6 to 10 adult females, some with offspring.

When the infants were between 22 and 33 weeks of age (mean 25.2 weeks), they were surgically instrumented with an implantable pulse amplitude modulated FM biotelemetry system of our design that transmits heart rate, body temperature, eye movement, muscle activity, and three channels of EEG.[3,4] Sutures were removed 10 days postoperatively, and physiological data collection began 11 days postoperatively.

After 3 to 5 days of normative baseline physiological and behavioral data collection, the mother was removed, leaving the infant in the otherwise intact group. There was no visual or auditory contact between the separated mother and infant.

Telemetered physiology was transmitted around the clock and recorded on both paper and magnetic tape. Behavioral data was obtained both by monitoring the infant on closed circuit TV and writing the ongoing behavior on the running paper record, and by systematic observation sessions which provided duration and frequency measurements of the various behaviors.[5,6]

BT was recorded 24 hours a day on a slow speed strip chart recorder. All night sleep records were hand scored; sleep stages included Drowsy, Stage 2, Stage 3–4 (combined), and REM. Heart rate was determined by measuring the time elapsed (from the paper record) during 25 heart beats and then converting to the beat per minute (bpm) rate. Samples were obtained at random during specific behaviors between 0900 and 1500 hours during the day; sleep samples were obtained at random during the various stages between 2200 and 0200 hours. One way analysis of variance was performed on the grouped HR values, over behaviors, for each animal separately. Multiple comparisons were performed on all behavior pairs.[7]

Results

Before separation BT circadian rhythms and sleep stage measures tended to show relatively little intersubject variability, while HR values were much more variable and individually characteristic of a given monkey infant.[8] As expected, HR was positively correlated with activity level. The range of daily minimum and maximum temperature in the 4 infants was 36.2 to 38.5°C.

Immediately following separation, the infants were behaviorally agitated, exhibiting increased motor activity of a restless 'searching' nature, and frequent "cooing," the plaintive distress call of the young macaque. The onset of agitation was accompanied by pronounced elevations of both HR and BT, lasting up to several hours.

During the first night following separation, sleep was markedly disturbed. All infants showed a marked decrease in REM sleep from normal values of about 100 minutes per night; one infant had *no* REM sleep at all. All animals showed significant ($p < .01$) decreases in HR during Stage 3–4 sleep in the first separation night; three of the four showed significant ($p < .01$) decreases in HR during Stage 2 sleep as well.

Sleep stage and heart rate values during baseline, the first separation night, and the next day, are tabulated in Table 14–1-a,b.

In three of the four infants, the BT during the first night of separation dropped to a value lower than the lowest baseline value; in one of the 2 youngest animals there was a precipitous drop to 33.5°C, a value of 2°C lower than the lowest baseline value recorded.

Table 14–1-a. Grouped mean sleep stage values during 3 baseline nights and the night following separation in the 4 infants. Standard deviations are in parentheses. T.S. = Total Sleep

	T.S. (minutes)	Drowsy, (%)	Stage 2, (%)	Stage 3–4, (%)	REM, (%)
Base	556 (33)	2.9 (1.5)	55.4 (3.9)	25.3 (4.2)	16.4 (3.7)
Sep	494 (55)	4.5 (2.7)	64.0 (5.9)	27.9 (4.2)	3.5 (2.3)

Table 14–1-b. Heart rate values in beats per minute in 4 infants during Baseline (Base.) and Separation (Sep.). N = number of samples; Obx = inanimate object exploration behavior. Significance levels are in parentheses.

Infant	Stage 2 Sleep			Stage 3–4 Sleep			Waking Obx		
	N	$\overline{X}$	S.D.	N	$\overline{X}$	S.D.	N	$\overline{X}$	S.D.
1 Base.	162	167	9	180	163	10	65	210	15
Sep.	80	146	21 ($<.01$)	76	138	9 ($<.01$)	39	182	12 ($<.01$)
2 Base.	126	182	8	114	173	8	30	222	19
Sep.	114	148	21 ($<.01$)	77	130	13 ($<.01$)	43	168	19 ($<.01$)
3 Base.	86	129	8	95	133	14	84	186	11
Sep.	86	127	9 (N.S.)	72	122	7 ($<.01$)	20	156	9 ($<.01$)
4 Base.	148	137	12	136	136	9	79	171	12
Sep.	83	102	5 ($<.01$)	93	101	5 ($<.01$)	75	134	8 ($<.01$)

The next morning, the two youngest infants were severely depressed behaviorally, exhibiting the characteristic slouched posture, retardation of movement with impaired motor coordination, and marked diminution of play behavior. The two older infants showed a diminution of play, and an increase in active exploration of inanimate objects, either manually, orally, or both (Obx behavior), but not the other depressive behavioral characteristics.

The relative bradycardia persisted, and in all four infants the maximum BT recorded the day following separation was lower than any daily maximum recorded during the baseline period.

Figure 14–1 shows an infant the morning after separation, with simultaneously recorded physiology. The infant exhibits the hunched-over posture characteristic of depression. HR is 115 bpm, whereas mean baseline HR at rest has been 144 (S.D. 9) bpm. Body temperature was 37.0°C, whereas at the same time of morning during the 3 baseline days, BT had been 37.9 (S.D. 0.15) degrees Celsius. The EEG shows the slouched infant to be awake and alert.

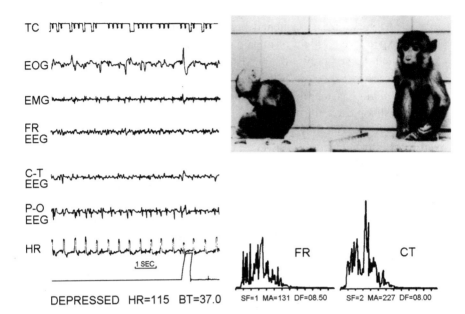

Figure 14–1. Depressed *M. nemestrina* infant the morning following maternal separation, with simultaneously telemetered physiology. The infant illustrates the characteristic hunched-over posture of depression while another adolescent female monkey sits unconcerned nearby. The low voltage fast EEG, presence of eye movements (and lambda waves in the P—O EEG), and the EEG power spectral distribution indicate that the infant is both awake and alert.

TC = time code; EOG = eye movement; EMG = muscle activity; FR EEG = frontal EEG; C—TEEG = central-temporal EEG; P—O EEG = parieto-occipital EEG; HR = heart rate; BT = body temperature. The photograph of the infant was taken at the leading edge of the square wave pulse in the bottom channel. Power spectral analysis of frontal (FR) and central-temporal (CT) EEG are shown at the lower right, and were performed on the illustrated EEG epochs prefiltered with a 2–40 Hz bandpass. Frequency resolution is from 0 to 32 Hz on the X axis (each small division is 2.5 Hz); relative power at each frequency on the Y axis. The spectral scale factor (SF), maximum amplitude (MA), and dominant frequency (DF) are plotted below each spectrum.

Discussion

The initial response of agitation with elevations in both body temperature and heart rate is compatible with a state of organismic hyperarousal and increased energy expenditure, and might be seen to function adaptively to re-gain the mother.

The nature of the subsequent depressive reaction is more complex. All four infants experienced a night of impaired sleep with profound hypothermia. Although the relative bradycardia persisted in all four, only two infants were severely depressed *behaviorally* the next morning.

One might consider this organismic state of behavioral depression and altered physiological activity as having adaptive value also, serving to conserve energy resources and prevent exhaustion, after the general form of the conservation-withdrawal theory of Engel.[9, 2]

An alternative hypothesis might consider the depressive reaction, with its prominent physiological disorganization, as intrinsically maladaptive, a manifestation of disturbed CNS physiology resultant from the stress of separation.

Bradycardia is an empirically well documented accompaniment of stress in man and lower animals.[10, 11] Data from lower species have implicated feeding as being important in the regulation of heart rate and body temperature.[12] The nature of our group living paradigm precluded our obtaining body weight or exact measurements of food consumption, but all of our separated infants were observed to eat usual amounts of food.

Depressive disorders in man have frequently been linked to disturbances in diencephalic function,[13–15] and certain of the physiological parameters affected in the depressed monkey infant are ultimately under diencephalic regulation. Our findings to date suggest that these regulatory mechanisms are influenced by the social stress of maternal separation. If confirmed, they would have important heuristic implications for psychobiology generally and depression specifically.

References

1. Harlow H, Gluck JP, Suomi SJ: Generalization of behavioral data between non-human and human animals. Am Psychol 27:709–716, 1972
2. Kaufman IC: Mother-infant separation in monkeys: an experimental model, in Separation and Depression. Edited by Senay E. AAAS, Chicago, IL, 1973, pp 33–52
3. Reite M, Walker S, Pauley JD: Implantation surgery in infant monkeys. Lab Primate Newslet 4:1–16, 1973
4. Pauley JD, Reite ML, Walker SD: An implantable multichannel biotelemetry system. Electroencephal Clin Neurophysiol 37:153–160, 1974
5. Kaufman IC, Rosenblum LA: A behavioral taxonomy for *Macaca nemestrina* and *Macaca radiata*. Primates 7:205–258, 1966
6. Reite ML, Pauley JD, Walker S, et al: A systems approach to studying physiology and behavior in infant monkeys. J Appl Physiol 37:417–423, 1974

7. Scheffe H: A method for judging all contrasts in the analysis of variance. Biometrika 40:87–104, 1953
8. Reite M, Pauley JD, Kaufman IC, et al: Normal physiological patterns and physiological-behavioral correlations in unrestrained monkey infants. Physiol and Behav 12:1021–1033, 1974
9. Engle G, Schmale A: Conservation-withdrawal: a primary regulatory process for organismic homeostatis, in Physiology Emotion and Psychosomatic Illness. London, CIBA Foundation Symposium, 1972, pp 58–85
10. Wolf S: Cardiovascular reactions to symbolic stimuli. Circulation 18:287–292, 1958
11. Richter CP: On the phenomenon of sudden death in animals and man. Psychosom Med 19:191–198, 1957
12. Hofer MA: The role of nutrition in the physiological and behavioral effects of early maternal separation on infant rats. Psychosom Med 35:350–359, 1973
13. Brown E, Barglow P: Pseudocyesis: a paradigm for psychophysiological interactions. Arch Gen Psychiat 24:221–229, 1971
14. Gellhorn E, Loofbourrow GN: Emotions and Emotional Disorders. Harper and Row, New York, 1963, p 295
15. Akiskal HS, McKinney WT: Depressive disorders: toward a unified hypothesis. Science 182:20–29, 1973

CHAPTER 15

Consequences of Social Conflict on Plasma Testosterone Levels in Rhesus Monkeys

ROBERT M. ROSE, M.D.,
IRWIN S. BERNSTEIN, PH.D., AND
THOMAS P. GORDON, M.A.

Prefatory Remarks

Robert T. Rubin, M.D., Ph.D.

The extent to which environmental circumstances can influence endocrine function has been studied by researchers for almost three-quarters of a century. Our understanding of the regulation of hormone secretion has progressed beyond the classical model, in which a series of negative feedback loops between the endocrine glands and their secretory products controls the output of the glands, to our current model of open-loop regulation of endocrine function, in which the brain plays a prominent role in determining patterns of hormone secretion. The major areas of discovery that underscore the importance of the brain in endocrine function include 1) the characterization of the hypothalamic releasing and inhibiting hormones for the anterior pituitary hormones, 2) the identification of brain neurotransmitters that influence the secretion of these releasing and inhibiting hormones, 3) elucidation of the contributions of specific regions of the hypothalamus and limbic system to the secretion patterns of specific pituitary hormones, and 4) elucidation of the changes in endocrine function resulting from environmental manipulation of intact subjects. These observations have been made both in humans and in other animals in laboratory and naturalistic settings. It is this last category to which the Rose et al. study makes a major contribution.

Twenty-five years ago, Mason et al.[1] performed seminal studies of multiple hormone secretion patterns in rhesus monkeys subjected to chair restraint in the laboratory. Two general components to the stress response occurred: an early catabolic phase in which hormones promoting increased glucose availability and utilization were secreted, and a later anabolic phase in which hormones promoting tissue repair, including gonadal steroids, were secreted. These studies indicated that multiple hormone responses to stress were organized and coordinated, providing an overall physiological influence that was consistent and appropriate to the stress and its duration.

Rose et al. demonstrated a similar logic in the endocrine response of the hypothalamo-pituitary-gonadal axis in male rhesus monkeys in a naturalistic setting. When four adult males were allowed to form a new social group, the subordinate monkey had a profound fall in plasma testosterone levels. When the four animals were placed in a larger breeding group and all became subordinate to the males in that group, plasma testosterone levels fell in all four of the newly introduced animals. The alpha male of the breeding group, who became dominant to all the males, experienced a large rise in testosterone level following successful defense of his status. These results give further credence to the concept of reciprocity between environment and physiology: Circumstances that call for subordination and passivity evoke a fall in testosterone, a hormone that promotes aggressive behavior and sexuality in males, and circumstances that call for continued aggression and that provide access to receptive females (i.e., becoming the dominant male) evoke a rise in testosterone.

Less clear is whether plasma testosterone concentrations prior to the environmental challenge contributed to individual behavior and outcome. The animals who became the dominant, alpha males in both group settings did not have the highest baseline testosterone concentrations. Therefore, other factors, such as physical strength, nonhormonal neurophysiological determinants of aggressiveness, and "personality" characteristics that may foster adaptability and affiliation with other males in the struggle for dominance become theoretically important. In human males, these other factors appear to be preeminent over testosterone levels in determining aggressive behavior. The Rose et al. study not only provides important information regarding the responsivity of testosterone in social situations in primates, it highlights aspects of hormone-environment interaction that continue to need further study.

Reference

1. Mason JW: Organization of psychoendocrine mechanisms. Psychosom Med 30:565–808, 1968

Four adult male rhesus monkeys formed a new social group with 13 adult females. The male who became dominant (alpha) showed a progressive increase in plasma testosterone. The male who became subordinate to the other three males showed an 80% fall in testosterone from baseline levels. After 7 weeks, this group was introduced to a well-established breeding group, and all 4 males became subordinate to all members of the breeding group. All four males evidenced a fall in testosterone during the first week after introduction, and within 6 weeks their levels were approximately 80% of pre-introduction values. The alpha male of the breeding group showed a large increase in testosterone (238%) 24 hrs. after he successfully defended his group and became the dominant animal of the larger, newly formed group. Thus, plasma testosterone levels appear to be significantly influenced by the outcome of conflict attendant to alterations in status of rhesus monkeys living in social groups.

Introduction

In recent years there has been a renewal of interest in the study of behavioral-endocrine interactions. Much of the emphasis of these studies has focused on assessing the influence of both gonadal and adrenal hormones on sexual and aggressive behavior.[1,2] Many investigations have examined the behavior of rodents, typically in a paired cage situation, and comparatively few studies have utilized social animals such as nonhuman primates in naturalistic settings. Thus, there is still considerable uncertainty about cause and effect relationships between altered endocrine levels and changes in primate social behavior. As has been noted by Beach,[3] as one moves to the study of nonhuman primates and man, it becomes difficult to differentiate hormonal influences on behavior from historical, social and learning variables. Nevertheless, there is a great deal of evidence to suggest that endocrine factors do affect both sexual and aggressive behavior in primates.[4-7] At the same time, many studies have documented that social and environmental factors significantly influence endocrine activity.[8-11] It thus seems possible that the changes in endocrine activity secondary to environmental stimuli may play a role in influencing future behavior, precisely the model proposed by Beach.[12]

In order to investigate both these dimensions of behavioral-endocrine interaction, we have chosen as a subject rhesus monkeys living in social groups. As with many other nonhuman primates, as well as man, rhesus macaques naturally live in social groups. The behavior of individuals is significantly influenced by others in the group, in large part as a function of the animal's position in the status or dominance hierarchy. Position in the social structure not only is predictive of the outcome of agonistic encounters, but may also influence the occurrence of maintenance behaviors such as feeding, mating or grooming. Social position is not fixed, and appears to be the product of many influences, past and present, including age, sex, size, fighting ability, alliances, social history and presence and rank of blood relatives in the social group. For example, a young male with a high ranking mother or older brother might himself hold high social rank, while a peer of equal size and strength but less formidable social bonds may be very low ranking or forced into a peripheral status. Thus, familiarity and acceptance by others is a crucial determinant of the individual's social status, which in turn greatly influences his existence in that group. A strange animal of the same species is not usually tolerated, let alone readily accepted, by other members of an established social group. Consequently, newly introduced animals, especially adult males, are subject to intense threat and attack by all other group members, including females, juveniles and even infants. After a period of time, sometimes requiring as long as a year or more, newly introduced animals are integrated into the group, e.g., adult males rise in the social hierarchy, exhibit consort behavior with sexually receptive females, engage more frequently in grooming interaction with the other animals, etc.

Because the animal's status in the group determines so much of his behavior, and because social status is greatly influenced by familiarity with other animals in the group, we have manipulated individual animals' exposure to different social groups. We have then measured both the endocrine and behavioral changes provoked by the social conflict accompanying these manipulations.

In an earlier study,[10] we reported that plasma testosterone levels rise in adult male rhesus monkeys following access to sexually receptive females. Each subject was placed individually with a group of 13 females for a 2-week period during which time each was observed to assume the dominant social position (alpha) and to engage in frequent copulations with various receptive females. All animals showed significantly increased testosterone levels, which returned to baseline after removal from the female group. At varying lengths of time following return to an individual cage, the males were introduced individually to a well-established group of 34 males. Each of the introduced males was vigorously attacked by the resident males and was removed from the group within 2 hrs. following introduction. During the following week, the four males averaged an 80% drop in plasma testosterone levels; two animals exhibited markedly depressed levels during the subsequent period. We concluded that access to sexually receptive females, along with assumption of dominance in a group, provoked an increase in testosterone secretion. Defeat was associated with a fall in testosterone secretion, but this interpretation is subject to several qualifications. Two of the four animals did suffer wounding extensive enough to require suturing. Thus, one might argue that injury, per se, could account for the fall in testosterone levels. Furthermore, all four animals were returned to individual cages following their brief exposure to and defeat by the group of adult males. This social isolation following defeat could function to enhance the depression of plasma testosterone, although baseline measures were also obtained in social isolation. Finally, sudden exposure of one animal to a well-established group without means of fleeing from this group is unusual and possibly artificial, in that it may rarely occur in the natural environment.

The two experiments reported in this study attempt to clarify the influence of social conflict on plasma testosterone levels, as well as to report on the behavior of animals maintained in a social context following defeat and fall in testosterone levels.

Methods

All the animals studied lived in two large outdoor compounds, each approximately 0.13 hectare (1/3 of an acre) in area. Animals had access to indoor quarters and were given food and water *ad lib*. The compounds were constructed to permit a clear view of all animals for observation and recording behavior. Behavior was recorded via standardized inventory based on dyadic interactions of who does what to whom. Also, during group introductions, the animals were observed as a group, as well as individually.

All the males who were studied had been experimental subjects previously, and all were accustomed to capture and venipuncture techniques. Blood samples had been obtained (average over 50 times) over the past several years and all had accommodated to the routine of placement in a squeeze cage and blood withdrawal from the saphenous vein. Analysis of plasma cortisol and testosterone samples taken immediately following capture and venipuncture failed to show significant changes that would reflect a persistent "stress" effect of the capture and venipuncture experience.

Plasma testosterone was analyzed with a modification of the Mayes and Nugent techniques.[13] Separation of testosterone from dihydrotesterone and other 17-beta hydroxysteroids that cross-react with sex steroid binding globulin was accomplished by column chromatography using Sephadex LH-20.[14] Coefficient of variation of samples from four different pools run repeatedly over an 8-month period averaged 10.1%.

Results

Experiment 1

Four males, Proco, Quid, Ribot and Strom, who had been studied previously, were released *simultaneously* into the same group of 13 females that they had been exposed to individually in the past. These 17 animals formed a new social group (R-7 formation). Plasma testosterone levels were determined from samples drawn at the same time of day (0900 to 1000) in the week prior to group formation when the animals were in individual cages, and on nine occasions over the 8 weeks following group formation. Systematic behavioral observations were made for 1 hr. each day during the 2-month period following group formation and stabilization.[1]

Experiment 2

On the 46th day after R-7 formation, immediately after blood was taken from the four males, this relatively recently formed group of four males and 13 fe-

---

[1] See Bernstein, Gordon and Rose[15] for details of this procedure.

males was merged with a larger, well-established breeding group consisting of two adult males, a subadult male, 34 females and 14 immatures. The groups were permitted access to one another by removing a partition in the wall separating the two compounds. Blood samples were taken from the two adult males and the subadult male in the breeding group, both before, as well as following, group formation, along with sampling from the four males from R-7. The animals in the newly formed R-9 group were studied extensively during the first week and for 2 hrs. daily for the subsequent 6 weeks of this study.

In the first hour of the R-7 formation, two of the four males, Proco and Ribot, engaged in serious fighting. The other males did not become involved in agonistic encounters, and in fact, avoided all social contact. The fight between Proco and Ribot continued throughout the day, with neither animal clearly dominant over the other, and both sustaining some wounds. All four males were placed in individual cages overnight to prevent serious wounding at a time when immediate attention was unavailable. On the morning of the second day (+1 day), after withdrawing blood samples, the animals were rereleased. This time, Proco formed an alliance with Quid and clearly became dominant over Ribot, who became subordinate to the three other males in the group. Proco became the alpha (dominant) male and remained in this position during the next 46 days prior to R-9 formation.

Table 15–1 contains each animal's plasma testosterone levels for R-7 formation. It is apparent that Ribot, who suffered defeat and became subordinate to the other males, showed a significant (87%) drop in plasma testosterone by the 8th day of R-7 formation. This is similar to the 80% drop in testosterone levels that all the males showed following individual defeat after they were exposed briefly to the all-male group. However, in contrast to this previous study, Ribot's

Table 15–1. R-7 formation; plasma testosterone (ng/100 ml)[a]

Baseline			Group formation							
Proco	540	590	640	850	1230	750	1260	1080	800	1940	2400
Quid	440	480	770	510	630	740	620	740	1080	750	610
Strom	420	300	—	900	540	440	320	660	500	440	980
Ribot	910	1300	800	160	140	590	660	630	730	960	800
Days	−6d	−3d	+1d	+3d	+8d	+11d	+23d	+30d	+36d	+45d	+46d

[a]Plasma testosterone responses of the four adult males to the R-7 group formation. Proco becomes the alpha male and had a significant rise in plasma testosterone. Ribot became subordinate to the other three males, had a brief drop in testosterone, but by the second week his values started back toward pre-group formation levels.

testosterone started to rise by the second week and approached pre-group baseline levels by the 45th day of the study. When he was kept in a cage following his earlier defeat, his testosterone levels were still depressed 41 days later.

Proco, who became the alpha male in the R-7 group, showed a rise in testosterone during the period following group formation. Of note is the fact that both Proco and Ribot were wounded during the first day of R-7 formation, with Proco sustaining the more serious wounds. It would seem that social outcome and not presence or severity of wounds is the significant factor in producing depressed testosterone output. It is also noteworthy that this period corresponds with the birth season in *Macaca mulatta,* and is usually associated with a fall in testosterone in males in well established groups.[10] However, mounting was observed during this period, especially by Proco. It does not appear as if the females were in fertile estrus during this period of time. Indeed, several of the 13 females were pregnant prior to the formation, and none were impregnated in the weeks following formation. Proco's rise in plasma testosterone, shown during this period, seems to be a product of social stimulation, possibly related to his becoming the alpha male. However, we cannot rule out the specific effect of access to females who did permit mounting, despite the fact that they did not appear to be in estrus.

R-9 Formation

When the partition between the two compounds was opened, both groups oriented to the partition and gradually approached. Gamma, the alpha male of the large breeding group (R-6), and Proco, the alpha male of the R-7 group, approached one another and fought across the threshold. Gamma, supported by other group members, forced his way into the R-7 compound as the R-7 group slowly gave ground. The R-7 group gradually fled to one small corner area of the compound, where group cohesion was maintained. As a group they were clearly subordinate to the larger group, as evidenced in the yielding of space and submissive behaviors of most individuals. However, the males continued to defend themselves and female group members from attack. During the rest of the day, there was continued agonistic interaction with an increasing percentage of aggression (expressed primarily as threat and chase) on the part of Gamma and Kodine, and declining percentage of aggression and increased submissive behavior shown by the R-7 males. In contrast to previous studies, there was no wounding of the R-7 males throughout the period of R-9 formation. This may reflect the fact that the two adult males in the breeding group, Gamma and Kodine, were without their canine teeth, which both had lost before they arrived at the Field Station.

Despite the clear dominance of the larger breeding group, the R-7 group remained intact and continued to defend against attack throughout the first week following the merger. On the 8th day, Gamma attacked and defeated each of the R-7 males, whose previously effective defensive behaviors were now replaced with submissive behaviors. This event seems to have marked the dissolution of the R-7 group, since cohesive defensive behavior was not observed again in the days following. Attacks upon R-7 males occurred frequently for a few days, then were replaced by milder forms of aggression (harassment), which could be directed to defeated R-7 group members by any member of the victorious R-6 group. In the months following merger the R-7 animals were gradually assimilated into the R-6 group without regard to their previous status. Indeed, the new relative rankings of the R-7 males placed Ribot above the other three and Proco at the bottom.

Plasma testosterone for the four males from R-7 during R-9 formation is shown in Figure 15–1. The last three values drawn on the 36th, 45th and 46th day of R-7 were used to determine a baseline or pre-R-9 formation average for each animal (shown as a dotted line). Every animal showed a drop in testosterone 24 hrs. after R-9 formation (the first value after the arrow, which depicts the day of formation). It is of note that on Day 10 after formation (May 6), Proco's testosterone level dropped to 210 ng/100 ml. This drop occurred after Proco, previously the alpha male of R-7, was clearly and unambiguously defeated (submitted repeatedly after being threatened) by Gamma (the alpha male of the breeding group who also became the dominant animal of the newly formed R-9 group). By the sixth week after R-9 formation, all four males showed much lower plasma testosterone levels, averaging 80% of the levels they showed while still in the R-7 group. The individual response of these four males is shown in Figure 15–2.

We also measured plasma testosterone levels in the two resident males from the breeding group, Gamma and Kodine, both before and after R-9 formation. The values for the alpha male, Gamma, are plotted in Figure 15–3. His plasma testosterone rose abruptly to 1260 ng/100 ml (a 238% increase) on April 27, 24 hrs. after his group was permitted access to the R-7 group. Although he did not clearly emerge as the alpha male of the larger combined R-9 group until 7 days later, he did engage in a great deal of aggressive behavior during this first day after group formation, and showed few submissive responses during this period. By the 8th day after group formation, and during the next 4 weeks, his testosterone values returned to the pre-group formation levels.

Gamma's relatively low, but stable, baseline during April and May is characteristic of males living in well-established social groups. We have recently measured plasma testosterone levels in several males over a 30-month period.

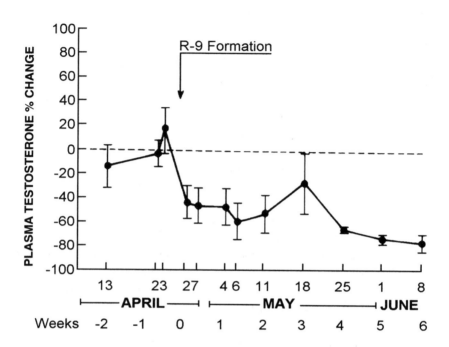

Figure 15–1. Plasma testosterone responses of the four males following merger of their group with the breeding group (R-9 group formation). All four males were defeated within the first week by the alpha male of the other group, during which time their plasma testosterone levels fell. They remained subordinate throughout the period under study, and showed consistently lower levels, -80% of baseline. Values plotted as mean ± SEM.

Testosterone peaks during the breeding season, during October and November, and falls to lower levels, averaging from 200 to 300 ng/100 ml during the birth season, approximately March through August. It is very unusual for plasma testosterone levels to exceed 1000 ng/100 ml in males during this period in well-established social groups. We therefore interpret this single abrupt elevation in testosterone levels to 1260 ng/100 ml in Gamma following group formation as possibly reflecting the stimulatory effect of increased aggression and his emergence as a dominant animal. This is in contrast to a rise in testosterone observed in Proco while he was in R-7. During this time, he emerged as the alpha male in a newly formed group, unlike Gamma, who was well-established as the alpha male in his group. In addition, Proco was sexually stimulated, engaging in frequent copulation, despite the fact that it was the birth season in the breeding group; Gamma engaged in no sexual activity during this time.

Social Conflict and Testosterone in Rhesus Monkeys 291

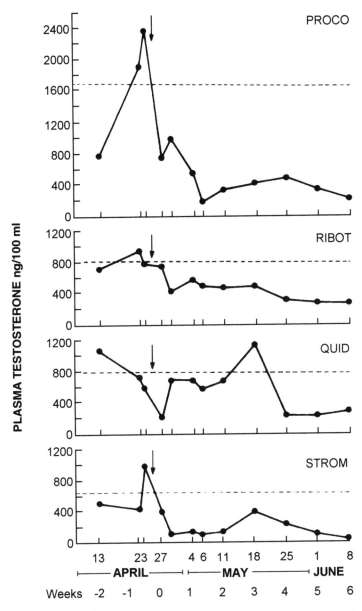

Figure 15–2. Individual responses of the R-7 males after R-9 group formation. All animals showed a drop in levels following defeat. Although there is some individual variability in the first 4 weeks after R-9 group formation, by the sixth week all males showed consistently lower levels.

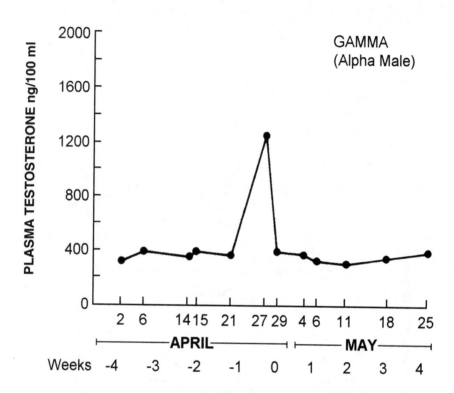

Figure 15–3. Plasma testosterone rise of the alpha male 24 hr. after the R-9 group formation. During this first day, he successfully defended his group against the animals from the R-7 group and emerged as the alpha male of the newly formed larger group.

The only other adult male in the breeding group was Kodine, who also showed some increase in testosterone following merger with the R-7 group. However, he was a low-status animal in the breeding group, and demonstrated relatively little threat or challenge to the R-7 males when they were introduced to the breeding group.

The integration of the defeated males into the social structure of the newly formed group was a gradual process without a discrete endpoint but certainly extending over a period of months. By the following mating season (6 months after formation) all four males were active participants in the social and sexual behavior observed at that time. It is of particular interest to attempt to characterize the behavior of the defeated males during the intervening months when plasma testosterone levels were so markedly depressed.

Behavioral observations were conducted before, during and for 8 weeks after the merger of the two groups, with the main focus upon the behavior patterns of the adult males. In the first hours after the group merger agonistic behavior was greatly increased, and most other social behaviors were not observed. In the days and weeks following the merger agonistic behavior fell, sharply at first, then more gradually, back to pre-merger levels. At the same time other social activities were observed with increasing frequency. Thus, a comparison of the activity patterns of the four males before and after defeat does not reveal any marked differences, except for an increase in aggressive attacks directed toward them, which was most pronounced in the days immediately following the group merger. The four males had access to food, water and shelter as they had had prior to merger, and continued to engage in such social behaviors as grooming, chiefly with other members of the defeated group.

More qualitative observations do suggest two aspects of the new situation that may relate to plasma testosterone levels. First, all the members of the R-7 group were subordinate to every member of the larger group, regardless of age/sex class. Some 60 animals could (and most did) reinforce this new status arrangement from time to time by mild harassing displays. Second, in the weeks following the merger the R-7 animals were severely limited in space. The males, in particular, spent most of the time in one corner of the compound, and any movement there from seemed to be a sufficient stimulus to provoke an attack by any R-6 group member who happened to be nearby. The R-7 males responded to all such attacks with submission and flight back to the corner. Naturally, movement away from the "safe" area became infrequent, as the defeated males attempted to avoid contact with or even proximity to R-6 group members.

The primary behavioral correlate of low plasma testosterone levels following defeat was low placement in the status hierarchy of a group that was newly formed and unsettled to the extent that minimal stimulus cues could provoke aggressive attack, which the males invariably responded to with submissive signals.

Discussion

These studies extend our previous findings that defeat of rhesus males provokes a fall in their plasma testosterone levels. They are also consistent with previous studies showing that testosterone secretion falls following a variety of stressful events, i.e., following surgery,[16] during Officer Candidate School[17] or during basic combat training.[18]

The studies reported here differ from previous work in several ways. The males were not introduced by themselves to a strange group, a relatively unnatural event, but along with other monkeys. They were permitted to remain in the group following defeat, and there was no significant wounding associated with group formation.

In the R-7 group formation, the four males quickly established a dominance hierarchy among themselves. Ribot, who became the most subordinate male, did show a significant drop in plasma testosterone. In contrast to his earlier defeat by the all-male group, after which he was placed in an individual cage, he showed a rapid return (within 2 weeks) to his pregroup plasma testosterone levels. Although he was clearly subordinate to the other males, he did interact with the females. He thus achieved some immediate integration into this newly formed group, and this may account, in part, for the rise in testosterone during the second week of R-7 formation. Ribot's rapid integration in R-7 is in contrast to what occurred to him and to the other males after R-9 formation.

Proco tended to increase his plasma testosterone levels from Day 1 to the end of the R-7 group (+46 days). This rise, clearly evident in the first week after R-7 formation, occurred despite the fact that he, as well as Ribot, was wounded in the first 24 hrs. of group formation. This observation casts doubt on the interpretation that wounding by itself during defeat by the all-male group could account for the fall in plasma testosterone. Proco's rise in testosterone appears related to both his assumption of alpha status in the R-7 group, as well as to the stimulation of the females present. The stimulating effect of the females, some of whom were receptive, outside the usual breeding season, may also account for the more modest rise in plasma testosterone observed in Quid and Strom at the end of R-7 (+36, +45 and +46 days).

During R-9 formation, the four males from R-7 were clearly defeated by Gamma, who became the alpha male of the newly formed group. Each of the four animals again showed a fall in plasma testosterone. After R-9 formation, the alliances between the four R-7 males broke down, and each animal interacted individually with the animals from the breeding group. There was no carryover of the original dominance hierarchy in R-7 for the four males when they were integrated into R-9. Proco no longer remained dominant to the other three males but instead fell below the other three in the new status hierarchy, and Ribot now had the highest rank of the four males.

By the beginning of June, the four males functioned as subordinate animals in the R-9 group. They submitted to almost all the other animals in Gamma's original group, including young juveniles. As noted, their defeat and subsequent subordinate status was paralleled by a drop in plasma testosterone, averaging 74% of their pre-group formation levels. The magnitude of the fall in plasma testosterone is similar to that observed for Ribot during R-7 formation and for all four animals when they were defeated individually in the earlier study. However, it is possible that some of this decrease in plasma testosterone levels could be due to seasonal influences. In stable groups, we have observed that plasma testosterone shows a significant drop during the birth season, rising again in the fall with the onset of the breeding season.[10] The reason that the four males did not show the seasonal decrease in plasma testosterone in March and April during R-7 formation may be due to the social stimulation of being in a new group with access to females, some of whom were sexually receptive, despite the time of year. Nevertheless, it is most likely that the fall in plasma testosterone in June for these four males is a consequence both of their defeat and subsequent subordinate status in the new group, as well as seasonal influences on testosterone secretion.

We now know that the four males began to improve their positions in R-9 during the fall. This social mobility and subsequent rise in status may be due in part to their consort behavior with receptive females of high rank. All four animals did show consort behavior with females in September and October of this same year, and plasma testosterone levels had increased in September prior to the onset of copulatory behavior, as is typical of all our group-living males.

It is possible that the assumption of dominance or success during intense agonistic encounters may also function as a stimulus to increase plasma testosterone. We observed a temporary increase in plasma testosterone in both resident males from the breeding group 24 hrs. after R-9 formation. We have also observed an increase in plasma testosterone in another animal, after he was exposed to a group of seven unfamiliar males. Instead of his defeat by this group, however, he successfully defended himself and did not show consistent submissive responses to others in the group following introduction. It is of note that 24 hrs. after his introduction, his plasma testosterone rose to 3030 ng/100 ml, from a baseline of 949 ± 285 ng/100 ml (mean $\pm$ SD, n = 4) during the preceding month. The evidence for agonistic encounters in which the male emerges as clearly dominant acting as a stimulus to increase plasma testosterone levels is only anecdotal. We have observed this on only a few occasions. This is because the event is relatively rare, and we have had only a few occasions on which we have measured plasma testosterone in animals who have emerged as clearly victorious over others in social encounters. We hope to investigate this more systematically in the future.

A summary of the present and past studies involving the effects of social stimulation and conflict on plasma testosterone for one animal is presented in graphic form in Figure 15–4. This figure plots the plasma testosterone responses of Ribot for 7 months.

Initially, in November of 1970, he was in an individual cage, and then permitted access, by himself, to a group of receptive females in December for a 2-week period. His plasma testosterone rose to a peak of 1940 ng/100 ml during this period. He was then returned to his individual cage for 4 weeks, and plasma testosterone levels fell to baseline. He was then exposed to the large all-male group for 2 hrs. and placed back in his individual cage. The week following this sudden and decisive defeat, his plasma testosterone fell to 160 ng/100 ml, and 5 weeks later, still remaining in the cage, his testosterone was still low, at

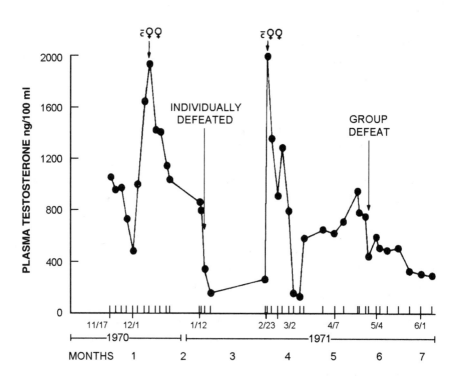

Figure 15–4. Plasma testosterone responses of Ribot over a 7-month period. He showed two distinct increases in testosterone following access to receptive females. He showed a fall in testosterone following defeat in three different circumstances. On the first occasion, he was defeated after a brief exposure to an all-male group of 34 animals. On the second occasion, he became the subordinate male in a newly formed group consisting of three other adult males and 13 females (R-7 group formation). On the last occasion he was defeated, along with the three other males, by a large, well-established breeding group (R-9 group formation).

270 ng/100 ml. Twenty-four hrs. after his reintroduction to the females, his testosterone rose to 2010 ng/100 ml. He was then placed back in his individual cage for 10 days, after which time he was released, with the other males, to the females, in R-7 formation. Three days after R-7 formation, and subsequent to his defeat and becoming the most subordinate male of the group, his testosterone again fell to 160 ng/100 ml, and at the end of the week was still low, at 140 ng/100 ml. Unlike previously, he remained in this group, interacting with the other animals, and his testosterone returned toward pre-group formation levels. His final defeat occurred, along with the other males from R-7, during R-9 formation. He again showed a fall in plasma testosterone subsequent to defeat.

These findings strongly suggest that testosterone is sensitive to both stimulation and suppression by appropriate social stimuli. It is possible that following defeat in a social group, the associated fall in testosterone is adaptive. We would invoke the feedback loop explanation to say that defeat produces the fall in testosterone and that this lower level decreases the probability of aggressive action on the part of the subject, thus precluding instigation of additional combat and repeated defeats.

References

1. Rose RM, Bernstein IS, Gordon TP, et al: Androgens and aggressive behavior: a review and recent findings in primates, in Primate Aggression, Territoriality and Xenophobia. Edited by Holloway RL. Academic Press, New York, 1974, pp 275–304
2. Rose RM: The psychological effects of androgens and estrogens: a review, in Psychiatric Complications of Medical Drugs. Edited by Shader RI. Raven Press, New York, 1972, pp 251–293
3. Beach FA: Evolutionary aspects of psychoendocrinology, in Behavior and Evolution. Edited by Roe A, Simpson GG. Yale University Press, New Haven, CT, 1958, pp 81–102
4. Vandenbergh JG, Vessey S: Seasonal breeding of free-ranging rhesus monkeys and related ecological factors. J Reprod Fertil 15:71–79, 1968
5. Wilson AP, Boelkins RC: Evidence for seasonal variation in aggressive behavior by *Macaca mulatta*. Anim Behav 18:719–724, 1970
6. Lindburg DG: Rhesus monkeys: mating season mobility of adult males. Science 166:1176–1178, 1969
7. Goy RW, Resko JA: Gonadal hormones and behavior of normal and pseudohermaphroditic nonhuman female primates. Recent Prog Horm Res 38:707–733, 1972

8. Mason JW: Organization of psychoendocrine mechanisms. Psychosom Med 30:565–808, 1968
9. Sade DS: Seasonal cycle in size of testes of free-ranging *Macaca mulatta*. Folia Primat 2:171–180, 1964
10. Gordon TP, Bernstein IS, Rose RM: Seasonal changes in sexual behavior and plasma testosterone levels of group living monkeys (abstract). Am Zool 13:1267, 1973
11. Rose RM, Gordon TP, Bernstein IS: Plasma testosterone levels in the male rhesus: influences of sexual and social stimuli. Science 178:643–645, 1972
12. Beach FA: Retrospect and prospect, in Sex and Behavior. Edited by Beach FA. John Wiley & Sons, New York, 1965, pp 558–563
13. Mayes D, Nugent CA: Determination of plasma testosterone by the use of competitive protein binding. J Clin Endocrinol Metab 28:1169–1176, 1968
14. Murphy BEP: Hormone assay using binding proteins in blood, in Principles of Competitive Protein-Binding Assay. Edited by Odell WD, Daughaday WH. JB Lippincott, Philadelphia, PA, 1971, pp 108–127
15. Bernstein IS, Gordon TP, Rose RM: Factors influencing the expression of aggression during introduction to rhesus monkey groups, in Primate Aggression, Territoriality and Xenophobia. Edited by Holloway RL. Academic Press, New York, 1974, pp 211–240
16. Matsumoto K, Takeyasu K, Mitzutani S, et al: Plasma testosterone levels following surgical stress in male patients. Acta Endocrinol 65:11, 1970
17. Kreuz LE, Rose RM, Jennings JR: Suppression of plasma testosterone levels and psychological stress: a longitudinal study of young men in Officer Candidate School. Arch Gen Psychiat 26:479–482, 1972
18. Rose RM, Bourne PG, Poe RO, et al: Androgen responses to stress, II. Psychosom Med 31:418–436, 1969

CHAPTER 16

From Explanation to Action in Psychosomatic Medicine
The Case of Obesity

ALBERT J. STUNKARD, M.D.

Prefatory Remarks

Bernard T. Engel, Ph.D.

Stunkard has made extensive and important contributions to the understanding of obesity and its treatment. In a number of studies he showed that body weight is determined in part by genetic predispositions and in part by environmental influences. However, the major focus of his research has been on the role of social and environmental factors in mediating weight gain and weight loss. In the midtown Manhattan study reported here, he showed that obesity was related to socioeconomic status. Women from the lowest socioeconomic group were seven times more likely to be obese (20% above ideal body weight based on prevailing insurance standards) than were women in the highest socioeconomic group; among men, the ratio was 1.5 to 1. Stunkard also studied the various programs for weight loss—fasting, behavior therapy, drugs, and surgery—and has shown that no matter what the intervention, most patients do not maintain their weight losses. Nevertheless, throughout his career, Stunkard has been a leading figure in identifying the most effective interventions for weight loss.

One should not only read this article for its intrinsic merit, but with an appreciation for the scholarship and analytical skills underlying the program of research Stunkard represents. The article is a model for programmatic research in psychosomatic medicine. The following references will enable the interested reader to pursue other aspects of this remarkable research effort.

Suggested Readings

Stunkard AJ, Pennick SB: Behavior modification in the treatment of obesity: the problem of maintaining weight loss. Arch Gen Psych 36:801–806, 1979

Sobal J, Stunkard AJ: Socioeconomic status and obesity: a review of the literature. Psychol Bull 105:260–275, 1989

Psychosomatic medicine began as a social movement within medicine, designed to counteract the mechanistic and impersonal features that had accompanied the introduction of science into medical education. In its early days, therapeutic inefficacy led to a concentration upon understanding the origins of disorders in which emotional determinants played a role. To a large extent, psychosomatic medicine is still identified with such understanding. Within recent years, however, the development of increasingly effective therapeutic techniques has changed the emphasis in psychosomatic medicine from understanding to action.

These developments are particularly well exemplified by the case of obesity. Social investigations have revealed that the prevalence of obesity within populations is determined to a very high degree by social factors, operating in an unplanned and uncontrolled manner. More planned social intervention, particularly by means of behavior modification, has improved the effectiveness of treatment of obesity by a factor of 2. Furthermore, this intervention has been subjected to research whose increasing effectiveness derives from the availability of both a powerful independent variable—specification of the precise behaviors of the therapeutic intervention—and a dependent variable of unprecedented reliability, validity and economy in psychotherapy research—

weight change in pounds. Some of the new experimental designs developed in this research are laying the groundwork for a truly cumulative science of psychotherapy.

The development of more effective treatment techniques leads to the question of how best to deliver them. The relative merits of medical auspices, patient self-help groups and commercial enterprises are discussed.

Introduction

"What is psychosomatic medicine, and where is it going?"

As I read the early writings, particularly of our journal, *Psychosomatic Medicine,* it seems as if the field had its origin 40 years ago as a social movement within the greater medical enterprise. It appears to have arisen as a response to the increasingly mechanistic and impersonal quality of medicine. This was one of the less happy outcomes of the generally favorable introduction of science in medical education, which followed the Flexner report. It sought to restore respect for the psychological, to humanize medicine in order to improve the care of patients.

Whatever its impact upon the humanization process, psychosomatic medicine did not give rise to effective treatments. We attempted to fill the void with explanations—of the meaning of symptoms we could not control and of the psychophysiological relationships of the diseases we could not treat.

In the past 6 years this state of affairs has changed significantly for the better. I will use the case of obesity to exemplify this change and to illustrate where psychosomatic medicine may be going. For obesity had proven as refractory to treatment as any of the so-called psychosomatic disorders. And now in these past 6 years we have learned how to apply psychological measures to improve the care of obese patients to a significant degree. We have learned how to go about making further progress in this direction. And it looks very much as if these psychological measures are going to improve the care of large numbers of patients suffering from conditions other than obesity.

The immediate result of this development is that the psychosomatic approach to obesity has moved dramatically from a concern with explanation to a focus on action. The old questions of "why" are being replaced by new questions of "how." The conceptual paraphernalia of the past—the explanations—are dropping by the wayside, and we are moving into new ways of proceeding and into new forms of action. I would like to suggest that this shift from explanation to action is a realization of the original goal of psychosomatic medicine and that what is happening in obesity today may presage developments in all of medicine.

The story of recent developments in obesity is a thrilling one.

No more than 15 years ago, attempts at explanation of obesity were the appropriate response to the state of the field. There was very little else that we could do. Treatment for obesity could be summarized by the following five propositions:

(1) Most obese people do not enter treatment for obesity.
(2) Of those who do enter treatment, most will not remain.

Figure 16–1 shows the attrition rate of 151 persons during outpatient treatment for obesity.[70] It was constructed from data in a report designed, ironically, to support the benign nature of dieting. A survey of the medical literature in 1959 revealed an attrition rate of from 20% to 80% in the outpatient treatment of obesity.[81]

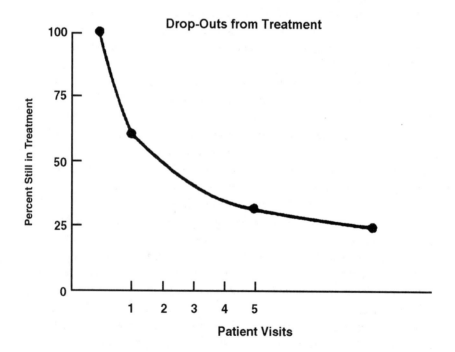

Figure 16–1. Attrition rate of 151 persons during outpatient treatment for obesity. After Shipman.[70]

(3) Of those who remain, most will not lose much weight. The literature survey noted above revealed that no more than 25% of persons entering outpatient treatment for obesity lost as much as 20 pounds and only 5% as much as 50 pounds.[81] More sophisticated mathematical treatment of the data of an even larger series the following year provided a more detailed picture of the patterns of failure.[17, 18] And a study of the results of routine medical treatment, as opposed to the results of physicians who wrote papers about their work, revealed an even more dismal story. Only 12% were able to lose as much as 20 pounds![81]

(4) Of those who lose weight, most will regain it. Of the unusual 12 patients in the foregoing study who were able to lose 20 pounds, only 2 had maintained their weight loss a year later.

(5) Many will pay a high price for trying. A recent resurvey of the medical literature of untoward responses to dieting has established that emotional symptoms occur with high frequency in outpatients treated for obesity and that such symptoms occur also during prolonged inpatient treatment, whether by dieting or by fasting.[88] Two careful outpatient studies are particularly revealing. The first was a retrospective one. One hundred consecutive persons referred to a nutrition clinic of a large general hospital from the medical clinics of the hospital were questioned as to any symptoms they had experienced during any *previous* attempts at weight reduction.[79] A retrospective method was used in order to deal with the problems of ascertaining symptoms of persons who dropped out of treatment (perhaps because of these very symptoms) and on whom information would thus be lost. Seventy-two had made serious attempts to diet in the past: of these, 54% said that they had suffered emotional symptoms at least once; 21% suffered "nervousness," 21% "weakness," 8% "irritability," 5% "fatigue" and 4% "nausea." (Some patients reported more than one symptom.)

A corollary prospective study with a dropout rate low enough (17%) not to distort seriously the results discovered a similar high incidence of symptoms[72] (Figure 16–2). Fifty percent reported either the onset or intensification of depression. Forty percent reported increases in anxiety. Again, some patients reported both symptoms.

This dismal picture has changed with striking rapidity—in less than 10 years—and we have moved from explanation to action.

For many years, attempts at understanding psychological and psychosomatic aspects of obesity focused on intensive studies of individual persons. At first these studies were almost exclusively psychotherapeutic.[11, 16, 32, 43, 64, 65, 97] Later, objective measures of other variables were correlated with the data col-

Symptoms During Outpatient Dieting

Retrospectively (All Efforts)

"Nervousness"	21 %
"Weakness"	21 %
"Irritability"	8 %
"Fatigue"	5 %
"Nausea"	4 %
Total Reporting	54 %

Stunkard, Am. J. Med. 23:77–86, 1957

Prospectively (One Diet)

Depression	50 %
Anxiety	40 %

Silverstone & Lascelles, Brit. J. Psychiat. 112:513–519, 1966

Figure 16–2. Symptoms reported by obese persons in two reports.

lected in psychotherapy: glucose tolerance tests,[86] pedometer[15, 80] and time-motion measurements[9] of physical activity, distorting lens[26] and mirror images[89] of the human body, and so on.

These studies taught us that most obese persons impute great importance to emotional factors in determining the status of their obesity. Many report that they overeat and gain weight when they are emotionally upset and that when an emotional upset subsides, they eat less and lose weight. Observers can frequently add supporting objective evidence for this phenomenon. Obese persons under stress frequently gain weight, which they lose when the stress is relieved. Falling in love seems to be a particularly effective weight loss agent, just as falling out of love—or losing a loved one—is a potent force for fatness.

Furthermore, it has been widely believed that obese persons are more neurotic than are nonobese persons.

Despite the widespread acceptance of the importance of emotional factors in human obesity, it has proved singularly difficult to proceed from these simple and provocative findings to a more precise understanding. Although heroic psychodynamic psychotherapeutic endeavors—lasting over a decade and more—by the author and by Bruch[10] revealed that some obese persons could be helped to lose weight, and even to keep it off, the results seemed rather the nonspecific effects of a reduction in tension than contributions to the practical management of obesity.

Three lines of investigation during the past 10 years have changed this state of affairs and have moved us from explanation to action. The first has been a series of studies examining the relationship of social factors to obesity. The series began, paradoxically, with an effort to answer an old question: are obese persons more neurotic than nonobese persons? And it ended with the discovery of what is probably the most powerful determinant of obesity yet discovered—social pressure.

The preliminary investigation of the extent of psychopathology of obese persons yielded important results, important in large part because of their negative quality and because they contrast so dramatically with the positive findings linking social factors and obesity.

The question "are obese persons more neurotic than nonobese persons?" can now be answered quite definitely—"yes." And the "yes" can be immediately qualified with, "but not much more neurotic."

The answer was obtained through the same study that revealed the strong influence of social factors—a reanalysis of the data of the Midtown Manhattan study, a comprehensive survey of the epidemiology of mental illness.[74] This study has been described in great detail elsewhere so that only a brief review of its methodology will be presented here. The population under study consisted of 110,000 persons, all adults, between the ages of 20 and 59 years of age in an area of Manhattan selected so that it represented extremes in socioeconomic status, from extremely high to extremely low. A cross-section of 1,660 persons was selected as representative of the 110,000 by systematic probability sampling. Two hour interviews were conducted with these subjects in their homes by trained interviewers, who obtained information about social and ethnic background, a number of items designed to assess psychological and interpersonal functioning and height and weight.

Eight psychological scores were derived from the interviews and in seven out of the eight, the obese subjects had higher scores for psychopathology.[82] Table 16–1 shows the overall, uncontrolled, scores of obese and nonobese persons.

When appropriate controls for age and social class are introduced, differences between obese and nonobese persons decrease dramatically. Table 16–2 shows that the differences for three of the items retain respectable levels of statistical significance, but the introduction of controls decreases markedly the overall effects.

Table 16–1. Comparison of obese and normal people on mental health indices[a]

Trait	Percentage making pathological scores	
	Obese	Normal
Immaturity	63	49
Suspiciousness	43	25
Rigidity	67	45
Frustration-depression	23	18
Withdrawal	40	30
Tension-anxiety	34	31
Neurasthenia	17	10
Psychiatrists' rating	30	22
Childhood anxiety	32	38

[a] Obese persons show higher pathological scores on 8 indices. These figures are not controlled for socioeconomic status (Stunkard[82]).

The Social Environment

In contrast to the relatively small differences in psychopathology between obese and nonobese persons, the differences in social factors are dramatic indeed. The first such difference to emerge and still perhaps the most important one is that of social class, or socioeconomic status.[27, 56] Socioeconomic status was rated by a simple score based upon occupation, education, weekly income and monthly rent, and the scores divided into "low," "medium" and "high."

There was a marked inverse relationship between socioeconomic status and the prevalence of obesity. Figure 16–3 shows that the prevalence of obesity among women of lower socioeconomic status was 30% falling to 16% among those of middle status and to only 5% in the upper status group. The prevalence of obesity in the lower class was thus 6 times that found in the upper class! And when socioeconomic status was divided into 12 classes, as the richness of the data permitted, the difference between the lowermost and uppermost social classes became even greater—from a low of less than 2% in the uppermost to a high of 37% in the lowermost class.

Among men the differences between social classes were similar, but of a lesser degree. Men of lower socioeconomic status, for example, showed a prevalence of obesity of 32% compared to that of 16% among upperclass men.

One notable feature of these studies was that they were designed to permit

Table 16–2. Comparison between obese and normals on mental health measures[a]

Sex	Status	Age	Immaturity	Suspiciousness	Rigidity	Frustration-depression	Withdrawal	Tension-anxiety	Neurasthenia	Psychiatric rating	Childhood anxiety
Male	Low	Yng.	+3	+3	+2	−2	−6	+6	+5	−1	−9
		Old	+1	+9	+2	+1	+24	+8	+6	−9	−17
Male	Middle	Yng.	+4	+7	+11	+4	+2	+1	−15	+6	−9
		Old	+15	+21	+27	+2	+11	−13	+5	+6	−8
Male	High	Yng.	+15	+21	+<1	+<1	+14	+24	+5	+11	+17
		Old	+25	+18	+13	+9	+14	−9	−3	+16	−6
Female	Low	Yng.	+3	+13	−9	−12	−8	+4	+3	−9	+19
		Old	+1	+6	+13	+10	−1	+4	+21	+7	+3
Female	Middle	Yng.	+38	+25	+46	+6	+11	+9	+13	+13	−3
		Old	+15	+20	+26	+9	+19	+7	+23	+12	−7
Female	High	Yng.	+1	+21	+13	+21	+5	+45	−13	−12	−5
		Old	+18	+5	+25	+6	−2	+4	+10	+9	−26
		P	<0.003	<0.003	<0.007	<0.055	<0.055	<0.108	<0.137	<0.204	<0.478

[a]Corrected for sex, age and socioeconomic status. Figures are the differences between percentages of normals and obese who responded pathologically (+ means a higher percentage of obese group fell into pathological category; − means that a higher percentage of normals did) (Moore et al.[56]).

causal inferences about the influence of socioeconomic status. Earlier studies, which had demonstrated associations between socioeconomic status and psychiatric disorder, had been unable to go beyond these correlations to any statements about cause. In Midtown, however, sufficient data were collected to make possible such statements. This was achieved by ascertaining not only the socioeconomic status of the respondents at the time of the study, but also that of their parents when they were 8 years old. Although a subject's schizophrenia, or obesity, might influence his social class, it is unlikely that his disability in adult life could have influenced his parents' social class. Therefore, associations between the social class of the respondent's parents and his disability can be viewed as causal. Figure 16-3 shows that such associations were almost as powerful as those between the social class of the respondents and their obesity.[27]

The impact of these findings increased as additional social variables were considered. For it is a remarkable fact that, in Midtown at least, every single social variable investigated was related to the prevalence of obesity, with the relationship usually stronger for women than it was for men. In addition to socioeconomic status and socioeconomic status of origin, these variables included social mobility, generation in the United States and ethnic and religious affiliation.

For example, Figure 16-4 shows that obesity was more prevalent among downwardly socially mobile subjects (22%) than among those who remained in the social class of their parents (18%) and far more prevalent than among those who were upwardly socially mobile (12%).[27]

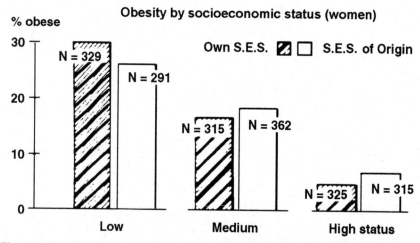

Figure 16–3. Decreasing prevalence of obesity with increase in socioeconomic status (SES) (Goldblatt et al.[27]).

Generation in the United States was also strongly linked to obesity.[27] Respondents were divided into one of four groups on the basis of the number of generations their families had been in this country. Generation I consisted of foreign-born immigrants; generation II of all those native-born respondents who had at least one foreign born parent; generation III of all those who are native-born and of native-born parents but had at least one foreign-born grandparent; and generation IV of all those who had no foreign-born grandparents and who otherwise met the qualifications for generation III.

Figure 16–5 shows that the longer a woman's family had been in this country, the less likely she was to be obese. Of first-generation respondents, 24% were overweight in contrast to only 5% in the fourth generation ($\chi^2 = 56.5$; $P < 0.001$).

Generation in the United States is closely linked to socioeconomic status. The data relating generation to obesity was therefore reanalyzed, holding socioeconomic status constant. This analysis showed that the inverse relationship between generation and obesity was independent of socioeconomic status.

The presence of nine different ethnic groups in the Midtown Study permitted an assessment of the influence of ethnicity upon obesity. Once again, a social factor was found to be closely linked to the prevalence of obesity. Table 16–3

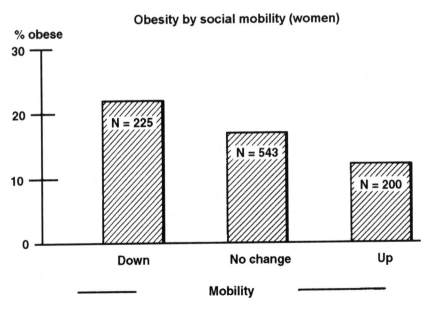

Figure 16–4. Decreasing prevalence of obesity with upward social mobility (Goldblatt et al.[27]).

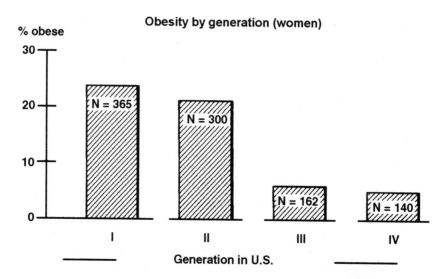

Figure 16–5. Decreasing prevalence of obesity with increasing length of time of family of respondent in United States (Goldblatt et al.[27]).

shows striking differences in the prevalence of obesity in the nine ethnic groups.[83] The sample size was not large enough to permit tests of statistical significance of the differences between all of the groups, when all essential controlling variables were utilized. Nevertheless, a striking picture emerges, particularly among women.

The strongest evidence of the influence of ethnic factors on the prevalence of obesity is found among persons of lower socioeconomic status, with wide variability about the mean of 30%. Ethnicity is not quite as strong a predictor of obesity as socioeconomic status, with its 6–1 differential between lower and upper classes. Nevertheless, when only lower class respondents are considered, the greater than 40% prevalence among Hungarian and Czech respondents means that there is a 3–1 differential between them and the least obese group, fourth generation Americans, who show a prevalence of only 13%.

There is a suggestion of an interesting interaction between ethnicity and socioeconomic status. Among both Hungarians and Czechs, for example, the prevalence of greater than 40% among the lower classes differs strikingly from the absence of obesity in the upper classes. By contrast, the similar differential between lower and upper class, fourth generation American, is only 13% compared to 4%.

Religious affiliation was still another social factor linked to obesity. Again, the sample size precluded control of all relevant variables. Nevertheless, the

Table 16-3. Distribution of obesity among nine ethnic groups (women)

	Socioeconomic status	Total	% Obese
American (fourth generation)	Low	15	13
	Medium	23	4
	High	102	4
Puerto Rican	Low	13	15
	Medium	4	25
	High	1	0
Russian, Polish, Lithuanian	Low	11	18
	Medium	25	12
	High	41	10
British	Low	13	23
	Medium	22	0
	High	21	10
Irish	Low	69	25
	Medium	51	16
	High	29	3
Italian	Low	31	32
	Medium	31	23
	High	5	20
German, Austrian	Low	82	35
	Medium	69	16
	High	55	4
Czech	Low	46	41
	Medium	17	29
	High	5	0
Hungarian	Low	16	44
	Medium	17	24
	High	11	0

findings closely fit the now-expected pattern. The greatest prevalence of obesity was among Jews, followed by Roman Catholics and Protestants. Among Protestants, the pattern is further exemplified. The largest amount of obesity is found among Baptists, with a decreasing prevalence among Methodists, Lutherans and Episcopalians.

Influence of Social Factors in Other Countries

Is the relationship between social factors and obesity an exclusively American phenomenon? Or does it apply more broadly—in other Western societies and in the developing nations? It should be noted at this point that all further data relating social factors to obesity are correlational. No other study has gone to the immense pains of the Midtown investigators to determine the social status of the respondents' parents. Nevertheless, the close correspondence between the socioeconomic status of respondents and that of their parents in Midtown makes it likely that causation underlies at least part of the correlations described below.

Two reports from England describe the same kind of relationship between socioeconomic status and obesity among women that had been discovered earlier in Manhattan. Silverstone et al. discovered nearly twice the prevalence of obesity in women of lower socioeconomic status as in those of upper socioeconomic status. Figure 16–6 makes it appear that prevalence of obesity is far higher in London than in New York. In fact, most of the difference is due to a more generous definition of obesity in the London Study.[71]

Among men, prevalence of obesity increased as one descended the socioeconomic ladder from upper to middle status. It fell again, however, among lower class men, thus providing the first exception to the emerging pattern. Accordingly, they were selected for special study. It was learned that the lower

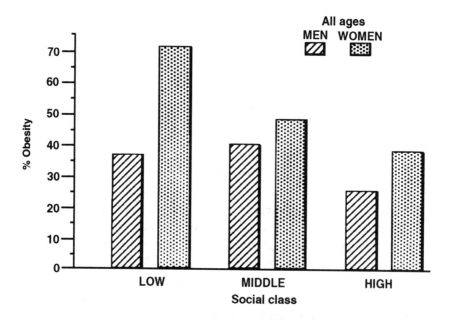

Figure 16–6. Prevalence of obesity by social class in London. Among women increasing social class is associated with decreasing prevalence of obesity. Lower class men provide an exception to this pattern (Silverstone et al.[71]).

prevalence of obesity among lower class men was accounted for entirely by older men; younger ones showed the expected pattern of very high prevalence. Study of the older, lower class men revealed that every member of this group was engaged in very heavy manual labor—porters, hod carriers, mailmen, etc. These men appeared to exemplify Mayer's position that very high levels of physical activity override other factors predisposing towards obesity and make it possible to regulate body weight.[51]

McLean Baird et al.[3] have recently confirmed the relationship between social class and obesity in London. Table 16–4 summarizes the results of their survey of 1,334 Londoners.

The criterion for obesity utilized in this study was closer to that of the Midtown Study than was that of Silverstone and permits a closer comparison of the prevalence of obesity by social class in the two cities. Obesity is more prevalent among upper class women in London than among the comparable group in New York, resulting in a social class differential of slightly more than 2:1 compared to the 6:1 ratio in Manhattan. As in Manhattan, the social class differential among men is considerably less than that among women—3:2. It appears that in a Western urban setting, social factors have more influence upon women than upon men. This inference is supported by the finding that women in the United States have become somewhat thinner during the last 20 years of mounting concern over obesity, while men have continued to become fatter.

The only comparable studies of the relationship of social factors to obesity among adults in Western society were carried out in Germany.[62] Among German women, socioeconomic status showed the now-expected negative correlation with obesity. Among German men, on the other hand, a positive correlation was found; the higher the socioeconomic status, the greater the prevalence of obesity.

Age of Onset of Social Influences

The consistent and striking relationship between social factors and obesity has led three groups to investigate the vital question of the age at which this influ-

Table 16–4. Social class and prevalence of obesity (%) in London Survey[a]

	Social class		
	A & B	C	D & E
Men	16	18	36
Women	12	16	18

[a]Figures are the percent of obese persons in each social class. A&B = upper, C = middle, D&E = lower social classes (Baird[3]).

ence makes itself felt. The first of these studies, by Huenemann,[38] found the same inverse relationship between socioeconomic status and obesity well established by adolescence. Table 16–5 shows the decrease in prevalence of obesity with increasing social class in 1,000 teenagers in Berkeley, California. Obesity was defined as 30% of total body weight as fat in girls and 25% in boys.

Whitelaw[92] also found a decrease in obesity with increasing social class in London schoolboys aged 7–15. Skinfold thickness measures revealed that 8.5% of lower class boys were obese, compared with 5.1% prevalence of obesity in middle class boys and 4.9% among upper class boys. Interestingly, he found no relationship between social class and mean skinfold thickness, suggesting that there is no general increase in fatness among lower class boys, but rather an increased proportion of definitely obese individuals. Whitelaw also reported an interesting and significant trend for obesity to be less frequent with increasing sibling number. The significance of this finding is still unclear.

A study of 3,344 white school children in three Eastern cities provided conclusive evidence for the influence of social class upon obesity in children, and further disturbing indications of just how early this influence is exerted.[85] Figure 16–7 shows the relationship between socioeconomic status and prevalence of obesity for girls ($\chi^2 = 70,83$, $P < .001$). At age 6, the lower socioeconomic group contained 8% obese girls, while the upper class group had no obese girls at either age 6 or 7. This difference was maintained until age 18, with an increase in the prevalence of obesity with increasing age in both groups. Figure 16–7 shows further that the slopes for the upper and lower classes differ, with a greater yearly increment in the percentage of obese among lower class girls. Obesity is thus not only more prevalent among poor girls, but its greater prevalence is established earlier and increases at a more rapid rate than among upper class girls.

In this study, obesity was defined as the 10% of each sex in the total population that had the thickest skinfolds, and the minimum skinfold thickness of this group was used to define obesity within each age group. These empirically derived values for obesity were 23 mm for girls and 18 mm for boys. Use of per-

Table 16–5. Social class and prevalence of obesity

	Percent who are obese			
	Low	Medium	High	
Girls	11.6	6.2	5.4	Huenemann[38]
Boys	6.3	6.0	2.3	
	8.5	5.1	4.5	Whitelaw[92]

centile criterion is favored over some others for purposes such as this study.[33]

Lower class boys showed a greater prevalence for obesity than did those of the upper class. Figure 16–8 shows differences comparable to those among girls through age 10. Unlike the pattern among the girls, however, the difference between the boys is not continuous to age 18. At age 12, for example, there is a curious and unexplained greater prevalence of obesity among lower class boys. Lower class boys showed a greater prevalence of obesity than did those of the upper class, but the differences were neither as large nor as consistent.

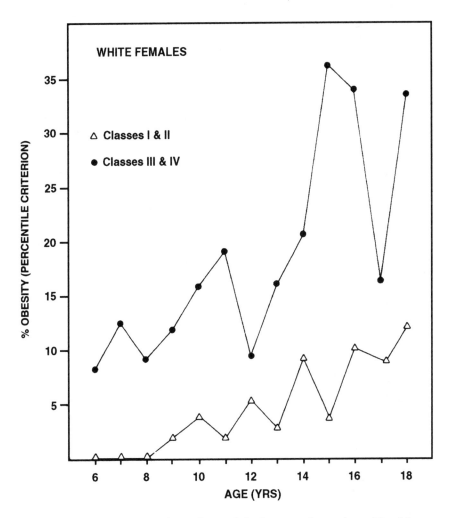

Figure 16–7. Greatly increased prevalence of obesity among lower class white girls compared to upper class white girls (Stunkard et al.[85]).

Influence of Social Factors in Less Affluent Societies

To what degree are these findings applicable also to other cultures? To answer this question, we must bear in mind that rarely, if ever, has an entire people had more than enough to eat for any prolonged period of time. As a result, throughout history, as in many underdeveloped areas today, obesity has been restricted to the privileged classes. In many cultures it is a status symbol, and the legendary yearly weighings of the Aga Khan suggest that the size of its leaders can represent a source of pride for an entire community. Under the circumstances,

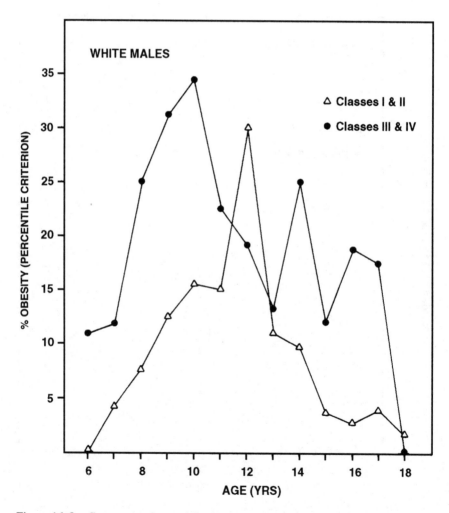

Figure 16–8. Greater prevalence of obesity among lower class boys compared to upper class boys (Stunkard et al.[85]).

one might expect obesity to be more prevalent among the privileged classes.

Until now, we have had no information on the relationship between social factors and obesity in a nonaffluent, developing society. This is most unfortunate, for such information is essential to an understanding of this most potent force. Are the obesity-controlling effects of increasing socioeconomic status in New York a general phenomenon or only a special case in an affluent society?

There is growing evidence that the relationship in New York *is* a special case. Scattered information on the relationship of social factors and mean body weight or mean skinfold thickness (not obesity) in developing countries reveals a relationship that is the precise opposite of that in Western urban societies. Figure 16–9, adapted from Mayer,[51] shows a strong positive correlation between

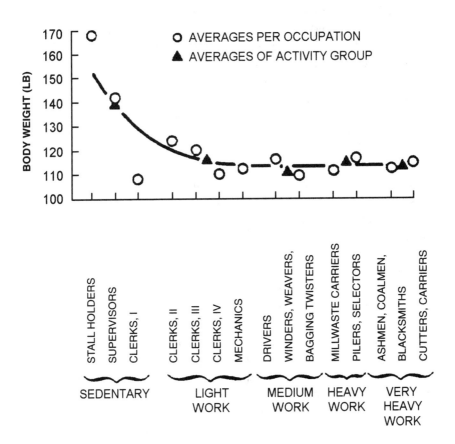

Figure 16–9. Decreasing mean body weight with decreasing affluence in a population in West Bengal (Mayer[51]).

relative affluence and mean body weight. Although Mayer related these findings to physical activity, they also represent the influence of social forces. Most people cannot afford to buy enough food to become obese. The opportunity of becoming obese is restricted by hard economic forces to the more affluent members of the society.

Similar findings have been reported among adults in Latin America and Puerto Rico and among children in South China and the Philippines; increasing standard of living is associated with increasing mean body weight or skinfold thickness.[2, 13, 91]

The first data on the relationship of social factors to obesity (as contrasted to mean body weights) in a less affluent society have been obtained recently. They show that in this setting, affluence is directly related to the prevalence of obesity, in sharp contrast to the relationship found in Western urban societies.[23] One of the most powerful social forces in Navaho society is acculturation to the surrounding "Anglo" (white) culture, a factor that correlates strongly with relative affluence. A reliable acculturation index was devised and administered to 690 Navaho children between the ages of 6 and 12. Figure 16–10 shows the relationship between acculturation to Western affluent society and prevalence of obesity in boys. From the ages of 7–11, obesity was significantly more prevalent among acculturated boys than among traditional ones, and this difference is statistically significant. Furthermore, also in contrast to the findings in Western urban societies, thinness was more common among the traditional children.

Comparison of the standard of living of these Navaho children and those in the study of Eastern city children revealed that the least affluent Eastern city children enjoyed a considerably higher standard of living than did the most acculturated (and affluent) Navaho children. These findings permit us to construct a general proposition relating affluence and its associated social factors to the prevalence of obesity. Figure 16–11 shows a maximum prevalence of obesity occurring among the poorer members of Western urban society. This prevalence decreases with both decreasing *and* increasing affluence, but the reasons for the decreases differ dramatically. With decreasing affluence, the constraint upon the development of obesity is the lack of food. With increasing affluence, fads and fashions exert the control. We do not currently have enough information to transform this qualitative model into a quantitative one, but that day may not be far off. It is of interest that, although less detailed, the information on the relationship of affluence to thinness shows a pattern that is the mirror image of that for obesity.

The full implications of these findings for our understanding of obesity and for its control have yet to be realized. For they mean that whatever its genetic determinants and its biochemical pathways, obesity is to an unusual degree

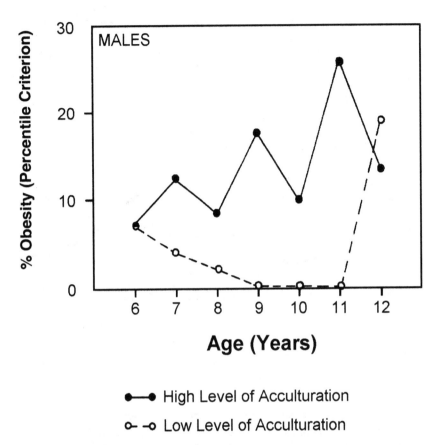

Figure 16–10. Greater prevalence of obesity among Navajo boys with high level acculturation (Garb et al.[23]).

under social environmental control. They set the next target of investigation—how does the social environment exert this control? And they suggest that a broad scale assault on obesity need not await further understanding of its biochemical determinants. Understanding of its social determinants may be sufficient.

The Immediate Environment

Further impetus towards the study of influence of the immediate, small group environment on eating behavior came from two sources: experimental obesity

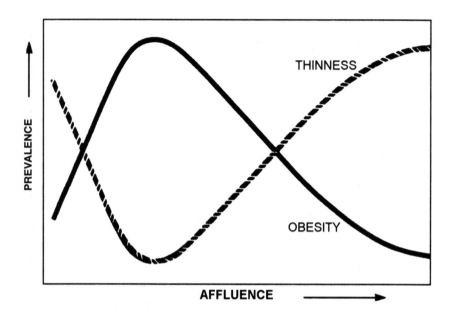

Figure 16–11. Schematic representation of the relationship between affluence and prevalence of obesity and thinness. (For description see text.)

in animals and psychotherapy of obese patients. Both sources suggested that obese persons might be unusually susceptible to the influence of their environment. These studies began with a paper in 1950 by Neal Miller[55] on "Decreased Hunger and Increased Food Intake in Hypothalamic Obese Rats." In this prescient study, Miller described for the first time the peculiar feeding behavior of rats made obese by hypothalamic lesions. A cardinal feature of this behavior was that obese rats overate when food was freely available, but when an impediment was placed in the way of their eating, food intake not only decreased, but actually decreased to a far lower level than that of control rats without hypothalamic lesions. Furthermore, it seemed to make little difference what kind of impediment was used. Motivation to work for food was impaired in every manner of task that could be devised. These tasks included lifting the covers of food cages, pressing levers for food, accepting the discomfort of crossing an electrified grid, or tolerating dilution of their food with quinine. These studies exploded our traditional views of "hunger" as a unitary phenomenon. Hunger defined by food intake can be a quite different matter from hunger defined by traditional instrumental criteria.

The study of the eating behavior of hypothalamic obese animals suggests that this behavior is characterized by an impairment in the mechanism of satiety. Of perhaps equal importance, because of its potential for therapy, is the likelihood of an impairment in the drive to eat, as this latter drive has been measured by traditional instruments. One could say that the food intake of these animals was not controlled by internal factors to the same degree as that of normal weight rats or, conversely, that it was to a far greater degree under the control of external, environmental, factors.

This view of the food intake of hypothalamic obese animals has proved congenial to clinicians who have dealt with obese persons. For a characteristic complaint is an inability to stop eating once they have started, and it is the exceptional obese person who presents a picture of voracious overeating or a desire for food that drives him in the way that a desire for narcotics drives the addict, or the need for drink, drives the alcoholic. Until the work of Stanley Schachter, however, such characterizations had been based primarily on self-reports, and the problem had not been approached experimentally. In recent years, however, Schachter and his associates have applied the tools of social psychology to deal with the disinclination of obese persons to adopt their usual eating habits under the special circumstances of the laboratory. These tools—especially the deception experiment—obscure the nature of the experiment and present plausible cover stories to distract the subjects still further from its real purpose.

In two lengthy review articles, Schachter[68, 69] had described a series of such studies demonstrating the susceptibility of human eating behavior to environmental cues. In an early study, obese subjects tended to eat either one or three sandwiches, depending upon the number (one or three) presented on a table in front of them, even though they were told that there were many more sandwiches in a conveniently placed refrigerator. A second study revealed what has been called dietary "finickiness" in lower animals with some forms of experimental obesity. When distracted from the purpose of the experiment, obese persons ate far more of a creamy, delicious ice cream than of an acrid, quinine-adulterated one. A third study utilized a clock that could be manipulated to run twice as fast, and twice as slow, as real clock time. Obese subjects ate twice as many crackers when they thought it was later than when they thought it was earlier than it really was.

In each study, Schachter and his associates reported that nonobese subjects were considerably less susceptible to these environmental cues than were the obese subjects. On this basis he elaborated a popular theory ascribing overeating by obese persons to their "externality," or peculiar susceptibility to environmental cues. More recent work from other laboratories has failed to confirm this theory.[63, 66, 73, 95, 96] The failures to replicate Schachter's earlier findings, however, seem to have arisen more from an unexpected responsiveness on the part of nonobese persons than from a lack of responsiveness on the part of the obese ones. Indeed, it now appears as if many persons, obese and nonobese alike, are far more "external" than we have had any reason to believe.

Even if susceptibility to food and eating cues in the environment is not peculiar to obese persons, it may still form a basis for therapy of obesity.

Special Therapeutic Environments

It may be unusual to view therapy as a form of social environment, but the introduction of behavior modification for the control of obesity in 1967 has made such a view entirely appropriate. For behavior modification is an attempt to construct a special kind of environment—social and material—that will help obese persons to gain control over their eating. If the food intake of obese persons is determined to such a great extent by unplanned environmental factors, could it not be controlled by planned and purposeful rearrangement of the factors?

It seems appropriate to begin this account with a disclaimer. The term therapy may imply the restoration to normal of a previously disordered function. Some of the more enthusiastic behavior modifiers are drawing such implications from their work with obesity. They are saying that because obese persons can lose weight by modifying their eating behavior, disordered eating behavior must have been the cause of their obesity. There is just no evidence for such a contention. It is equally plausible that behavior modification may simply be helping someone who biologically should be obese to live in a semistarved condition. Such a state of affairs is no reflection on the potency of behavioral techniques. In fact, it could be accounted a greater therapeutic triumph to overcome such a biological gradient than simply to improve bad habits. In any event, the effects of the special therapeutic environment described below reflect no presumptions as to the etiology of obesity. They do, however, teach us something about the social control of a biological function. And they raise the tantalizing possibility of establishing a purposeful control over eating and obesity, in contrast to the unplanned and often erratic control exerted by the large-scale social environment.

The distinguishing characteristic of the various methods called behavior modification is the belief that behavior disorders of the most divergent types are learned responses, and that modern theories of learning have much to teach us regarding both the acquisition and extinction of these responses. Furthermore, proponents of behavior modification have been distinguished by their explicit statements of methods and goals and by their willingness to put their results on the line for comparison with other forms of treatment. For example, behavior therapists were among the first to recognize the power, as a dependent variable in psychotherapy research, of weight change in pounds, and they have turned to the treatment of obesity in increasing numbers in order to utilize this measure. It is ironic that psychiatry, so sorely in need of measures to evaluate therapeutic effectiveness, has taken so long to recognize the sensitivity, reliability and validity of weight change as such a measure.

In the past it was fairly easy to assess any outpatient treatment for obesity because the results were so uniformly poor and the treatments so obviously inadequate. (Inpatient treatment, with its potential for greater control of the patient, has, of course, been more successful in weight reduction. Its usefulness has been limited, however, because patients almost invariably regain the lost weight after discharge.) Only 25% of persons entering treatment lose as much as 20 pounds and 5% as much as 40 pounds.[81]

A Landmark in the Treatment of Obesity

Against this background, Stuart's[77] 1967 report on "Behavioral Control of Overeating" stands out. It describes the best results ever reported for the outpatient treatment of obesity and constitutes a landmark in our understanding of this disorder. Even the absence of a control group does not vitiate the significance of its findings.

Stuart's results are summarized in Figures 16–12 and 16–13, which show the weight losses, over a 1-year period, of eight patients who remained in treatment out of an original 10 who started. Three, or 30% of the original sample, lost more than 40 pounds and 6 lost more than 30 pounds. All were women, six were married and two had children. All had been referred for private treatment.

Certain features of the report deserve attention. First, the expenditure of time was not exorbitant. In fact, time spent in treatment was no greater than that in a number of other studies that achieved far poorer results. At the beginning of the treatment period, patients were seen in 30-min sessions held three times a week, for a total of 12 to 15 sessions. Thereafter, treatment sessions were scheduled as needed, usually at 2-week intervals, for the next 3 months. Subsequently, there were weekly sessions and finally, "maintenance" sessions as needed. The total number of visits during the year varied from 16 to 41.

The program utilized by Stuart[78] formed the basis for an increasingly sophisticated "package" of behavioral techniques. Stuart's program was derived in large part from an earlier study by Ferster et al.,[20] which described in great detail the rationale and procedures of a behavioral approach to obesity. Ferster never

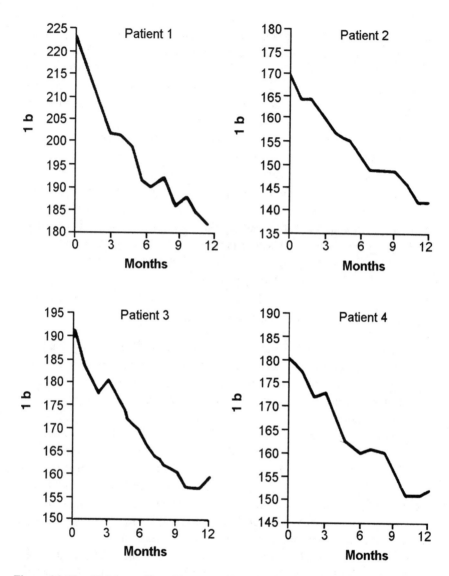

Figure 16–12. Weight profiles of four women undergoing behavior therapy for obesity (Stuart[77]).

reported the results of treatment, and a personal communication revealed negligible weight losses. A critical feature of Ferster's and Stuart's approach is the specification of a rigid set of "how to do it" instructions for each of the 10 or 12 patient contacts. Within this framework, there is a surprising opportunity for the exercise of creativity by both patient and therapist. For example, Stuart noted

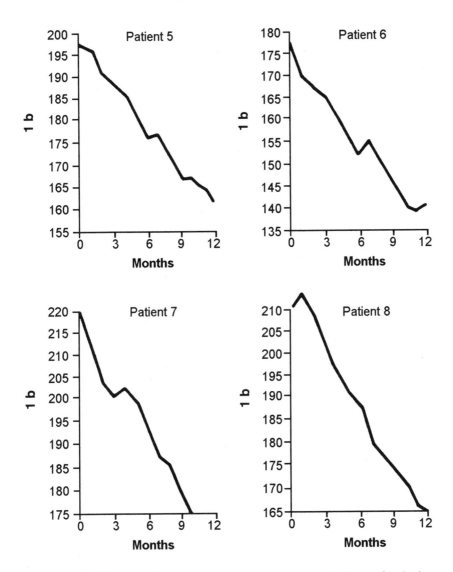

Figure 16–13. Weight profiles of four women undergoing behavior therapy for obesity (Stuart[77]).

that, for patients suffering from a "behavioral depression," eating may be the only available reinforcer. Effective treatment depends upon helping them develop a reservoir of positively reinforcing responses. Two persons in Stuart's program were helped to develop such responses: an interest in growing violets and in caring for caged birds.

There was no evidence of untoward responses to the program or of "symptom substitution." Seven of the eight patients reported that they had developed an increased range of social activities, and three of the six married patients reported more satisfying relationships with their husbands. Furthermore, three of the eight who were also compulsive smokers applied the same general program to smoking and either substantially reduced or eliminated it.

These results were so good that control subjects were not needed to establish the power of the method. But it was not long before carefully controlled studies began. The first appeared in 1969.

Introduction of No-Treatment Controls

The possibility of rigidly specifying treatment conditions, and the availability of a dependent variable—weight change in pounds—of unprecedented reliability, validity and economy, has produced a veritable explosion of research on behavioral control of obesity. Soon after Stuart's trailblazing study, Harris[35] reported excellent results in a controlled study that utilized a behavioral program based upon Stuart's. Subjects were mildly overweight college students. Two treatment groups of three male and five female students each were compared with a control group of eight students. In order not to discourage the latter, and thereby bias the results, the control subjects were told that they could not enter treatment at once because of a conflict in schedules, but that they would receive treatment later. Treatment sessions were held twice weekly for the first 2 months and then on an irregular basis for the second 2 months.

The results are illustrated in Figure 16–14. The mean weight loss for the experimental group was 10.5 pounds compared with a weight *gain* of 3.6 pounds for the control group, a highly significant difference ($P < 0.001$).

Although the results in the treatment group are clearly far superior to those in the no-treatment control group, they are not as good as others reported in the literature when judged by the criteria mentioned earlier: only 21% of Harris' subjects lost 20 pounds and none lost as much as 40 pounds. A major reason for these results was that her subjects were considerably less obese than those studied by Stuart.

There were two important features of this study other than the demonstration that behavior modification was more effective than no treatment. The first important feature was the finding that weight loss continued for the 16 weeks following the end of treatment. As we have noted earlier, under traditional conditions, most obese persons regain most of the weight they have lost in treatment. For an obese person to continue to lose weight following treatment is uncommon; for a group to do so may well have been unprecedented. Harris'

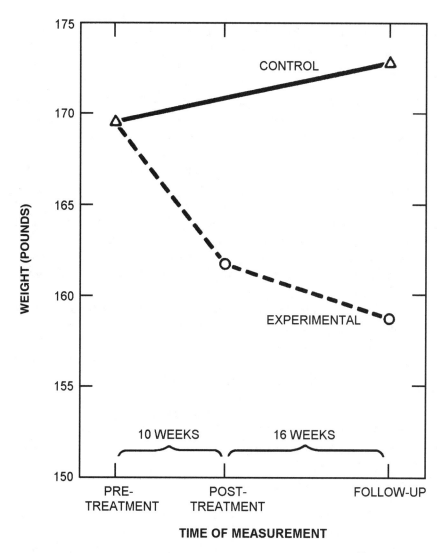

Figure 16–14. Weights for behavior therapy and control subjects (Harris[35]).

follow-up results, almost as much as Stuart's weight-loss results, represent a landmark in the treatment of obesity. These follow-up results were not an isolated occurrence. Half of subsequent broadly based behavioral programs have produced similar results. Three of the more carefully reported studies, it is true, noted weight gain during the follow-up period.[19, 30, 93] Interestingly, all three studies were of mildly overweight college students. Two others, on the other hand, confirmed Harris' finding of continuing weight loss following treatment.[45, 61] Each utilized moderately to severely obese subjects and reported follow-ups of substantial duration—1 year.

The second important feature of the study was that it highlighted the problem of controls in psychotherapy research. Harris' control group consisted of subjects who were promised treatment, but received it later. This procedure was quite acceptable, indeed, it was methodologically advanced for psychotherapy research in 1969. Yet the use of a no-treatment control group has serious disadvantages. Refusing treatment to someone who has come seeking it is far from a neutral event. Deterioration in the condition of members of a control group that has been disappointed in its expectation of a treatment could give the false impression that a treatment was effective. The mere attention given to the treatment group might prevent their deterioration and explain their relative improvement as compared to the no-treatment control group. Such a possibility may seem remote, yet it was precisely the weight gain in Harris' no-treatment control group that rendered statistically significant the modest weight losses in her active treatment condition.

The problem calls for the use of a placebo control condition to match the attention and interest that is received by patients in the active treatment condition. It has long been an article of faith in psychopharmacology that adequate evaluation of a therapeutic agent requires the use of placebo controls. The need for similar controls in the assessment of psychotherapy is every bit as great. For the positive expectations elicited by a charismatic practitioner of a popular therapy may well be even greater than those evoked by a new drug. Yet until very recently, the problem of providing a placebo control for psychotherapy had seemed an insurmountable obstacle.

The Introduction of Placebo Controls

A scant 2 years after Harris' study posed the problem of placebo controls in psychotherapy research, a graduate student at the University of Illinois took a giant step towards solving it. In an elaborate factorial design, Janet Wollersheim[93, 94] introduced one of the first, and perhaps the finest, example to date of placebo controls. This design opened up new vistas in psychotherapy research. It deserves careful consideration.

Wollersheim's study contained four experimental conditions based upon Stuart's and described below in detail.

(1) "Focal" (behavioral) treatment.
(2) "Nonspecific therapy" to control for factors such as increased attention, "faith," expectation of relief and presentation of a treatment rationale. This

rationale was compatible with common current beliefs about obesity, purporting to "develop insight into the real and not readily recognizable underlying reasons" for the patients' behavior and to "discover the unconscious motives" underlying their "personality make-up." Each subject was told that as she obtained insight into the "real motives and forces" operating within her personality, she would find it easier to lose weight. This rationale helped the therapist to divert subjects away from discussion of ways of modifying eating patterns that might inadvertently duplicate measures of the behavioral treatment. When such discussions began, the therapist simply directed the groups' attention away from such "superficial" issues back to the "real . . . underlying causes" of their behavior.

(3) "Social pressure" condition was patterned after that of the self-help group TOPS (Take Off Pounds Sensibly) and included such TOPS procedures as a weigh-in, followed by praise for weight loss and encouragement for failure to lose weight.

(4) A no-treatment-wait control condition of persons promised treatment but receiving it later.

The study thus contained three treatment conditions—(1), (2), (3)—and three control conditions—(2), (3), (4)—for behavior modification. The 80 subjects were mildly (29%) overweight female college students. Four therapists each treated one group of five subjects in each of the three treatment conditions for a total of 10 sessions during the 3-month period.

Wollersheim's findings are illustrated in Figure 16–15. At the end of treatment, and at 8 weeks' follow-up, subjects in the focal treatment condition had lost far more weight than those in the no-treatment condition. In addition, they had lost significantly more weight than those in the two placebo control conditions who had themselves achieved respectable weight losses. The behavioral treatment clearly contributed something to the outcome that was over and above the usual effects of psychotherapy.

This contribution seemed to have resulted from the specific effects of the behavioral intervention. For not only did this condition produce greater weight loss, but it also produced major changes in self-reports dealing with eating behaviors. Statistically significant differences between the "focal" therapy and the other three conditions were found in four of the six factors assessed by the questionnaire: "emotional and uncontrolled eating," "eating in isolation," "eating as a reward," and "between-meal eating." Whatever caused the weight loss in the two placebo control conditions apparently did so without affecting these behaviors. The "focal" therapy apparently produced weight loss by means of its proposed rationale.

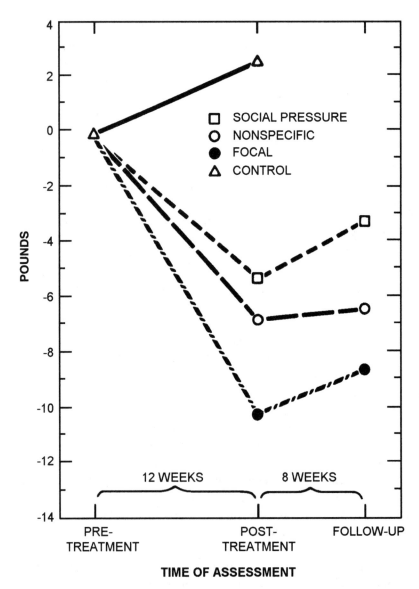

Figure 16–15. Mean weight loss of the focal (behavioral) treatment group, the two alternative treatment control groups, and the no-treatment control group (Wollersheim[93]).

Before leaving Wollersheim's study, let us consider a flaw that arose from the very advances in her experimental design. It is the problem of experimenter bias, a problem that had seemed mercifully distant in psychotherapy research. In such research, unlike the situation in psychopharmacology, it is still not apparent how one can obscure from the person administering a treatment the precise nature of the treatment. The identically-appearing placebo capsule of psychotherapy has yet to be devised. And although Wollersheim's placebo treatments controlled for the patient's expectations of treatment, they could not control for the therapist's. This is hardly a trivial matter. A large measure of therapeutic effectiveness is that conveyed by the therapist's expectations. Development of the methodology of the double-blind experiment in psychopharmacology has shown how powerful this influence can be when dealing with drugs. It is surely more powerful in the more emotional case of the psychotherapies. And therapists' expectations of the effectiveness of behavioral approaches must have been at a peak of optimism in the behaviorally-oriented department at the University of Illinois where Wollersheim conducted her research. It would have been hard to find a potential therapist who had any doubt about the efficacy of the behavioral approach; it would have been even harder for a therapist to report that his patients fared less well on a behavioral regimen. It is a tribute to the sophistication of Wollersheim's experimental design that psychotherapy research has finally achieved the maturity of coming face-to-face with a problem of mature research fields—the problem of experimenter bias.

Another Method of Controlling Bias: Its Use in the Treatment of Severe Obesity

It is unlikely that psychotherapy research will ever attain to the elegance and economy of the double-blind methodology of the psychopharmacologist. The control of experimenter bias will require methods tailored to the special needs and opportunities of this kind of research. One such method, deceptive in its simplicity, was introduced by Penick et al.[61]

The essence of this ingenious study was to give up at the start the notion that therapists could be unbiased in the use of therapies that they favored and disfavored. Instead, therapists were selected on the basis of their commitment either to a behavioral or a traditional approach to therapy. Penick further biased the outcome against the behavioral approach by selecting therapists of vastly different experience for the two conditions. For the behavioral treatment, the therapists were beginners; for the control condition, they were experts.

Therapists for the behavioral treatment were a male experimental psychologist with a strong background in learning theory but little clinical experience and a female research assistant with no previous experience in therapy. The control therapy was carried out by Penick himself, an internist who at that time had had 10 years of experience in the treatment of obesity, and who was completing a psychiatric residency that had given him considerable additional training in group therapy. The female co-therapist was a research nurse who had worked with Penick for several years. They utilized supportive psychotherapy, instruction about nutrition and dieting, and, upon request, appetite suppressants.

Each therapeutic team began with the conviction that its method was superior and sought, in a competitive way, to prove it. For, despite his curiosity about behavioral methods, Penick was convinced that inexperienced practitioners could not match his own highly accomplished performance.

In addition to its ingenious method of attempting to control for bias, Penick's study is worthy of note for the character of its patients. A great many of the trials of behavior modification have been carried out with mildly overweight college students. By contrast, the patients in Penick's study were severely obese—78% overweight. Two cohorts, of eight and seven persons respectively, were treated in weekly group meetings lasting 2 hours for a period of 3 months.

What were the results? The weight losses for each subject are plotted in Figures 16–16 and 16–17. They show that subjects treated with behavior modification lost more weight than those treated by the full armamentarium of traditional therapy. In each cohort, the median weight loss for the behavior modification group was greater than that of the control group: 24 pounds versus 18 pounds for the first cohort; 13 versus 11 for the second.

The weight losses of the control group are comparable to those found in the medical literature—none lost 40 pounds and only 24% lost more than 20 pounds. By contrast, 13% of the behavior modification group lost more than 40 pounds and 53% lost more than 20 pounds. Although the differences between the experimental and control groups for these weight losses did not reach statistical significance, that for weight losses of over 30 pounds did—$P = 0.015$ by the Fisher exact probability test.

Two further points should be noted. First, the variability in the weight losses of the behavior modification subjects was considerably greater than that of the patients treated by traditional methods ($F = 4.38$, $P < 0.005$). The five best performers were patients in the behavior modification condition as was the single least effective patient, the only patient who actually gained weight during treatment. Such greater variability has in other circumstances been associated with greater specificity of the treatment, and this explanation of the findings seems reasonable. It would appear that for half of the patients, behavior modification seems to offer something specific that results in greater weight loss than usual. For about another half, it seems of considerably less value. By contrast, the results of traditional treatment seem much more homogeneous, reflecting, perhaps, such nonspecific effects of therapy such as attention, support and encouragement.

The Case of Obesity

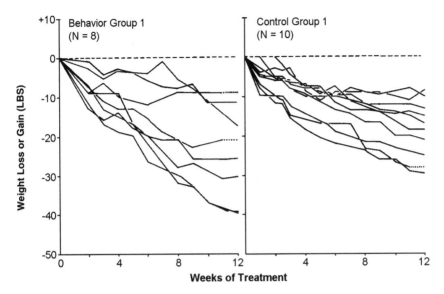

Figure 16–16. Weight changes of severely obese persons in two cohorts. Dotted lines represent interpolated data based upon weights obtained during follow up. Note greater weight loss of behavior modification groups and greater variability of this weight loss as compared to the control group (Penick et al.[61]).

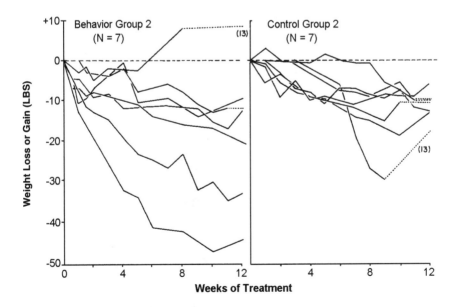

Figure 16–17. Same as Figure 16–16.

The second point is illustrated in Figure 16–18. At 1 year follow-up, weight losses of the behavior modification group had not only continued, they had actually increased.[84] All subjects who had lost more than 20 pounds during treatment had maintained that loss, and fully one third of the subjects had lost more than 40 pounds. Clearly, weight loss achieved by behavior modification was maintained and extended. Those who did not lose weight during treatment, did not lose weight during the follow-up. This finding, too, speaks to the specificity of the treatment. It is worthy of note that these results—both of treatment and follow-up—have been replicated by the successors of Penick et al. in purely clinical therapeutic work with over 100 patients of comparably severe obesity.

What then is the significance of Penick's study? Quite simply it showed that behavior modification, devised by a team with little experience in the modality, was more effective in the treatment of obesity than was the best alternative program that could be devised by a research team with long experience in treatment of this disorder.

This result flies in the face of one of the most cherished beliefs about psychotherapy: the experience of the psychotherapist is of greater importance than the nature of his psychotherapy. Although it is true that this belief is supported by a minimum of experimental evidence, it has been shared by some of our wisest thinkers, and there had been no strong reason to question their collective wisdom on this point. Therefore, if a behavior modification program contains

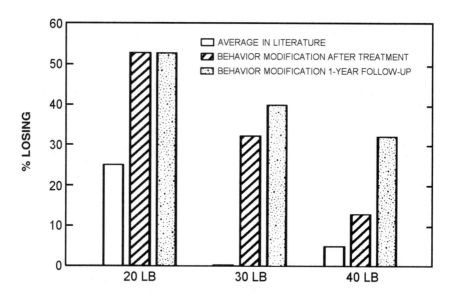

Figure 16–18. Weight loss after treatment and at one year follow up of the foregoing study.

sufficient content to override the venerable variable of therapist experience, it is news. It is also evidence of a different kind for the efficacy of a behavioral approach.

Something New in Psychotherapy Research: Therapy Without a Therapist

The next act in this unfolding drama followed closely upon the demonstration that the therapeutic content of a program could outweigh the experience of the therapist. Audacious to a fault, it raised a question that had been, until then, hardly conceived, let alone asked. If the therapist's experience is of less value than the content of a (behavioral) therapy, what is the function of the therapist in the conduct of psychotherapy? And, further, is it a necessary function?

Until quite recently this question would have been heretical. For the relationship between therapist and the patient has long been viewed as the heart of the psychotherapeutic process. Only once had this view been challenged, and then in a modest way. Melamed and Lang,[52] in 1967, reported a study, which, while not entirely excluding personal contact, suggested that a "Device for Automated Desensitization" was as effective as a therapist in the systematic desensitization of persons suffering from phobias. But beyond this isolated and specialized effort, the field was wholly barren.

Richard Hagen, then a graduate student at the University of Illinois, dared to question the function of the psychotherapist in psychotherapy. In reviewing the work of his fellow graduate student Janet Wollersheim, he recognized that the behavioral program had been significantly more effective than traditional programs, and that it contained something over and above the interpersonal influence of the therapist. Was it possible that this special something could even substitute for the interpersonal influence of a therapist? The program had been spelled out in sufficient detail that he could conceive of prescribing it without the actual presence of the therapist. He could thereby ask the question, "Is it possible to carry out psychotherapy without a doctor-patient relationship? Can there be therapy without a therapist?"

Hagen[29, 30] devised a study to find out. Specifically, he asked two questions: (1) Can a written presentation of materials previously found effective in the treatment of obesity produce significant weight reduction without a personal relationship with a therapist or a therapy group? (2) Does attendance in a therapy group, which includes personal contact, make a contribution to treatment over and above the same principles provided through written communication?

Hagen compared three treatment conditions with each other and with a no-treatment-wait-control condition similar to Wollersheim's. The first treatment condition, *Contact Only,* consisted of an exact replication of Wollersheim's Focal (Behavioral) Therapy program. The second, critical, treatment condition, *Manual Only* or "bibliotherapy," consisted of a manual of 10 lessons, which was mailed weekly to the subjects. The manual was constructed from that utilized by the therapists in the first treatment condition. It took the form of a programmed text, with homework assignments that the subjects returned each week by mail to the investigator, who corrected them and returned them promptly to the subjects. The third treatment condition, *Manual Plus Contact,* also presented the 10 lessons on a weekly basis, but the exchange of lessons and of homework took place at the therapy sessions instead of by mail.

The 90 subjects in the study were mildly (25%) overweight women college students, randomly assigned to one of the four treatments. Three therapists treated six subjects each in the *Contact Only* and *Manual Plus Contact* conditions. Ten treatment sessions were held over a 3-month period.

The results of treatment are shown in Figure 16–19. The greatest weight loss occurred in the *Manual Plus Contact* condition, with subjects losing an average of 15 pounds during treatment. The difference in weight loss produced by this condition and the other two did not reach statistical significance. All treatments, however, were more effective than the No-Treatment-Wait-Control condition. There was no difference between the Contact Only and Manual Only conditions, not only in weight lost, but also in the response to Wollersheim's eating-patterns questionnaire. And the 12.0 pound weight loss in the Manual Only or "bibliotherapy" condition compared most favorably with the 10.3 pound weight loss of Wollersheim's most effective, behavioral, treatment condition.

Hagen exuberantly concluded: "the present investigation demonstrates that it is possible to treat obesity effectively, using a written manual, and that this treatment is apparently as effective as any yet evaluated in a controlled study." He went on, "in terms of practical significance, the findings of the present investigation point to the possibility of offering an effective treatment for obesity, without the involvement of costly and scarce professional time."

It was an exciting prediction, but as it has developed, a premature one.

Further Refinements: The Therapist Is Not Wholly Dispensable

During the time that Hagen was carrying out his study of "bibliotherapy," one of the program's therapists, Edward Craighead, developed particular interest in it that he later followed up. For he had noted that Hagen's Manual Only condition included more therapist contact than the name of the condition implied. For example, Hagen interviewed all of the subjects at the beginning of the study, and presumably made them aware of the importance of the study to the comple-

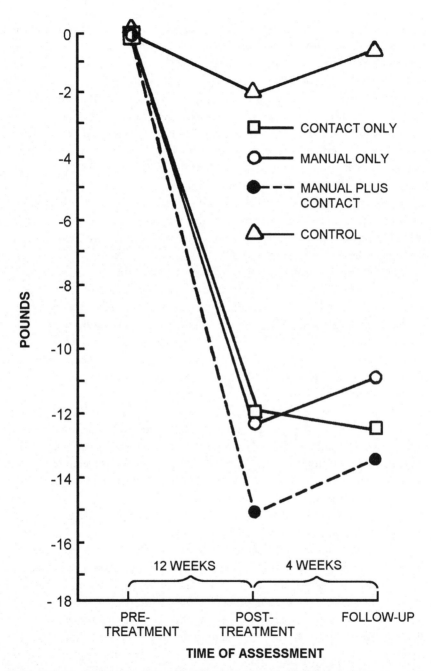

Figure 16–19. Weight loss of the three treatment groups and of the no-treatment control groups. The former three lost significantly more than the latter one, but there was no significant difference in weight loss between the three treatment groups (Hagen[30]).

tion of his Ph.D. The subsequent weekly critiques that he mailed to his subjects, and the telephone calls that he made to them when they failed to send in their homework, may have conveyed a significantly greater measure of interpersonal influence than one would have expected from the somewhat impersonal conditions described in his report. In an attempt to evaluate the effects of some of this apparent "minimal" therapist contact, William Fernan, a graduate student working with Craighead, carried the evaluation of bibliotherapy of obesity a significant step further. The importance of this study was underscored by the publication of bibliotherapy manuals such as those of Stuart and Davis,[78] which are designed to be used without therapist contact.

In effect, Fernan replicated elements of Hagen's study, just as Hagen had replicated elements of Wollersheim's. For this purpose he utilized the same manual in lesson form that Hagen had devised for his study. He presented it, however, under the two different conditions.[19]

Fernan's first—Lessons Without Contact—condition was perhaps even more severe than that of Hagen's manual only condition. Essentially all interpersonal contact was eliminated, including returning of the homework assignments. By contrast, the Lessons With Contact condition precisely replicated Hagen's manual only condition. Subjects received the same lessons on a weekly basis, mailed in their weekly homework assignments, received back weekly comments in writing as well as telephone calls from the experimenter whenever necessary to ensure return of the homework.

The study was embedded in an elaborate design that involved 90 mildly (28%) overweight women college students, who were stratified on the basis of percent overweight and randomly assigned from blocks of five to one of five experimental conditions. The three conditions that concern us were the Lessons With Contact of 10 subjects, the Lessons Without Contact of 11 subjects and a No-Treatment-Wait-Control of 8 subjects.

The results are illustrated in Figure 16–20. The Lessons With Contact subjects lost an average of 11.8 pounds, almost exactly replicating the 12.0 pounds lost in Hagen's "manual only" condition. Subjects in the Lessons Without Contact group lost only 4.9 pounds, even less than the 5.2 pounds lost by subjects in the No-Treatment-Wait-Control condition. The difference between the Lessons With Contact condition and the other two was significant ($P < 0.05$), despite small number of subjects and the large variability. Clearly, doing what Hagen did is an effective weight loss procedure; doing what he said he did is far less effective.

Two further comments seem in order. The remarkable similarity in the weight loss in Fernan's Lessons With Contact condition (11.8 pounds) and that in Hagen's Manual Only condition (12.0 pounds) adds significantly to the con-

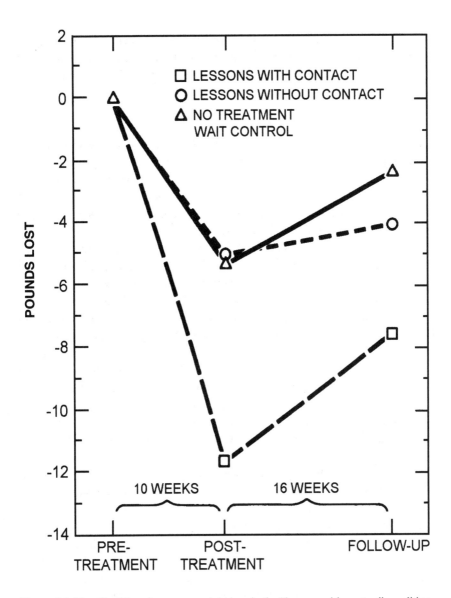

Figure 16–20. Significantly greater weight loss in the "lessons with contact" condition over "lessons without contact" (Fernan[19]).

fidence that we can have in the positive findings of Fernan's study. The second point deals with the large weight loss in Fernan's No-Treatment-Wait-Control condition. Investigating the subjects in this condition at the end of the study to try to understand this unusual result, he learned that five of the eight subjects in this condition had, in fact, actively participated in the program by utilizing the manuals of friends in the active treatment conditions. These five subjects had lost 39 of the 46 pounds lost collectively by subjects in this condition. They might with reason, therefore, be excluded from the No-Treatment-Wait-Control group.

Fernan's study thus significantly amplified Hagen's earlier findings by demonstrating that therapist contact may be of critical importance, even though it does not occur in a face-to-face setting. By defining with increasing precision the minimal amount of contact that may be necessary, Fernan has made it possible to focus ever more precisely upon what is the effective element in therapist contact. And this work poses a heretofore unasked question: Is such slight therapist contact of importance because of its effect upon motivation or because of its effect upon feedback? Does the therapist's encouragement and support increase the subject's motivation, or does the therapist's feedback lead to more effective application of weight loss principles, or do both occur?

In addition to its theoretical implications, bibliotherapy has important practical implications. For the first time we have the suggestion of an alternative to the traditional labor-intensive psychotherapeutic approach to problems of human behavior. Until now, the high cost of a trained psychotherapist's time and the critical shortage of therapists have restricted psychotherapeutic services to the treatment of a privileged few. Even the use of therapist-extenders, such as paraprofessionals and mental health aides, and even the application of therapy in groups, have made only modest inroads into this problem. The potential of bibliotherapy, by contrast, points to the possibility of treatment at nominal cost to all who can read.

Let us reflect on this extraordinary progress in psychotherapy, progress that has been made in no more than 7 years as a result of research on behavioral treatment of obesity. What has been the origin of this following, of this remarkable productivity? The answer lies in two areas, a powerful independent and a powerful dependent variable. It would be hard to overestimate the power, as a dependent variable, of weight change in pounds. Compared to every other dependent variable that has ever been used in psychotherapy research, weight change in pounds is unprecedented in its reliability, validity and economy. There is every reason to believe that psychotherapy research will increasingly value this variable of weight change, and that what we have surveyed here is only the beginning of what may bring us, far earlier than we had any reason to hope, to a cumulative science of psychotherapy.

The independent variable, which has played an equally significant role in the productivity of this research, has been the specification, in exquisite detail, of the precise behaviors that comprise the therapeutic intervention. We have referred many times to the program that was initially proposed by Ferster et al.[20] and that was refined and made to work by Stuart.[77] Of what does this program consist? Let us briefly describe the Stanford program, which shares with so many others this common origin.

A Description of the Basic Behavioral Program for Treatment of Obesity

The program consists of four elements: (1) description of the behavior to be controlled; (2) control of stimuli that precede eating; (3) development of techniques to control the act of eating; and (4) modification of the consequences of eating.

(1) Description of the behavior to be controlled. Patients are asked to keep careful records of the food that they eat. Each time they eat, they write down precisely what it was, how much, at what time of day, where they were, who they were with, and how they felt. The immediate reaction of many patients to this time-consuming and inconvenient procedure was grumbling and complaints. In retrospect, such reactions occurred far more frequently when we were starting the program and may well have been due to our own uncertainty about the techniques. More recently, since we have ourselves become convinced of its effectiveness and stress its importance in a wholehearted manner, patients have responded more positively. Many come to the view that record-keeping may be the single most important part of the behavioral program. It vastly increases patients' awareness of their eating behavior. Despite their years of struggle with the problem, once patients begin to keep records they are surprised at how much they eat and the circumstances of their eating.

Three examples illustrate the effectiveness of record-keeping. A middle-aged traveling salesman came to realize for the first time that he overate only in his car, which he kept liberally stocked with candy bars, peanuts and potato chips. He thought over the problem, stopped keeping food in the car and promptly lost weight. After 2 weeks of record-keeping, a 30-year-old housewife reported that, for the first time in her life, she recognized that anger stimulated her eating. She acted promptly upon this discovery. Whenever she found herself getting angry she would try to leave the kitchen or wherever food was available and write down how she felt. She became increasingly able to avoid eating in response to anger and she, too, began to lose weight. A striking example of the effects of record-keeping was described by a middle-aged obese woman who had undergone 3 years of intensive psychotherapy, adjudged by her and her psychiatrist as fairly successful. She said that 2 weeks of record-keeping taught her more about the therapeutically important aspects of her eating than had her entire previous treatment.

(2) Control of the stimuli that precede eating. A behavioral analysis traditionally begins with a study of the events antecedent to the behavior to be controlled. So-called stimulus control involves many of the kinds of measures that are traditional in weight-reduction programs. Every effort is made to limit the amount of high-calorie food kept in the house and to limit accessibility to food that must be kept in the house. For times when eating cannot be resisted, adequate amounts of low-calorie foods, such as celery and raw carrots, are available.

In addition, the behavioral program introduced new and distinctive measures. For example, most patients reported that their eating took place in a wide variety of places and at many different times during the day. Some noted that if they ate while watching television, it was not long before watching television made them eat. It was as if the various times and places had become so-called discriminative stimuli signalling eating.

The concept of a discriminative stimulus comes from the animal laboratory where such stimuli as the flashing of a light or the sounding of a tone may signal to an animal that pressing a lever will produce food pellets or other rewards. Since the reward never occurs without the discriminative stimulus, in the language of learning theory, the stimulus comes to "control" various forms of behavior. In an effort to decrease the number and potency of discriminative stimuli that controlled their eating, patients were encouraged to confine all eating, including snacking, to one place. In order not to disrupt domestic routines, this place was usually the kitchen.

A parallel effort is made to develop new discriminative stimuli for eating and to increase their power. For example, patients are encouraged to use distinctive table settings, perhaps an unusually colored place mat and napkin, and special silver. No effort is made to decrease the amount of food the patients eat, but they are encouraged to use the distinctive table settings whenever they eat, even for a small between-meals snack. One middle-aged housewife, convinced of the importance of this measure, went so far as to take her distinctive table setting with her whenever she dined out. She was one of our earliest successes.

(3) Development of techniques to control the act of eating. Specific techniques are utilized to help the patients decrease their speed of eating, to become aware of all the components of the eating process and to gain control over these components. Exercises include counting each mouthful of food eaten during a meal, or each chew, or each swallow. Patients are encouraged to practice putting down their eating utensils after every third mouthful until that mouthful is chewed and swallowed. Then longer delays are introduced, starting with 1 min towards the end of the meal when it is more easily tolerated, and moving to more frequent delays, longer ones and ones earlier in the meal.

Patients are encouraged to stop pairing their eating with such activities as reading the newspaper and watching television, and to make conscious efforts to make eating a pure experience. They are urged to do whatever they can to make meals a time of comfort and relaxation, particularly to avoid old arguments and new problems at the dinner table. They are encouraged to savor the food as they eat it, to make a conscious effort to become aware of it as they are chewing and to enjoy the act of swallowing and the warmth and fullness in their stomachs. To the extent that they succeed in this endeavor, they eat less and enjoy it more.

A mammoth, Burl Ives kind of man who greeted such admonitions with condescension, reported a month later, "you know—it's amazing, when I did those things I really tasted food for the very first time in my life. I *really tasted food!* I can't get over it. When somebody used to ask me if I liked food, I would always say 'sure, I like it.' But I had never really tasted it before. Now I eat one spoonful of ice cream and really taste it and it gives me as much pleasure as a whole half-gallon used to."

(4) Modification of the consequences of eating. In addition to the informal and incidental rewards that patients receive from the behavioral program, a system of formal rewards is also used. The one we use differs from earlier ones in that it establishes separate reward schedules for changes in behavior and for weight loss. Of the two, rewards for changing behavior seem the more effective.

In order to decrease the time between the exercise of a specific behavior and the attendant reward, we developed a system to award the patient a certain number of points for each of the activities that he is learning: record-keeping, counting chews and swallows, pausing during the meal, eating in one place, and so forth. Not only do patients receive a certain number of points for each activity, but they can earn extras, such as double the number of points, when they devise an alternative to eating in the face of strong temptation.

These points, which serve to provide immediate reinforcement of a behavior, are cumulated and converted into more tangible rewards, often in concert with the spouse. For example, a popular reward was trips to the movies and relief from housekeeping chores, while a more impersonal one was conversion of points into money, which patients brought to the next meeting and donated to the group. In our very first program, our first cohort donated its savings to the Salvation Army, the second to a needy friend of one of the members.

Promptness of the reinforcement seemed the key to success. One middle-aged housewife said, "My husband was always offering to buy me a car if I lost 50 pounds. I used to work away at it and knock myself out and lose 30 pounds, which was a lot of weight, but what did it get me? I didn't get half a car. I got nothing. I've only lost eight pounds in this program and he's done all sorts of good things for me."

A Flood of Research

Behavioral research on obesity appears to be assuming the character of a cumulative science of psychotherapy. We have proposed that the reasons for this event are the power of the dependent variable—weight change—and of the independent variable—clearly specified behavioral operations—used in the research. The immediately preceding section gave an indication of the nature of the behavioral operations. How are these operations, this independent variable, being developed through research?

Behavioral research on obesity has proceeded in two quantitatively different ways. One way has been by leaps of the imagination as in the six more salient studies described above. But it has also proceeded by less dramatic research, by the kind of research that characterizes the vast majority of studies in the more developed sciences. This is the kind of research that clears the underbrush and prepares the way for the critical experiment and the grand synthesis. Such research has, until now, been rare in psychotherapy. The presence of this kind of research is the surest indication of the scientific status of behavioral investigation of obesity. The method of proceeding is instructive.

Stuart's original program consisted of a complex and many-faceted "package" of procedures. Once the general effectiveness of this package had been demonstrated, the major research strategy was to subject its constituent parts to study, both in isolation and in various combinations. For example, just how important is record-keeping? Of what kind should it be and how should it be combined with other elements of the program? This process is now proceeding with an accelerating tempo in laboratories and clinics throughout the nation and, in fact, throughout the world. The 30 papers on behavioral control of eating reviewed here may well constitute the largest body of systematic research yet carried out on any aspect of psychotherapy.

For purposes of exposition we will review these studies according to the format just used to describe the program: (1) description of the behavior to be controlled; (2) control of stimuli that precede eating; (3) development of techniques to control the act of eating; and (4) modification of the consequences of eating.

(1) Description of the behavior to be controlled (research findings). When detailed record-keeping was introduced, it was solely for the purpose of obtaining information that might then be utilized in the construction of a behavioral control program. More recently, increasing attention has been paid to such record-keeping, now called self-monitoring, as a therapeutic modality in its own right. There is growing evidence that self-monitoring is of use in a number of behavioral control programs, especially when it is combined with social reinforcement.[44] Six different studies have already been directed to the influence of self-monitoring in the control of obesity. The largest number maintain that the effect is weak,[48, 76] or of only short duration.[46, 78] One study confirms the ineffectiveness of monitoring of body weight, while touting the effectiveness of monitoring of caloric intake.[67] The other found no effect of monitoring of caloric intake in the conventional manner, but a strong effect of "premonitoring"—in writing down what is about to be eaten, rather than what has been eaten.[4]

The discovery that self-monitoring has therapeutic effectiveness in its own right, even limited effectiveness as seems likely, is a kind of bonus that had not been anticipated in the first studies. Furthermore, we have observed that self-monitoring can be of considerable value in the period of weight maintenance, following termination of all contact with the program. Several patients have noted that reinstitution of self-monitoring of food intake at the point when their weight has begun to rise has been sufficient to regain control over their eating.

(2) Control of the stimuli antecedent to the eating (research findings). Stimulus control has been a part of almost every behavioral control program.[20, 30, 31, 35, 36, 45, 61, 78, 93] It is of interest, therefore, that there are no studies that we know of, similar to those of self-monitoring, which have been carried out to elucidate the effectiveness of stimulus control or of its various elements. What could be considered a special method of stimulus control—training in relaxation in the presence of "induced anxiety"—has been reported to be more effective than relaxation training alone.[8]

(3) Development of techniques to control the act of eating (research findings). Studies of the various measures designed to control the act of eating have been similarly sparse and unrevealing.

(4) Modification of the consequences of eating (research findings). In striking contrast to the foregoing, studies of the consequences of eating behavior have been both well designed and extensive. They are making a significant contribution to our understanding of the processes of reward and punishment of eating behavior.

A number of single case studies have strongly supported the early evidence for the effectiveness of rewards and punishments in the control of obesity. Reports of weight losses by individual patients of 102, 35 and 96 pounds, respectively, have been reported to follow rewards,[5, 57, 75] while a weight loss of 40 pounds has followed punishment.[58]

Positive reinforcement has been a major component in most programs and much of their effectiveness has been attributed to it,[19, 30, 31, 34, 42, 46, 49] but few specific studies have been carried out to test this effectiveness. Only one, for example, has systematically removed positive reinforcement to assess its efficacy.[48] It reported that there was little or no effect of the rest of the program unless positive reinforcement was also present.

Specific aspects of positive reinforcement have been investigated by a number of groups. Two, for example, have shown that self-reward is more effective in producing weight loss than is self-punishment.[40, 48] Furthermore, when the two sources of reward—behavior and weight loss—were examined for their separate efficacy, it was learned that reinforcement of behavior was more effective than reinforcement of weight loss.[46] The general impression that support by members of the patient's family is a key factor in the success of any program has been investigated in a systematic manner only once. This investigation produced strong support for the view.[47] A special form of positive reinforcement, contingency contracting, has proven to be a reliable measure for the control of eating.[34, 36, 49, 50, 75] Another practical issue—the relative efficacy of self-administered versus experimenter-administered rewards—has produced conflicting results.[31, 41]

Punishment as a method of suppressing behavior is generally viewed with considerably less favor than is positive reinforcement. It has, nevertheless, been utilized with surprising frequency and considerable effectiveness in the control of eating. One reason for its effectiveness may be the relative ease with which specific taste aversions can be developed. It is well established that the rat can develop a severe, lifetime aversion to a particular taste following even one exposure to that taste paired with a poison that produces a generalized illness. We have recently demonstrated that such taste aversions occur in man in the course of the usual vicissitudes of life.[25]

Attempts to produce aversions to high calorie foods by means of electric shock as the punishment produced inconstant or weak effects.[54, 76] Others, which utilized the kind of aversive consequences that give rise to bait shyness, were surprisingly effective.[25] When foul odors were paired with specific high calorie foods, stable taste aversions were produced that purportedly resulted in major weight losses in six persons.[21] More recently, cigarette smoke was utilized in a similar manner to produce specific aversions to three hard-to-control high calorie foods and a 40 pound weight loss in a young woman.[58] More simply, "doctoring" of certain high calorie foods with a combination of mineral oil and castor oil was utilized, with reported effectiveness, as part of a larger treatment package.[61]

The technique of "covert sensitization"—imagined aversive consequences—which was developed by Cautela,[12] and which can be viewed as a form of punishment, has been used to develop food aversion in no less than eight studies. Three reported that it was effective, but did not isolate the technique in such a way as to prove its unique efficacy.[12, 77, 93] Of the five controlled trials, three reported some effectiveness;[37, 39, 50] two others did not.[35, 90]

What Do We Do With This New Knowledge?

Health Consequences of Obesity and of Weight Reduction

Behavioral research on obesity has had a profound effect upon research in psychotherapy, to the extent, very probably, of transforming an art into a science. Has it done more? And, if so, has it gone beyond the satisfying of cosmetic concerns? Has the developing technology of weight reduction had an impact upon health? Has it, or can it, affect mortality and morbidity?

The traditional answer to these questions is a resounding "yes," and recent developments in the pattern of mortality in this country affirm this view. For today cardiovascular disease accounts for well over one half of all deaths in this country. Any suggestion that a condition may contribute to cardiovascular disease must be given the utmost consideration. The contribution of obesity to cardiovascular disease is far more than suggestive. The Framingham study, for example, has demonstrated an accelerating increase in both coronary heart disease and stroke with increasing degrees of overweight.[28] An increase of no more than 50% over ideal weight increases the risk of these disorders among men by over 100% and among women by over 150%. Two of the leading risk factors for coronary artery disease, hypertension and hypercholesterolemia, are similarly influenced by obesity. Chiang et al.[14] have reviewed 31 studies from all parts of the world that showed positive correlation between overweight and hypertension and 19 that showed reduction in blood pressure consequent upon weight reduction. Two excellent reports have similarly documented the relationship of obesity to diabetes with its attendant hypercholesterolemia.[1, 6]

To these traditional evidences of the adverse consequences of obesity must be added a singularly persuasive study of the effects of weight reduction.[60] This study is particularly credible, since its subjects showed only modest correlations between degree of obesity and metabolic indices. Its results thus do not depend upon any assumptions as to the effects of obesity upon these metabolic indices. It speaks to nothing more than the effects of weight reduction, pure and simple.

The subjects were mildly overweight (21%) men and women, unselected except to exclude frank diabetics, who lost an average of 24 pounds, a figure comfortably within the range of results of behavioral studies reviewed here. This modest weight loss initiated profound metabolic consequences. The best known consequence is improvement in glucose tolerance. Figure 16–21 shows the effect of weight reduction on plasma glucose levels following a test dose of 40 gm/m^2 of body surface area. In this case, the improvement, a 12% decrease in the area under the curve, while statistically significant, is less than is usually found, and far less than would be the case had frank diabetics been included in the sample.

Despite this small improvement in glucose tolerance, weight reduction produced a major decrease in insulin response to the glucose load. Figure 16–21 shows this striking 37% reduction in the area under the curve. Furthermore the reduction in insulin in response to a liquid meal, a closer approximation to real life than a glucose load, was a remarkable 48%!

Such hypersecretion of insulin, especially in response to carbohydrate ingestion, is believed to play a major role in the hyperlipemias associated with coronary artery disease. The effects of weight reduction upon the production of very low density lipoproteins was therefore assessed. Figure 16–22 shows the highly significant 40% decrease in the production of these lipoproteins, which are increasingly ascribed a critical role in coronary atherosclerosis.

Finally, this modest weight reduction had a powerful impact upon plasma triglycerides and cholesterol. Figure 16–23 shows the fall in plasma triglyceride levels from 319 mg% to 180 mg%, a decrease of 44%. Plasma cholesterol levels fell from 282 mg% to 223 mg%, a decrease of 21%.

Delivery Systems

A significant impact upon obesity in this country will require an intervention that is sufficiently effective and sufficiently economical to affect large segments of the population. Behavior modification meets both these criteria. Within 4 years of its introduction it was achieving a two-fold increase in the effectiveness of treatment. Far smaller increases in effectiveness have resulted in profound changes in the treatment of other disorders. Furthermore, the treatment is one that can be carried out by nonprofessional workers at a fraction of the cost of traditional medical efforts. What means exist, or can be developed, for the delivery of this new treatment? Three major possibilities exist: medical auspices, patient self-help groups and commercial enterprises.

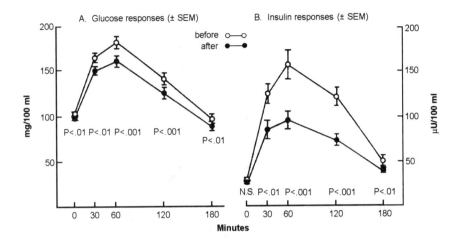

Figure 16–21. Improved glucose tolerance and greatly improved insulin tolerance following weight loss of 24 lbs. (Olefsky et al.[60]).

Medical Auspices

A preliminary report suggests that behavior modification can play a significant part in large-scale medical efforts, not only to control obesity but also the personal habits and lifestyles conducive to cardiovascular disease. Efforts by the Stanford Heart Disease Prevention Program have been centered in three California towns with populations of 15,000 each, carefully matched on a variety of demographic variables.[53] Two of these towns were subjected to a year-long multimedia campaign designed to provide information about reduction of cardiovascular risk factors. Significant increase in information was achieved in both towns as compared with the third, control, town. Furthermore, this information was translated into significant change in dietary habits. In town 1, 87 subjects at high risk of cardiovascular disease received, in addition, a behavior modification program designed to reduce still further these risk factors. These efforts were successful.

Table 16–6 shows a linear trend towards decreasing cardiovascular risk factors in the three towns, with town 1, where behavior modification supplemented the media campaign, showing greater effects than town 2, which received only the media campaign. Town 2, in turn, showed greater risk reduction than town 3, which received no intervention. The difference between towns in each of the four factors assessed was significant, $P < 0.01$. Behavior modification under medical auspices resulted not only in significant weight reduction, but also in cardiovascular risk reduction. Does the interest and energy

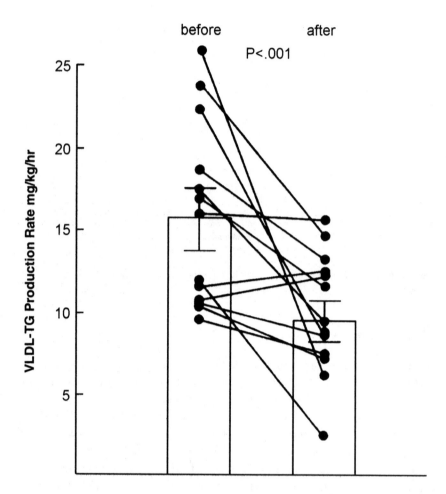

Figure 16–22. Highly significant fall in very low density lipoproteins following 24 lb. weight loss (Olefsky et al.[60]).

exist to capitalize upon this demonstrated capability?

The response of the medical profession to the development of behavioral treatments for obesity gives little grounds for optimism. Even psychiatry, which would seem the most hospitable environment within medicine, has been slow to accept developments in behavior modification. The field has grown up largely outside the purview of psychiatrists and, at times, in the face of their opposition. The extent of the failure of medical leadership is nowhere better illustrated than in the behavioral studies reviewed here. In only four of the 30 were physicians involved!

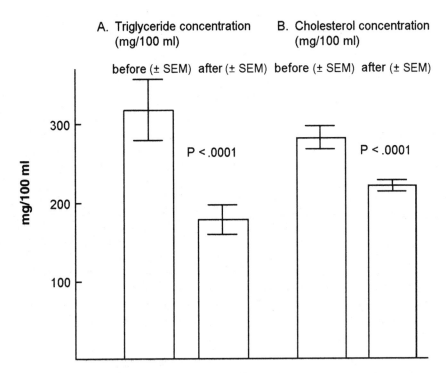

Figure 16–23. Marked falls in serum triglyceride and cholesterol concentration following 24 lb. weight loss (Olefsky et al.[60]).

Are there alternative vehicles for the introduction of behavior modification? The great American love affair with weight reduction suggests one—the patient self-help group.

Patient Self-Help Groups

A century and a half ago, de Tocqueville described the proclivity of Americans to organize in informal groups to achieve ends that are the responsibility of government in other societies. Nowhere is this proclivity more impressively expressed than in the organization of patients to cope with common illnesses. Patient self-help groups, pioneered by Alcoholics Anonymous, are favored by increasing numbers of persons suffering from a wide variety of conditions. One of the largest and most effective of these groups is TOPS (Take Off Pounds Sensibly), a 25-year-old organization that enrolls over 300,000 members in 12,000 chapters in all parts of the country.[24, 87] Figure 16–24 shows the growth of the organization, which is composed almost entirely of women. TOPS would

Table 16–6. Altered cardiovascular risk factors in three towns subjected to differing intensity of intervention

	Town		
	#1 Behavior modification Media	#2 — Media	#3 — —
Cholesterol	−11.4*	−1.2	3.9 mg %
Systolic blood pressure	−9.5*	−6.3	1.5 mm Hg
Relative weight	−5*	−1	−2%
Consumption of eggs	−63*	−37	−13%

*Between group comparison $P < 0.01$.

appear to offer a promising vehicle for the introduction of behavioral techniques. A recent feasibility study confirmed this promise.[45]

The study involved all 298 female members of 16 TOPS chapters, situated in West Philadelphia and its adjacent suburbs. Four treatment conditions, each utilizing four TOPS chapters, were employed. Two of the treatment conditions were experimental ones: (1) behavior modification carried out in four chapters by psychiatric residents and (2) behavior modification carried out in four chapters by the chapter leader and co-leader, each of whom had received brief training in the procedures and who used the same manual as that used by the professional therapists. The third treatment condition, also carried out in four chapters, consisted of nutrition education provided by chapter leaders and co-leaders who had received an amount of training in this area comparable to that provided the chapter leaders in behavior modification. The fourth treatment condition, also involving four chapters, used a continuation of the standard TOPS self-help techniques. Treatment of all 16 chapters lasted for 12 weeks.

The average subject was a 45-year-old woman who had been a member of TOPS for 3 years and who had lost 11 pounds during her membership. She currently weighed 180 pounds, 42% above her ideal weight. The homogeneity of TOPS membership permitted remarkably close matching of subjects in the different conditions.[24, 87]

TOPS shares with the medical treatment of obesity the problem of a very high dropout rate. An earlier study of the chapters involved in the current intervention trial revealed that 47% of TOPS members dropped out in 1 year and 70% within 2 years.[24] The results of the intervention trial thus involved two parameters—attrition rates and weight loss.

The first major finding was that far fewer subjects dropped out of the be-

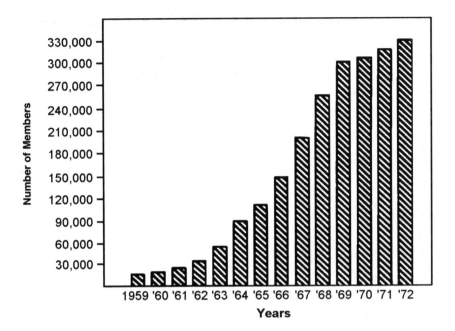

Figure 16–24. Growth in TOPS over a 13-year period.

havior modification programs. Figure 16–25 shows that the attrition rate in the two behavior modification conditions was lower during treatment, and significantly lower at 1 year follow-up. At 1 year, 38% and 41% of subjects had dropped out of the behavior modification programs, compared to 55% for the nutrition education and 67% for the standard TOPS program.

This differential attrition rate biased the weight reduction results against the behavior modification treatments. For poor weight losers drop out at a more rapid rate than do those who lose greater amounts, and decreasing the attrition rate means retaining less successful members. Despite this bias, behavior modification produced significantly more weight loss than did the control conditions ($F = 10.7$, $P < 0.001$). Figure 16–26 shows that professionally led chapters lost 4.2 pounds compared to the loss of 1.9 pounds in the TOPS leader-led chapters. The nutrition education chapters lost only 0.2 pounds and the groups receiving the standard TOPS program actually gained 0.7 pounds.

The relative superiority of the behavioral treatments increased at 1 year follow-up. The chapters that had had professional leadership continued to show lower attrition rates and also to lose weight, to a total of 5.8 pounds. The initial weight loss of subjects in the behavior modification program conducted by TOPS leaders was not maintained during follow-up, but these subjects did better

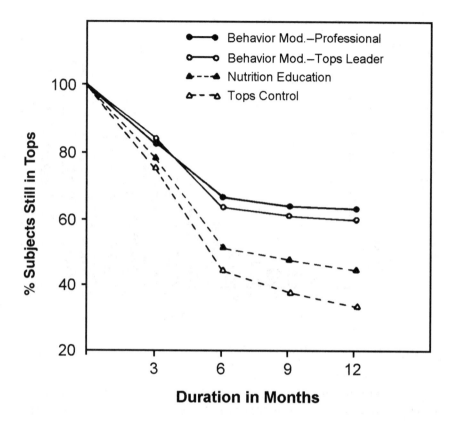

Figure 16-25. Attrition rate of TOPS subjects over a 1 year period under four experimental conditions (Levitz and Stunkard[45]).

than those in the nutrition education and control groups, who gained weight.

Clearly, both experimental and control groups performed less effectively than in previous studies, although the differential between the two was statistically significant. Several reasons may account for this finding: (1) the demographic characteristics of TOPS members are those usually associated with poor outcome; (2) The subjects had already lost weight (mean = 11 pounds) whereas other behavior modification studies used subjects new to treatment; (3) members who had reached or approximated their ideal weight before the intervention were excluded from the study, thus starting with a sample selected for difficulty in losing weight; and (4) probably most important, each TOPS group was considerably larger than those in earlier studies, which had rarely exceeded 10 members. By contrast, the chapter size, which averaged 19 members, made it impossible to individualize treatment.

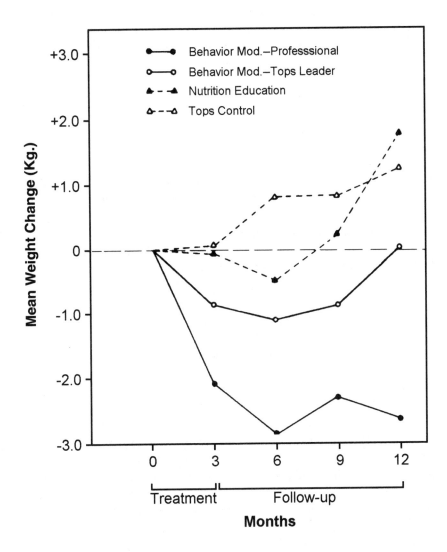

Figure 16–26. Weight loss of TOPS subjects over a 1 year period under four experimental conditions (Levitz and Stunkard[45]).

This has been an important feasibility study. We now know that behavior modification can be introduced into large population groups through appropriate institutional auspices. What we need is to improve the performance under these conditions and to find institutions receptive to introduction of the technique.

We have not yet found such an institution. Even TOPS, which helped to pioneer this approach, has made no effort to capitalize upon the program to which it made such a significant contribution. Ironically, the chief beneficiary may well be TOPS' arch rivals, commercial organizations such as Weight Watchers.

Commercial Enterprises

There has been essentially no scientific investigation of commercial weight reduction enterprises, and what we know about them is largely anecdotal and impressionistic. This situation is now changing and it is likely that the next few years will bring us an objective appraisal of this rapidly developing area. The two facts that we do know about the most prominent of these enterprises, Weight Watchers, suggests that private industry may be the most effective vehicle for the introduction of behavioral techniques for the widespread control of obesity.

First, Weight Watchers has already begun to develop behavioral techniques for its programs, under the direction of the same Richard Stuart who ignited the explosion of behavioral research in obesity 8 years ago.[77] Second, the appeal of Weight Watchers to obese persons is apparently far stronger than that of either medical auspices or self-help groups. Table 16–7 shows the growth of Weight Watchers, which during an 11 year period, has reached a size seven times that of TOPS.

It seems likely that other profit-making organizations will challenge Weight Watchers' virtual monopoly of the commercial weight reduction field and the next 5 years may well see a massive change in the social environment of obese persons as the genius of private industry is focused upon the enlistment of obese persons in large-scale programs of behavioral control. If this development is coupled, as it probably will be, with further improvement in the effectiveness of measures of behavioral control, we may well witness a phenomenon unprecedented in the history of medicine: a major medical problem delivered by the medical profession to private industry.

Table 16–7. Growth of Weight Watchers

1962	Start
1965	0.25 million
1968	0.8 million
1971	1.5 million
1973	2.4 million

Conclusions

In no more than 10 years we have become aware of the enormous influence of the social environment on the production and control of obesity. First we learned of the unplanned and uncontrolled influence of the fads and fashions of such factors as social class. Then social psychological experiments made it possible to begin the direct study of the specific factors involved in food intake. Finally, we have begun to study the effects of deliberately engineered changes—therapeutic interventions—into the social environment of obese persons. This therapeutic movement makes it appear that the powerful social influences upon obesity that occur in an unplanned and often erratic manner may be matched by purposeful and carefully controlled endeavors. In the process, we may be observing a model for the future of medical care and health maintenance.

References

1. Abrams ME, Jarrett RJ, Keen H, et al: Oral glucose tolerance and related factors in a normal population sample, II: interrelationship of glycerides, cholesterol and other factors with the glucose and insulin response. Br Med J 1:599–602, 1969
2. Baily K: The study of human growth in the framework of applied nutrition and public health nutrition programs in the western Pacific region, in Physical Growth and Body Composition: Papers From the Kyoto Symposium on Anthropological Aspects of Human Growth. Edited by Brozek J. Monographs of the Society for Research in Child Development, Vol 35 (No 7). University of Chicago Press, 1970
3. Baird I McLean, Silverstone JT, Grimshaw JJ, et al: The prevalence of obesity in a London borough. Practitioner 212:706–714, 1974
4. Bellack AS, Rozensky R, Schwartz J: A comparison of two forms of self-monitoring in a behavioral weight reduction program. Behav Ther 5:523–530, 1974
5. Bernard JL: Rapid treatment of gross obesity by operant techniques. Psychol Rep 23:663–666, 1968
6. Bierman EL, Bagdade JD, Porte D Jr: Obesity and diabetes: the odd couple. Am J Clin Nutr 21:1434–1437, 1968
7. Blinder BJ, Freeman DMA, Stunkard AJ: Behavior therapy of anorexia nervosa: effectiveness of activity as a reinforcer of weight gain. Am J Psychiat

126:1093–1098, 1970
8. Bornstein PH, Siprelle CN: Group treatment of obesity by induced anxiety. Behav Res Ther 11:339–343, 1973
9. Bullen BA, Reed RB, Mayer J: Physical activity of obese and non-obese adolescent girls appraised by motion picture sampling. Am J Clin Nutr 14:211–223, 1964
10. Bruch H: Eating Disorders: Obesity, Anorexia Nervosa and the Patient Within. Basic Books, New York, 1973, pp 309–387
11. Bychowski G: On neurotic obesity. Psychoanal Rev 37:301–319, 1950
12. Cautela J: Covert sensitization. Psychol Rep 20:459–468, 1967
13. Chang KS, Lee MM, Low WD, et al: Height and weight of Southern Chinese children in Hong Kong. Am J Phys Anthropol 21:497–509, 1963
14. Chiang BN, Perlman LV, Epstein FH: Overweight and hypertension. Circulation 39:403–421, 1969
15. Chirico AM, Stunkard AJ: Physical activity and human obesity. N Engl J Med 263:935–940, 1960
16. Conrad SW: The psychologic implications of overeating. Psychiatr Q 28:211–224, 1954
17. Feinstein AR: The measurement of success in weight reduction: an analysis of methods and new index. J Chronic Dis 10:439–456, 1959
18. Feinstein AR: The treatment of obesity: an analysis of methods, results, and factors which influence success. J Chronic Dis 11:349–393, 1960
19. Fernan W: The role of experimenter contact in behavioral bibliotherapy of obesity. Unpublished master's thesis, Pennsylvania State University, 1973
20. Ferster CB, Nurnberger JI, Levitt EB: The control of eating. J Mathetics 1:87–109, 1962
21. Foreyt JP, Kennedy WA: Treatment of overweight by aversion therapy. Behav Res Ther 9:29–34, 1971
22. Fry EI, Chang KS, Lee MM, et al: The amount and distribution of subcutaneous tissue in Southern Chinese children from Hong Kong. Am J Phys Anthropol 23:69–79, 1965
23. Garb JL, Garb JR, Stunkard AJ: The influence of social factors on obesity and thinness in Navaho children. Abstracts, First International Congress on Obesity, Royal College of Physicians, London, October 9–11, 1974
24. Garb JR, Stunkard AJ: A further assessment of the effectiveness of TOPS in the control of obesity. Arch Intern Med 134:716–720, 1974
25. Garb JL, Stunkard AJ: Taste aversions in man. Am J Psychiat 131:1204–1207, 1974
26. Glucksman ML, Hirsch J: The response of obese patients to weight reduction, III: the perception of body size. Psychosom Med 31:1–7, 1969
27. Goldblatt PB, Moore ME, Stunkard AJ: Social factors in obesity. JAMA 192:1039–1044, 1965
28. Gordon T, Kannel W: The effects of overweight on cardiovascular disease.

Geriatrics 28:80–88, 1973
29. Hagen RL: Group therapy versus bibliotherapy in weight reduction. Unpublished doctoral thesis. University of Illinois, 1970
30. Hagen RL: Group therapy versus bibliotherapy in weight reduction. Behav Ther 5:222–234, 1974
31. Hall SM: Self-control and therapist control in the behavioral treatment of overweight women. Behav Res Ther 10:59–68, 1972
32. Hamburger WW: Emotional aspects of obesity. Med Clin North Am 35:483–499, 1951
33. Hammond WH: Measurement and interpretation of subcutaneous fat, with norms for children and young adult males. Br J Prev Soc Med 9:201–211, 1955
34. Harmatz MG, Lapuc P: Behavior modification of overeating in a psychiatric population. J Consult Clin Psychol 32:583–587, 1968
35. Harris MB: Self-directed program for weight control: a pilot study. J Abnorm Psychol 74:263–270, 1969
36. Harris MB, Bruner CG: A comparison of a self-control and a contract procedure for weight control. Behav Res Ther 9:347–354, 1971
37. Horan JJ, Johnson RG: Coverant conditioning through a self-management application of the Premack Principle: its effect on weight reduction. J Behav Ther Exp Psychiat 2:243–249, 1971
38. Hueneman RL: Factors associated with teenage obesity, in Obesity. Edited by Wilson NL. F A Davis Company, Philadelphia, PA, 1969
39. Janda LH, Rimm DC: Covert sensitization in the treatment of obesity. J Abnorm Psychol 80:37–42, 1972
40. Jeffrey DB: Self-control versus external control in the modification and maintenance of weight loss, in Application of Behavior Therapy to Health Care. Edited by Katz RC, Zluntnick SI. Pergamon, New York, 1973
41. Jeffrey DB: Unpublished data.
42. Jeffrey DB, Christenson ER: The relative efficacy of behavioral therapy, will power, and no-treatment control procedures for weight loss. Paper presented at the 6th Annual Meeting, Association for Advancement of the Behavioral Therapies, New York, October, 1972
43. Kaplan HI, Kaplan HS: The psychosomatic concept of obesity. J Nerv Ment Dis 125:181–201, 1957
44. Kazdin AE: Self-monitoring and behavior change, in Self-Control: Power to the Person. Edited by Mahoney MJ, Thoresen CE. Brooks/Cole, Monterey, 1974
45. Levitz L, Stunkard AJ: A therapeutic coalition for obesity: behavior modification and patient self-help. Am J Psychiat 131:423–427, 1974
46. Mahoney MJ: Self-reward and self-monitoring techniques for weight control. Behav Ther 5:48–57, 1974
47. Mahoney MJ: Clinical issues in self-control training. Paper presented to the

American Psychological Association, Montreal, August 1973
48. Mahoney MJ, Moura NGM, Wade TC: The relative efficacy of self-reward, self-punishment, and self-monitoring techniques for weight loss. J Consult Clin Psychol 40:404–407, 1973
49. Mann RA: The behavior-therapeutic use of contingency contracting to control an adult behavior problem: weight control. J Appl Behav Anal 5:99–109, 1972
50. Manno B, Marston AR: Weight reduction as a function of negative reinforcement (sensitization) versus positive covert reinforcement. Behav Res Ther 10:201–207, 1972
51. Mayer J: The role of exercise and activity in weight control, in Weight Control. Edited by Eppright ES, Swanson P, Iverson CA. Iowa State College Press, Ames, IA, 1955
52. Melamed B, Lang P: Study of the automated desensitization of fear. Paper presented at the Midwestern Psychological Association Convention, Chicago, IL, May, 1967
53. Meyer AJ, Maccoby N, Farquhar JW, et al: A multifactor education campaign to reduce cardiovascular risk in three communities: results in high risk subjects. Abstracts, 47th Scientific Session, American Heart Association, Dallas, TX, 1974
54. Meyer V, Crisp AH: Aversion therapy in two cases of obesity. Behav Res Ther 2:143–147, 1964
55. Miller N, Bailey CJ, Stevenson JAF: Decreased hunger but increased food intake resulting from hypothalamic lesions. Science 112:256–295, 1950
56. Moore ME, Stunkard AJ, Srole L: Obesity, social class and mental illness. JAMA 181:962–966, 1962
57. Moore CH, Crum BC: Weight reduction in a chronic schizophrenic by means of operant conditioning procedures: case study. Behav Res Ther 7:129–131, 1969
58. Morganstern KP: Cigarette smoke as a noxious stimulus in self-managed aversion therapy for compulsive eating. Behav Ther 5:255–260, 1974
59. Nisbett RE, Storms MD: Cognitive and social determinants of food intake, in Thought and Feeling: Cognitive Alteration of Feeling States. Edited by London HS, Nisbett RE. Aldine, Chicago, IL, 1974
60. Olefsky J, Reaven GM, Farquhar JW: Effects of weight reduction on obesity. J Clin Invest 53:64–67, 1974
61. Penick SB, Filion R, Fox S, et al: Behavior modification in the treatment of obesity. Psychosom Med 33:49–55, 1971
62. Pflanz M: Medizinische-soziologische Aspekte der Fettsucht. Psyche 16:575–591
63. Price JM, Grinker J: The effects of degrees of obesity, food deprivation and palatability on eating behavior of humans. J Comp Physiol Psychol 85:265–271, 1973
64. Rascovsky A, Rascovsky MW de, Schlossberg T: Basic psychic structure of

the obese. Int J Psychoanal 31:144–149, 1950
65. Richardson HB: Obesity as a manifestation of neurosis. Med Clin North Am 30:1187–1202, 1946
66. Rodin J: Effects of obesity and set point on taste responsiveness and ingestion. J Comp Physiol Psychol (in press)
67. Romanczyk RG: Self-monitoring in the treatment of obesity: parameters of reactivity. Behav Ther 5:531–540, 1974
68. Schachter S: Obesity and eating. Science 161:751–756, 1968
69. Schachter S: Some extraordinary facts about obese humans and rats. Am Psychol 26:129–144, 1971
70. Shipman WG, Plesset MR: Anxiety and depression in obese dieters. Arch Gen Psychiat 8:530–535, 1963
71. Silverstone JT, Gordon RP, Stunkard AJ: Social factors in obesity in London. Practitioner 202:682–688, 1969
72. Silverstone JT, Lascelles BD: Dieting and depression. Br J Psychiat 112:513–519, 1966
73. Spiegel T: Caloric regulation of food intake in man. J Comp Physiol Psychol 84:24–37, 1973
74. Srole L, Langner TS, Michael ST, et al: Mental Health in the Metropolis: The Midtown Manhattan Study. McGraw-Hill, New York, 1962
75. Steffy RA: Service applications: psychotic adolescents and adults. Paper presented at the American Psychological Association, San Francisco, September, 1968
76. Stollak GE: Weight loss obtained under different experimental procedures. Psychother Theory Res Practice 4:61–64, 1967
77. Stuart RB: Behavioral control of overeating. Behav Res Ther 5:357–365, 1967
78. Stuart RB, Davis B: Slim Chance in a Fat World: Behavioral Control of Obesity. Research Press, Champaign, IL, 1972
79. Stunkard AJ: The dieting depression: incidence and clinical characteristics of untoward responses to weight reduction regimes. Am J Med 23:77–86, 1957
80. Stunkard AJ: Physical activity, emotions and human obesity. Psychosom Med 20:366–372, 1958
81. Stunkard AJ, McLaren-Hume M: The results of treatment of obesity: a review of the literature and report of a series. Arch Intern Med 103:79–85, 1959
82. Stunkard AJ: Obesity, in Comprehensive Textbook of Psychiatry, 1st Edition. Edited by Freedman AM, Kaplan HI, Kaplan HS. Williams & Wilkins, Baltimore, MD, 1967, pp 1059–1062
83. Stunkard AJ: Environment and obesity: recent advances in our understanding of the regulation of food intake in man. Fed Proc 27:1367–1373, 1968
84. Stunkard AJ: New therapies for the eating disorders: behavior modification of obesity and anorexia nervosa. Arch Gen Psychiat 26:391–398, 1972
85. Stunkard AJ, d'Acquili E, Fox S, et al: The influence of social class on obesity

and thinness in children. JAMA 221:579–584, 1972
86. Stunkard AJ, Blumenthal SA: Glucose tolerance and obesity. Metabolism 21:599–602, 1972
87. Stunkard AJ, Levine H, Fox S: The management of obesity: patient self-help and medical treatment. Arch Intern Med 125:1067–1072, 1970
88. Stunkard AJ, Rush J: Dieting and depression reexamined: a critical review of reports of untoward responses during weight reduction for obesity. Ann Intern Med 81:526–533, 1974
89. Traub AC, Orbach J: Psychophysical studies of body image: the adjustable body distortive mirror. Arch Gen Psychiat 11:53–66, 1964
90. Tyler VO, Straughan JH: Coverant control and breath-holding as techniques for the treatment of obesity. Psychol Rec 20:473–478, 1970
91. West KM: Epidemiology of adiposity, in Regulation of the Adipose Tissue Mass. Proceedings of the IV International Conference Meeting of Endocrinology, Marseilles, 1973. Excerpta Medica, Amsterdam, 1974, pp 202–207
92. Whitelaw GL: Association of social class and sibling number with skinfold thickness in London school boys. Hum Biol 43:414–420, 1971
93. Wollersheim JP: The effectiveness of group therapy based upon learning principles in the treatment of overweight women. J Abnorm Psychol 76:462–474, 1970
94. Wollersheim JP: The effectiveness of group therapy based upon learning principles in the treatment of overweight women. Unpublished doctoral dissertation. University of Illinois, 1968
95. Wooley OW: Long-term food regulation in the obese and non-obese. Psychosom Med 33:436–444, 1971
96. Wooley SC: Physiologic versus cognitive factors in short-term regulation in the obese and non-obese. Psychosom Med 34:62–68, 1972
97. Wulff M: Ueber einen interessanten oralen Symptomenkomplex and seiner Beziehung zur Sucht. Int Z f Psychoanal 18:281–302, 1932

CHAPTER 17

Behaviorally Conditioned Immunosuppression

ROBERT ADER, PH.D., AND
NICHOLAS COHEN, PH.D.

Prefatory Remarks

Bernard T. Engel, Ph.D.

Psychosomatic medicine is built on the principle that the natural history of most diseases includes behavioral elements. But behavior can act in either of two ways: first, it can have an indirect influence on pathophysiology—that is, it can be a risk factor; or second, it can have a direct influence—that is, it can be a causal mechanism. The former concept is universally accepted and is the basis for much of consultation psychiatry practice. The latter is much more controversial because the mechanism by which behavior can actually cause an antigen to overcome an antibody reaction is unclear.

Volume 37, 1975, pp. 333–340.

From the Departments of Psychiatry and Microbiology, University of Rochester School of Medicine and Dentistry, Rochester, New York 14642.

Presented at the Annual Meeting, American Psychosomatic Society, March 23, 1975, New Orleans.

This research was supported by Grants K5-MH-06318 to RA and K4-AI-70736 and 9R01-HDA1-07901 to NC from the United States Public Health Service and by funds generously provided by Mr. Arthur M. Lowenthal of Rochester, New York.

The authors acknowledge with gratitude the technical assistance of Elsje Schotman, Sumico Nagai, Darbbie Mahany, and Betty Rizen.

Received for publication November 27, 1974; revision received February 14, 1975.

To understand the significance of this article by Ader and Cohen, one first needs to understand the nature of behavior. *Behavior* is defined as the interaction between an effector system and the environment. An effector system includes the effector and the neural and humoral mechanisms that control its actions; the environment includes all of the stimuli impinging upon the organism around the time that the effector responds. Clearly this definition is complex because it requires not only an understanding of the nature of the effector system, but also an understanding of the temporal relationships between the occurrence of antecedent and consequent stimuli and their relationship to the consequent response. A true understanding of such relationships requires knowledge about the physiological mechanisms controlling the effector system and about the behavioral mechanisms that mediate stimulus-response bonds. It is remarkable how few articles addressing these mechanisms appear in the psychosomatic medicine literature (or even in *Psychosomatic Medicine*).

This article is truly extraordinary. For philosophers of science, the finding that immunosuppression can be classically conditioned raises (and suggests answers to) such questions as how experience modulates physiological function; how one can examine the relationship of brain and body without invoking the demon of mind-body dualism; and why science is a continuum and not a collection of disparate disciplines. For teachers, this study provides a vehicle for showing students why one needs to understand both physiology and behavior if one expects to carry out meaningful research at their interface; and it provides a model for the design of such experiments. For physicians, the existence of conditioned immunosuppression makes clear that they must understand the learning history of a patient if they expect to provide the patient with comprehensive and preventive care. The only way one can obtain such insight is by spending the time needed to collect requisite data; above all else, to collect relevant data, one must know how to observe behavior.

This article should be read, discussed, and reread.

An illness-induced taste aversion was conditioned in rats by pairing saccharin with cyclophosphamide, an immunosuppressive agent. Three days after conditioning, all animals were injected with sheep erythrocytes. Hemagglutinating antibody titers measured 6 days after antigen administration were high in placebo-treated rats. High titers were also observed in nonconditioned animals and in conditioned animals that were not subsequently exposed to saccharin. No agglutinating antibody was detected in conditioned animals treated with cyclophosphamide at the time of antigen administration. Conditioned animals exposed to saccharin at the time of or following the injection of antigen were significantly immunosuppressed. An illness-induced taste aversion was also conditioned using LiCl, a nonimmunosuppressive agent. In this instance, however, there was no attenuation of hemagglutinating antibody titers in response to injection with antigen.

Introduction

The hypothesis that immunosuppression might be behaviorally conditioned was invoked to explain certain incidental observations made in a study of illness-induced taste aversion.[1] In the illness-induced taste aversion paradigm[2-4] an animal is given a distinctively flavored drinking solution such as saccharin, which is followed by a toxic agent capable of eliciting temporary gastrointestinal upset. Lithium chloride, apomorphine, and cyclophosphamide are but a few of the toxins that are effective in inducing a taste aversion after a single trial in which the toxin (the unconditioned stimulus or US) is paired with a novel drinking solution (the conditioned stimulus or CS). By pairing different volumes of a preferred saccharin solution with a single intraperitoneal (ip) injection of 50 mg/kg cyclophosphamide (CY), rats acquired an aversion to the saccharin solution; the magnitude of the reduction in saccharin intake and the resistance to extinction of this aversion were directly related to the volume of saccharin consumed on the day of conditioning. It was also observed that some of the cyclophosphamide-treated animals died and that mortality rate tended to vary directly with the volume of saccharin originally consumed.

In order to account for this observation, it was hypothesized that the pairing of a neutral stimulus (saccharin) with cyclophosphamide, an immunosuppressive agent,[5] resulted in the conditioning of immunosuppression. If the conditioned animals that were exposed to saccharin every 2 days over a period of 2 months responded to this conditioned stimulus by becoming immunologically impaired, they would have been more vulnerable to the superimposition of latent pathogens that may have existed in the environment.

We report here our initial documentation of behaviorally conditioned immunosuppression.

Methods

Ninety-six male Charles River (CD) rats, approximately 3 months old, were individually caged under a 12 hr. light-dark cycle (light from 5 AM to 5 PM) and provided with food and water ad libitum. During a period of adaptation the daily provision of tap water was slowly reduced until all animals were provided with and consumed their total daily allotment during a single 15 min period (between 9 and 10 AM). This regimen was maintained throughout the experiment. The first 5 days under this regimen provided data on the baseline intake of water under these conditions.

On the day of conditioning (Day 0), animals were randomly distributed into conditioned, nonconditioned, and placebo groups. Conditioned animals received a 0.1% saccharin chloride solution of tap water during their 15 min drinking period and 30 min later were given ip injections of CY (50 mg/kg in a volume of 1.5 ml/kg).[*] Nonconditioned animals were, as usual, provided with plain tap water and 30 min after drinking were similarly injected with CY. Placebo animals received plain water and ip injections of an equal volume of vehicle (distilled water). On the following two days all animals were provided with plain water during their 15 min drinking period.

Three days after conditioning all animals were injected ip with antigen, 2 ml/kg of a 1% thrice washed suspension of sheep red blood cells (SRBC; approximately 3×10^8 cells/ml). Thirty minutes later randomly selected subgroups of conditioned and nonconditioned animals were provided with saccharin or plain water and/or received ip injections of CY or saline according to the treatment schedule outlined in Table 17–1.

One group of conditioned animals received a single drinking bottle containing the saccharin solution and drinking was followed by a saline injection; these animals constituted an experimental group. Two additional groups of conditioned animals received plain water; one of these groups was subsequently injected with CY (in order to define the unconditioned response produced by the immunosuppressive drug) while the second received saline (as a control for taste aversion conditioning, per se). Following antigen administration a nonconditioned group was provided with saccharin and injected with saline. These animals provided a control for the effects of saccharin consumption and the ip injections. Placebo animals remained unmanipulated and received plain water

---

[*]Cyclophosphamide was generously supplied by the Mead Johnson Research Center, Evansville, Indiana.

Table 17-1. Experimental treatments

Group	Day 0				Day 3		Day 6	
	Drnk. Soln.	Inj.	Subgroup	N	Drnk. Soln.	Inj.	Drnk. Soln.	Inj.
Conditioned	Sacch	CY	CS_1	11	Sacch	Sal	H_2O	—
($N = 67$)				9	H_2O	—	Sacch	Sal
			CS_0	10	H_2O	Sal	H_2O	—
				9	H_2O	—	H_2O	Sal
			US	10	H_2O	CY	H_2O	—
				9	H_2O	—	H_2O	CY
			CS_2	9	Sacch	Sal	Sacch	—
Nonconditioned	H_2O	CY	NC	10	Sacch	Sal	H_2O	—
($N = 19$)				9	H_2O	—	Sacch	Sal
Placebo ($N = 10$)	H_2O	Placebo	P	10	H_2O	—	H_2O	—

during the 15 min drinking period. On Day 6 of the experiment, conditioned and nonconditioned animals that had received antigen but had not been manipulated on Day 3 were first treated as described for Day 3, i.e., one conditioned group received the saccharin drinking solution, one conditioned group received water and CY, and one conditioned group received neither saccharin nor CY; a nonconditioned group also received saccharin. In addition, there was one experimental sample of conditioned animals that was provided with saccharin on Days 3 *and* 6. All animals remained unmanipulated on Days 7 and 8. Throughout this period the volume of plain water or saccharin consumed was measured daily.

On Day 9 (6 days after injection with SRBC), all animals were sacrificed. Trunk blood was collected in heparinized tubes for subsequent analysis of plasma corticosterone[8] and in nonheparinized tubes for the collection of sera to be used in the hemagglutinating antibody assay. Serum from each rat was heat inactivated (56°C for 30 min) and divided into aliquots some of which were stored at −70°C and others of which were refrigerated and assayed for hemagglutinating antibody activity within 24 hr of collection. Antibody titrations were performed according to standard procedures in microtiter trays and hemagglutination was assessed under the microscope. Titers were recorded as reciprocals of the endpoint dilutions expressed as powers of the base.[2]

The provision of plain water or saccharin and the injections of CY or placebo were conducted from coded data sheets. Similarly, antibody titrations and plasma corticosterone determinations were conducted without knowledge of the group to which an animal belonged.

Results and Discussion

Cyclophosphamide treatment administered 30 min after the ingestion of a novel saccharin drinking solution resulted in an aversion to the saccharin solution (Figure 17–1). Conditioned animals provided with saccharin on Day 3, on Day 6, or on Days 3 and 6 showed a reduced intake of the distinctively flavored solution on those days.

With regard to antibody responses, the following pattern of results was predicted. Sera from placebo-treated animals were expected to be relatively high titered. Nonconditioned animals, although subsequently presented with a saccharin drinking solution, were also expected to show high antibody levels. However, it was anticipated that the titers of sera from nonconditioned animals might be somewhat lower than those of placebo animals as a result of the CY administered 3 days before injection with SRBC.[6,7] Sera from conditioned animals that were given antigen but never again exposed to either saccharin or CY were expected to have antibody titers equivalent to those of unconditioned animals. Conditioned animals that were given a second injection of CY, an unconditioned stimulus for immunosuppression, were expected to show a minimum antibody response to SRBC. The critical groups for testing the hypothesis that immunosuppression can be behaviorally conditioned were the conditioned animals that were given one or two exposures to saccharin, the conditioned stimulus, following exposure to SRBC. Evidence in support of the hypothesis would be provided by an attenuation of the antibody response in these animals.

Antibody titers from the several groups are shown in Figure 17–2. Conditioned animals exposed to saccharin on Day 3 or Day 6 did not differ and were combined to form a single conditioned group (group CS) that received only one exposure to the conditioned stimulus, saccharin. Similarly, the conditioned animals that remained unmanipulated (group CS_0), the conditioned groups treated with CY on Day 3 or 6 (group US), and the nonconditioned animals given saccharin on Day 3 or 6 (group NC) were combined into single groups.

The results were as we had predicted. Placebo-treated animals showed the highest antibody titers. Conditioned animals that received neither saccharin nor CY and nonconditioned animals that were subsequently exposed to saccharin after antigen treatment showed similar hemagglutination titers that were also relatively high, although significantly lower than the titers of immune sera from

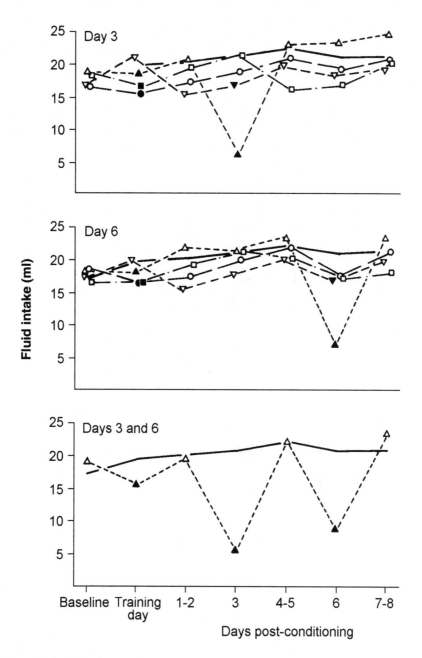

Figure 17–1. Mean intake of plain water (open symbols) and saccharin (filled symbols) for placebo (———) and nonconditioned (▲) animals, and conditioned animals that received saccharin (△), cyclophosphamide (□), or neither (○) on Day 3, Day 6, or Days 3 and 6. As a point of reference, the placebo-treated animals are shown in each panel.

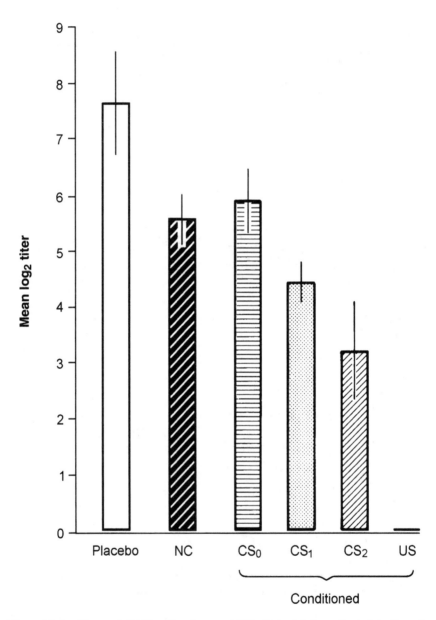

Figure 17–2. Hemagglutination titers (means ± SE) obtained 6 days after ip injection of antigen (SRBC). NC = nonconditioned animals provided with saccharin on Day 3 or Day 6; CS_0 = conditioned animals that did not receive saccharin following antigen treatment; CS_1 = conditioned animals given one exposure to saccharin on Day 3 or Day 6; CS_2 = conditioned animals exposed to saccharin on Days 3 and 6; US = conditioned animals injected with cyclophosphamide following treatment with antigen.

placebo animals in the case of both unconditioned ($t = 2.07$, $P < 0.05$) and conditioned ($t = 1.71$, $P < 0.10$) animals.** As expected, the hemagglutination tests revealed that administration of CY after SRBC caused complete immunosuppression. Conditioned animals that experience a single exposure to saccharin following antigen treatment (group CS_1) showed an antibody response that was significantly lower than that of placebo as well as nonconditioned animals ($t = 1.96$, $P < 0.05$) and conditioned animals that were not exposed to saccharin ($t = 2.14$, $P < 0.05$). The conditioned animals that experience two exposures to saccharin also showed an attenuated antibody response that was significantly below all other groups with the exception of the conditioned animals that received only one exposure to the conditioned stimulus.

Relative to placebo-treated animals, the reduction in hemagglutinating antibody titers shown by nonconditioned animals (group NC) and conditioned animals that were not given either saccharin or CY after antigen treatment (group CS_0) is most simply explained as resulting from some residual effect of CY administered on the day of conditioning (3 days prior to injection with SRBC).[9] These groups, then, become the relevant control condition against which to assess the antibody responses of the conditioned animals exposed to saccharin following antigen treatment. This latter condition did not result in complete suppression of the immune response, but conditioned animals exposed to saccharin did show a significant attenuation of the antibody response relative to these control groups. The attenuation would not appear to have resulted from saccharin, per se, since a comparable exposure to saccharin in association with and following antigen treatment was experienced by the nonconditioned animals for whom saccharin was not a conditioned stimulus. Also, behavioral conditioning, per se, did not result in antibody titers that differed from those of nonconditioned animals. The results, then, support the notion that the association of saccharin with CY enabled saccharin to elicit a conditioned immunosuppressive response.

The present study yielded little additional data that would be of direct importance in suggesting an explanation for this phenomenon. There were no differences among the several groups in body weight measured prior to the adaptation period, on the day before conditioning, or at the time that animals were sacrificed. Also, in conditioned animals exposed to saccharin there were nonsignificant correlations ranging from −0.34 to 0.16 between hemagglutination titer and volume of saccharin consumed. The correlation between plasma

---

**The significance levels reported in the text are based on two-tailed t-tests. Based on the specific differences that were predicted, however, it would be appropriate to report one-tailed probabilities and the reader may wish to interpret the results in this light.

corticosterone level sampled at the time that animals were sacrificed and antibody titer was virtually zero, and there were no group differences in steroid levels at this time.

Consistent with the known immunosuppressive properties of adrenocortical steroids and despite the failure to observe differences in plasma corticosterone levels *at the time of sacrifice,* it could be postulated that the attenuated antibody response observed in conditioned animals is a reflection of a nonspecific "stress" response to the conditioning procedures, or, perhaps, of a behaviorally conditioned elevation in steroid level in response to saccharin. Further support for such an explanation might be derived from the relationship between immune processes and physical and socioenvironmental "stress" or emotional responses[11-19] which, presumably, act through the hypothalamus, and from the several studies[20, 21] that suggest that hypothalamic lesions may influence some immune responses.

In order to evaluate the possibility that an elevation in adrenocortical steroids was responsible for the attenuation of antibody titers in conditioned animals, a second study used lithium chloride instead of cyclophosphamide as the US in inducing a taste aversion. Whereas lithium chloride also produces noxious gastrointestinal effects, it is not immunosuppressive. In this study, antigen was injected 5 days after conditioning, and the population of conditioned animals that was subsequently provided with the saccharin drinking solution (Group CS, $N = 10$) was exposed to the CS three times: at the time of injection with SRBC, and 2 and 4 days later. As in the first experiment, all animals were sacrificed 6 days after treatment with antigen.

The association of LiCl with saccharin was effective in inducing an aversion to the saccharin solution. Conditioned animals showed a 66% reduction in consumption of the saccharin solution on the initial test day relative to the intake measured on the day of conditioning. This corresponds closely to the 61%–68% reductions shown by animals conditioned with cyclophosphamide. Antibody titers for the conditioned animals and for the several control groups are shown in Figure 17-3. As indicated by the high titers found in animals injected with LiCl at the time of injection with SRBC, LiCl is not an unconditioned stimulus for suppression of the immune response. Although conditioning was effective in inducing an avoidance of the CS solution, antibody titers were similar in all groups.

It is not unreasonable to assume that an elevation in steroid levels might accompany the conditioning of a taste aversion. Nevertheless, the present data provide no support for the hypothesis that such an elevation in steroid levels could have been solely responsible for the attenuated immune response that was observed when conditioned animals were exposed to a CS previously associated

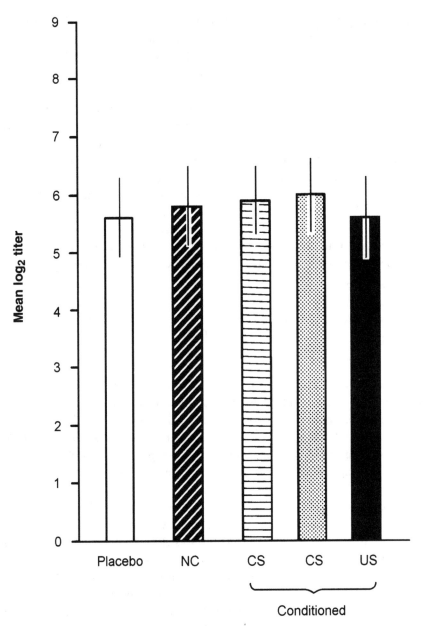

Figure 17-3. Hemagglutination titers (means ± SE) obtained 6 days after ip injection of SRBC in animals conditioned with LiCl as the US. NC = nonconditioned animals; CS_0 = conditioned animals that did not receive saccharin following antigen treatment; CS = conditioned animals given three exposures to saccharin; US = conditioned animals injected with LiCl following treatment with antigen.

with the administration of an immunosuppressive agent. The probability of an interaction between the magnitude and/or duration of an elevation in steroid level and the residual effects of cyclophosphamide, however, remains as a viable hypothesis.

The present results suggest, again, that there may be an intimate and virtually unexplored relationship between the central nervous system and immunologic processes and that the application of behavioral conditioning techniques provides a means for studying this relationship in the intact animal. Confirmation of the capacity of behavioral conditioning procedures to suppress (or elicit) immune responses would raise innumerable issues regarding the normal operation and modifiability of the immune system in particular and the mediation of individual differences in the body's natural armamentarium for adaptation and survival in general. Such data also suggest a mechanism that may be involved in the complex pathogenesis of psychosomatic disease and bear eloquent witness to the principle of a very basic integration of biologic and psychologic function.

Summary

The present study was designed to examine the possibility that behavioral conditioning techniques could be used to modify immune processes.

An illness-induced taste aversion was conditioned in rats by pairing saccharin (CS) with cyclophosphamide (CY), an immunosuppressive agent (US). Three days after conditioning, animals received ip injections of SRBC; 30 min later, subgroups of conditioned animals were (a) supplied with the CS solution, (b) provided with water but injected with the US, or (c) given neither CS nor US. A nonconditioned group was provided with the saccharin drinking solution, and a placebo group was injected with antigen but was otherwise unmanipulated.

The association of saccharin and CY was effective in inducing an aversion to the CS when it was presented 3 days after conditioning (at the time of antigen administration). Hemagglutinating antibody titers measured 6 days after injection of SRBC were high in placebo-treated rats. Relatively high titers were also observed in nonconditioned animals and in conditioned animals that were not subsequently exposed to the CS. No agglutinating antibody was detected in conditioned animals treated with CY at the time of antigen administration. In contrast, conditioned animals exposed to the CS when injected with SRBC (and/or 3 days later in additional samples of conditioned animals) were significantly immunosuppressed.

Similar procedures were used in a second experiment in which LiCl, a nonimmunosuppressive agent, was used as the US. While LiCl was effective in inducing a taste aversion, conditioned animals showed no attenuation of hemagglutinating antibody titers.

The results are interpreted as providing evidence for behaviorally conditioned immunosuppression. Further, it is suggested that this phenomenon is not mediated directly by nonspecific elevations in adrenocortical steroids that may be presumed to accompany an illness-induced taste aversion.

References

1. Ader R: Letter to the editor. Psychosom Med 36:183–184, 1974
2. Garcia J, Ervin RF, Koelling RA: Learning with prolonged delay of reinforcement. Psychon Sci 5:121–122, 1966
3. Garcia J, Kimmeldorf R, Koelling R: Conditioned aversion to saccharin resulting from exposure to gamma radiation. Science 122:157–158, 1955
4. Garcia J, McGowan BK, Ervin RF, et al: Cues: their relative effectiveness as a function of the reinforcer. Science 160:794–795, 1968
5. Gershwin ME, Goetzl EJ, Steinberg AD: Cyclophosphamide: use in practice. Ann Intern Med 80:531–540, 1974
6. Santos GW, Owens HA Jr: A comparison of selected cytotoxic agents on the primary agglutinin response in rats injected with sheep erythrocytes. Bull Johns Hopkins Hosp 114:384–401, 1964
7. Makinodan T, Santos GW, Quinn RP: Immunosuppressive drugs. Pharmacol Rev 22:198–247, 1970
8. Friedman SB, Ader R, Grota LJ, et al: Plasma corticosterone response to parameters of electric shock stimulation in the rat. Psychosom Med 29:323–329, 1967
9. Miller TE, North JDK: Host response in urinary tract infections. Kidney Int 5:179–185, 1974
10. Zurier RB, Weissman G: Anti-immunologic and anti-inflammatory effects of steroid therapy. Med Clin North Am 57:1295–1307, 1973
11. Brayton AR, Brain PF: Studies on the effects of differential housing on some measures of disease resistance in male and female laboratory mice. J Endocrinol 61:xlviii–xlix, 1974
12. Fessel WJ: Mental stress, blood proteins, and the hypothalamus. Arch Gen Psychiatry 7:427–435, 1962
13. Gisler RH: Stress and the hormonal regulation of the immune response in mice. Psychother Psychosom 23:197–208, 1974
14. Hamilton DR: Immunosuppressive effects of predator induced stress in mice

with acquired immunity to *Hymenolepsis nana.* J Psychosom Res 18:143–153, 1974
15. Hill OW, Greer WE, Felsenfeld O: Psychological stress, early response to foreign protein, and blood cortisol in vervets. Psychosom Med 29:279–283, 1967
16. Solomon GF, Amkraut AA, Kasper P: Immunity, emotions and stress. Psychother Psychosom 23:209–217, 1974
17. Solomon GF, Moos RH: Emotions, immunity, and disease. Arch Gen Psychiatry 11:657–674, 1964
18. Vessey SH: Effects of grouping on levels of circulating antibodies in mice. Proc Soc Exp Biol Med 115:252–255, 1964
19. Wistar R, Hildemann WH: Effect of stress on skin transplantation immunity in mice. Science 131:159–160, 1960
20. Korneva EA, Kahl LM: Effect of destruction of hypothalamic areas on immunogenesis. Fed Proc 23:T88–T92, 1964

CHAPTER 18

Social Support as a Moderator of Life Stress

SIDNEY COBB, M.D.

Prefatory Remarks

Stanislav V. Kasl, Ph.D.

Sidney Cobb's 1976 Presidential Address and the resulting article, "Social Support as a Moderator of Life Stress," have been unquestionably a major influence on theory and research in psychosomatic medicine in the last 15 years. The article provided an integrating concept, a broad theoretical formulation, a tantalizing review of some of the evidence, and a stimulus and challenge to fellow colleagues doing research in psychosomatic medicine and in related or overlapping fields of psychosocial epidemiology, behavioral medicine, health psychology, and medical sociology.

The developments and redirections in psychosomatic medicine up until the mid-1970s have been best described by Lipowski (1976).[1] Basically, psychosomatic medicine was freed from intentional or unintentional doctrinaire moorings in a particular theoretical framework or particular methodology (e.g., intrapsychic conflict, psychoanalytic theory) and from any commitment to study certain diseases because they are "psychosomatic." Changes in health and illness were seen as multiply determined, and increasingly, *social-environmental* factors were included, along with the more traditional biological and psychodynamic factors. The research theme of "stress and disease," with the emphasis on stressful life experiences, was the hallmark of these developments in the field. Sidney Cobb's article, together with the publication that same year by John Cassel (1976),[2] broadened immensely the scope of the socioenvironmental factors that were being examined in the etiology of disease. In addition, the article also broadened the scope of the "disease process," which was linked to social support mechanisms: incidence (new events) of disease, recurrence, course of recovery, case fatality, medical care seeking, symptom experience, and so on. The invitation was to examine these from a broad life-cycle perspective so that the psychosocial dynamics of social support could be firmly embedded in a developmentally specific context.

Sidney Cobb's article is a marvelous mixture of specific concepts and hypotheses, offered in a broad cross-disciplinary context for studying health and illness. Investigators who have been influenced by this article have not necessarily adopted his specific definition of social support or his primary emphasis (albeit tentatively proposed) on its buffering role. But researchers have been inspired by his lucid and compelling scholarly invitation to begin to address this uniquely important human dimension of health and illness.

References

1. Lipowski ZJ: Psychosomatic medicine: an overview, in Modern Trends in Psychosomatic Medicine, Vol 3. Edited by Hill OH. London, Butterworths, 1976, pp 1–20
2. Cassel J: The contribution of the social environment to host resistance. Am J Epidemiol 104:107–123, 1976

> "I assure you it is much wholesomer to be a complaisant, good humored, contented Courtier, than a Grumbletonian Patriot, always whining and snarling."
> —John Adams to his wife Abigail. The Hague, July 1, 1782

Social Support as a Moderator of Life Stress

Social support is defined as information leading the subject to believe that he is cared for and loved, esteemed, and a member of a network of mutual obligations. The evidence that supportive interactions among people are protective against the health consequences of life stress is reviewed. It appears that social support can protect people in crisis from a wide variety of pathological states: from low birth weight to death, from arthritis through tuberculosis to depression, alcoholism, and the social breakdown syndrome. Furthermore, social support may reduce the amount of medication required, accelerate recovery, and facilitate compliance with prescribed medical regimens.

Everybody talks about health, but nobody does much about it. The issue was stated cleary by Stephen Smith,[53] the first president of the American Public Health Association. He said, ". . . the customs of society must be so changed that the physician is employed to prevent rather than cure disease." Only recently has this concept begun to be implemented in the United States as a part of the Health Maintenance Organization movement.[37] It is, therefore, timely to address ourselves to preventive issues. As the title suggests, this essay will focus on social support. It will examine some of the areas in which social support has been demonstrated to have dramatic health-related effects and identify some in which it seems to have had no effects. It will not attempt to review all the diverse literature on this subject, for exhaustive bibliographies are available.[23, 30, 49] Rather, it will emphasize the way that social support acts to prevent the unfortunate consequences of crisis and change.

Before proceeding, we must come to some mutual understanding of the concept of social support. For the present discussion, social support is conceived to be information belonging to one or more of the following three classes:

1. Information leading the subject to believe that he is cared for and loved.
2. Information leading the subject to believe that he is esteemed and valued.
3. Information leading the subject to believe that he belongs to a network of communication and mutual obligation.

Let us examine each in turn.

Information that one is cared for and loved or, as the Greeks might say, information about agapé, is transmitted in intimate situations involving mutual trust. In a dyadic relationship, this information meets Murray et al.'s[43] need succorance for one person, need nurturance for the other, and need affiliation for both. It is often called emotional support.

Information that one is valued and esteemed is most effectively proclaimed in public. It leads the individual to esteem himself and reaffirms his sense of personal worth. It may be called esteem support.

Information that one belongs to a network of mutual obligation must be common and shared. It must be common in the sense that everyone in the network has the information and shared in the sense that each member is aware that every other member knows. The relevant information is of three kinds. The first answers the questions: What is going on and how did it begin? What is the relationship between us? How and when did we get here? These questions are the essence of history. The second pertains to goods and services that are available to any member on demand and includes information about the accessibility of services that are only occasionally needed, e.g., equipment, specialized skills, technical information. The third contains information that is common and shared with respect to the dangers of life and the procedures for mutual defense. In this last sense, the knowledge that a competently staffed hospital is available in case of need is socially supportive.

The present meaning of social support does not include the activities of the hospital in repairing a broken leg. Those activities are material services and are not of themselves information of any of the major classes mentioned above. This does not mean that the deferential manner of the intern may not provide esteem support or that the tender care of the nurses may not communicate emotional support. It is only to say that the services do not in themselves constitute such support because social support, being information, cannot be measured as mass or energy. This distinction is important, for goods and services may foster dependency, while the classes of information listed above do not. In fact, they tend to encourage independent behavior.

This set of dimensions is hardly new. Angyal,[1] Antonovsky,[2] Fromm,[22] Leighton,[34] Weiss,[56] and many others have illustrated and illuminated them. Perhaps the most notable illumination is the novel *Come Near* by Alexander Leighton.[35] Gerald Caplan[9] and his colleagues have taught the importance of these concepts in community mental health. But let's face it, these notions have been expressed over the millenia in the writings of most of the world's religious leaders. I have only added some precision and emphasized that it is information rather than goods or services that is central to the concept.

The first group, emotional support, was initially expressed in the need terms of Murray.[43] The second can similarly be expressed as need recognition from the Murray lexicon. The third is clearly akin to at least two of Leighton's[34] essential striving sentiments: "Orientation in terms of one's place in society . . ." and "The securing and maintaining of membership in a definite human group." This means that the whole concept can be expressed in person-environment fit terms[21, 41] or as the extent to which the relevant needs are met.

Social support begins *in utero,* is best recognized at the maternal breast, and is communicated in a variety of ways, but especially in the way the baby is held (supported). As life progresses, support is derived increasingly from other members of the family, then from peers at work and in the community, and perhaps, in case of special need, from a member of the helping professions. As life's end approaches, social support, in our culture, but not in all cultures, is again derived mostly from members of the family.

As will be seen in the section on the mechanism of this effect, it is my current opinion that social support facilitates coping with crisis and adaptation to change. Therefore, one should not expect dramatic main effects from social support. There are of course some main effects simply because life is full of changes and crises. The theory says that it is in moderating the effects of the major transitions in life and of the unexpected crises that the effects should be found. This theory is supported by the work of Pinneau,[49] who found few effects in cross-sectional studies.

With this background, it is time to turn to a careful examination of the extent to which this social support protects an individual as he passes through the various transitions and crises of the life cycle. We will begin with the infant *in utero* and end with death.

Pregnancy, Birth, and Early Life

The elegant study of Nuckolls et al.[44] is a good place to start this review. This was a study of 170 army wives delivered at a large military hospital. Data on life change scores before and during pregnancy and on psychosocial assets were collected. The measure of psychosocial assets (TAPPS) covers all three of the areas described above as the main components of social support in a subjective way and relatively little else except for some assessment of affect, which we know from other studies to be associated with support.

A recalculation of the data of Nuckolls et al.[44] is presented in Table 18–1. Those women who are designated as having high life change scores are those

Table 18–1. Percent of women with complications of pregnancy by life change score and social support (TAPPS) [recalculated from data of Nuckolls et al.[44]]

Life change score	Social support		t	P
	High	Low		
High[a]	33% (15)[b]	91% (11)	3.87	< 0.001
Low	39% (72)	49% (72)		NS

Interaction $t = 2.24$ $P < 0.05$.
[a]High both before and during pregnancy.
[b]Numbers in parentheses are the numbers of women in the respective cells.

who were above the median both before and during pregnancy. All other women have been included in the low category. The measure of social support (TAPPS) is split at the median. As can readily be seen, the proportion of women having complications is excessive (91%) only in the high life change/low social support cell. However, the upper left-hand cell (high life change and high support) is the really interesting one, for here 15 women were exposed to the same high frequency of life changes but had no increase in complications, presumably because of some protective effect exerted by the high level of social support. One useful point about this study is that, if the association is causal, the direction is clear, for the complications cannot have influenced the TAPPS score, which was measured at the first visit, or the life changes, almost all of which occurred well before the complications. This kind of moderating effect will appear again and again as this review progresses.

Another approach to social support in pregnancy is reported by Morris et al. in 1973.[42] The data came from a study of wantedness of babies in 60 major hospitals in 17 cities. A simplified presentation of their findings is to be seen in Table 18–2. It is clear that, at least for women who have completed high school, the reporting that a baby was wanted at the time it was conceived is associated with a significant decrease in the frequency of low birth weight. This is true for both blacks and whites. Over against this, one must set a Swedish study that did not find a difference in birth weight between babies for whom abortion was requested but refused and other babies.[27] However, education was not used as a control variable in this study. It is not reasonable to suppose that "wantedness" is information that is transmitted from mother to fetus and influences growth rate. Rather, it seems likely that the most common reason that a woman rejects her baby is that she herself feels inadequately socially supported. The societal reaction to illegitimate pregnancy is a case in point. In this instance, the causal direction is not so clear, for the inquiry was made the day after delivery and it is

Table 18–2. Percent of babies with birth weight < 2500 g by education, race, and wantedness [recalculated from data of Morris et al.[42]]

	Wanted or did not matter		Timing error or unwanted		
	N	%	N	%	P
Less than 12 years education					
Black	867	10.7	1657	11.5	NS
White	2118	4.9	1434	6.1	NS
12 or more years education					
Black	227	3.1	257	10.5	< 0.001
White	875	2.4	359	6.4	< 0.01

possible that babies known to be small were less likely to be declared to have been wanted than those known to be large.

Moving on to the first major social demand that the child faces, namely, achievement of sphincter control, Stein and Susser[54] tell us that control of bladder function at night was significantly delayed for those children whose mothers went out to work while the children were in the second six months of life. This was not true if the mother went to work earlier or later in the child's life nor was it true of the small number of children who had a substantial parental separation. These data are open to a variety of possible interpretations, so further study is indicated, but it seems at least possible that social support given by the mother during the time when toilet training is beginning is important to the early acquisition of sphincter control.

When we get to the important area of later social development, there are two studies. Forssman and Thuwe[20] have shown that wanted children adapt to and/or cope with the stresses of growing up better than those who started out with a parental request for abortion that was denied, in a study that followed a matched series of 120 cases and 120 controls until age 21. The cases fared worse with respect to juvenile delinquency and need for psychiatric treatment. Particularly striking was the distribution with respect to educational achievement. This is presented in Table 18-3. It is of special interest that the authors point out that the negative effects were essentially wiped out for those cases that were reared by their two natural parents together. The force of simple economic factors in this situation cannot be neglected.

The more recent study by Dytrych et al.[17] of the children of Czech mothers who had been twice refused abortion for the relevant pregnancy has an appropriately matched control group but is subject to the criticism, on the material so far presented, that the number of significant findings does not seem to exceed

Table 18–3. The educational achievement of unwanted children compared with that of controls. [Data of Forssman and Thuwe [20]]

	Unwanted	Controls	Total
Advanced study	17	40	57
Completed required schooling	90	74	164
Retarded	13	6	19
Total	120	120	240

$\chi^2 = 13.4$; $P < 0.005$.

the number to be expected by chance. However, the findings in the area of socialization into school are quite suggestive because, of the 15 performance and behavioral items presented, all are in the predicted direction and two are significant. We will all look forward to the full report with interest. The possibility that social support increases the efficiency of socialization in school must be kept in the forefront of our minds.

Transitions to Adulthood

There seems to be little information about the effects on the transitions to college, to first job, and to marriage. This is an area in which the literature must be more thoroughly combed and in which specific research is indicated.

Hospitalization

The effects of social support on an individual in relation to hospitalization for mental and physical illness are widespread, but much of the evidence is inferential. That is to say, the several studies in question imply differences in social support without measurement. The social breakdown syndrome, which is so intimately intertwined with admission to mental hospital, can be largely prevented.[24] This prevention is accomplished by a community-oriented service providing continuing care from the same team with hospitalization held to the minimum. Surely, that which is provided is mostly social support, although some specific services are included.

Moving on to hospitalization of children for tonsillectomy, there is a considerable volume of clinical literature. Much of this was summarized by Jessner and her colleagues back in 1952.[29] It indicates that supportive behavior on the part of parents and staff is helpful in preventing post-hospital psychological reactions. Recalculation of Jessner's own data indicates that the simple provision, by the parents, of adequate information about the anticipated hospitalization has a significant effect in preventing postoperative reactions.

In concluding this section, we should take note of the evidence that treating patients with myocardial infarcts at home carries no greater, and perhaps less, risk of death than treating them in the hospital intensive care unit. This is despite all the intensive care and fancy equipment that is available in the hospital. Mather and his colleagues[38, 39] deserve congratulations for their foresight and courage in setting up this field experiment. The mechanism by which staying at home exerts its protective effect was presumably identified by Leigh et al. in 1972,[33] when they pointed to the association of cardiac arrhythmias with high separation anxiety and the direction of hostility inward rather than outward. Both of these psychological sets are presumably reduced in the supportive atmosphere of the home. Obviously, network support is particularly at issue. However, Engel[19] suggests that the effect may be due simply to protection from environmental insults.

Recovery From Illness

This section shows the importance of the supportive physician in recovery from congestive heart failure and from surgical procedures and the importance of psychosocial assets in the recovery from psychosomatic illness, especially tuberculosis and asthma. Then the evidence that social support keeps the patient in treatment and promotes compliance with prescribed regimens will be reviewed.

In 1953, Chambers and Reiser[10] described the association of emotionally significant events with the onset of episodes of cardiac failure. In addition, they demonstrated the extraordinarily beneficial effects that emotional support from the physician could have on the course of the disease. A related finding is reported by Egbert et al.[18] They took two comparable groups of surgical patients. One group was given special supportive care by the anesthetist and the other served as a control. The surgeons managing the patients did not know which patient was in which group. The patients in the special care group needed substantially less medication for pain and were discharged on the average 2.7 days earlier than the control group. Both findings were statistically highly significant.

This same kind of effect must be demonstrable for a variety of other conditions involving fragile equilibrium. It points to the fact that social support is an important component of the therapeutic process. As Francis Peabody[47] stated in his essay *The Care of the Patient*, "One of the essential qualities of the clinician is interest in humanity, for the secret of the care of the patient is in caring for the patient." More recently, Lambert[32] and Caplan[9] have emphasized the importance of social support in the psychiatric management of life crises.

Some years ago, Berle, working with Harold Wolf and others,[4] developed an index of social and psychological characteristics of the patient, which had substantial prognostic value with regard to recovery from psychosomatic illness. Over half of the score on this index is easily codable to the categories of social support enumerated above. Holmes et al.[26] showed that this scale was highly predictive of the outcome of sanatorium treatment for tuberculosis, in that all the treatment failures were in the lowest third of the scores on this index. This is consonant with the evidence reviewed by Chen and Cobb,[11] suggesting that tuberculosis is a disease of social isolation, i.e., low social support.

More recently, de Araujo and van Arsdel, working with Holmes and Dudley[16] in Seattle, used this Berle Index to show a remarkable interaction of social support with life change with respect to the need for steroid therapy in adult asthmatics. Table 18–4 summarizes their data. The figures in the cells are average daily doses of steroids (prednisone or equivalent). It is clear that those with low life change scores needed only small doses of steroids and that those with a lot of life changes and a low Berle Index needed three to four times as much. The important point about this table is that those with a high Berle Index were protected from the need for high doses of steroids that presumably would be generated by a high life change score. It is this interaction between life change and support, in a way that suggests a protective effect of support, that is the focus of this review.

Table 18–4. Average daily steroid dosage in milligrams per day for patients with asthma by life change score and social support (Berle Index). [de Araujo et al.[16]]

Life change score	Berle Index	
	High	Low
High	5.6 (12)[a]	19.6 (11)[b]
Low	5.0 (10)	6.7 (4)

[a]Number of cases.
[b]This cell is significantly different from each of the other cells ($P < 0.01$).

There are a lot of pathways to the above mentioned effects. They fall into two major classes. The first is a direct effect through neuroendocrine pathways. This is the one that we in psychosomatic medicine are most apt to emphasize. The second is through promoting compliant behavior on the part of the patient. There is a large quantity of very consistent evidence pointing to the fact that those patients who are not socially isolated and are well supported are, in our casual lingo, good patients, in that they stay in treatment and follow our recommendations. The evidence on dropping out of treatment is summarized by Baekeland and Lundwall,[3] who state, "The importance of social isolation and/or lack of affiliation was indicated in 19 out of 19 studies (100%) that considered them." In a review of compliance with therapeutic regimens that does not overlap with the above, Haynes and Sackett[25] indicate that only one of 22 articles in which social support-relevant variables were measured gave evidence contrary to the hypothesis that social support is positively associated with compliance. Six of the 22 articles found no evidence either way. As data on such matters go, this association of cooperative patient behavior with various components of the social support complex is one of the best established facts about the social aspects of medical practice.

Life Stress

Here data will be presented on the dangers of stopping drinking without social support and the way in which social support protects against depression in the face of extensive life changes. After that, we will go on to two particular life changes: job loss and bereavement.

Joan Jackson, in a chapter in Sparer's book *Personality, Stress and Tuberculosis*,[28] presented some truly remarkable data, the significance of which did not receive adequate recognition at the time. I have recalculated her data in Table 18–5. She compared the men sent to the police farm for alcoholism with the alcoholics admitted to the tuberculosis sanatorium with respect to the frequency of men attempting to stop drinking in the preceding year with and without the support of an institutionally based program and/or Alcoholics Anonymous. As you can see, the frequency distributions are highly significantly different ($P < 0.005$). The relative risk calculation says in essence that men who tried to stop drinking on their own, i.e., without the support of an organized program, had 20 times the likelihood of being admitted to the tuberculosis sanatorium as their peers who did not try to stop or who tried with support. In fact, the numbers suggest that the risk of tuberculosis is reduced for those who try with support, but they are too small to be convincing. This is an impressive difference and deserves attention from those who work with alcoholics. Again, the social support dimension emerges as especially important for tuberculosis.

Turning to the work of George Brown and his collaborators,[7] one finds another striking datum. In Table 18–6 is shown the percent of a random sample of women classified as having a severe affective disorder. They are divided by whether or not they had a confidant. A confidant was defined as a person, usually male, with whom the woman had "a close, intimate and confiding relationship." The table makes it clear that those women who had severe events and lacked a confidant were roughly 10 times more likely to be depressed than those in any of the other three cells. If one assumes that the events had some causal relationship here, one is forced to the conclusion that the intimate relationship is somehow protective. Although one must be cautious about interpreting the effect of life events on depression because depressed people over-report unpleasant events, I have seen no evidence that depressed people tend to deny their confidants.

Alcoholism is related to depression, so it is not surprising that Quinn[50]

Table 18–5. The risk of tuberculosis to men stopping drinking in the preceding 12 months without social support [recalculated from data of Jackson[28]]

	Alcoholic admissions to	
	Police farm	TB Sanatorium
Stopped drinking during past 12 months		
Without support	1	18
With support	5	2
Did not stop drinking	28	27
Total	34	47

$\chi^2 = 14.8$; $P < 0.005$; relative risk $= 18 \times 33 / 1 \times 29 = 20$.

Table 18–6. Percentage of a random sample who had a recent onset of affective disorder by life stress and social support [Brown et al.[7]]

	Social support	
Life stress	Confidant	No confidant
Severe event or major difficulty	4% (2/45)	38% (17/45)[a]
Neither	1% (1/82)	3% (1/34)

[a] Significantly different from each of the other cells ($P < 0.001$). Interaction: $t = 3.60$, $P < 0.001$.

found that escapist drinking, but not other forms of drinking, is significantly elevated only among those who have high job stress and are not supported by their supervisors. These data come from the National Quality of Employment Survey, 1972–73.[50]

Employment Termination

This is a major life crisis for most men, particularly if they have dependents and have been stably employed for some years. My colleagues and I have made a special study of this matter. The doctoral dissertation of Susan Gore[23] was specifically focused on the moderating effect of social support on a selected set of outcome variables. Our total study examined a wide variety of economic, social, psychological, and medical variables in 100 men whose jobs were abolished and 74 men whose employment was stable. The men were visited by public health nurses before the termination, soon after the termination, and then at 6, 12, and 24 months after the plant closings. The men were all married blue-collar workers with about 19 years of seniority. In this study, the measure focused almost entirely on network support, although there was one item on subjective emotional support. This measure had moderating effects on some physiological variables and some indicators of illness, but not with regard to others. Cholesterol and uric acid levels in the serum were higher during the weeks surrounding the termination for those with little support than for those with adequate support. No such differences were observed with respect to norepinephrine in the urine or creatinine in the serum, although important changes over time were noted with respect to each and both were modified by the level of psychological defense.[12] The changes in level of complaints noted on a symptom check list was significantly moderated by high social support, but no effect was noted on hypertension or, surprisingly enough in view of the findings of Cobb et al.,[13] on peptic ulcer. At the other end of the social support scale, the finding that marital hostility is associated with ulcer disease was replicated.

When it came to arthritis, the data presented in Table 18–7 emerged. Here it can be seen that there was a 10-fold increase in the proportion of men found to have two or more joints swollen as one went from the highest to the lowest quartile of the social support dimension. This was not predicted in advance, so the matter was examined with some care and the finding stands up no matter how you look at it.

Table 18–7. The effect of social support in preventing joint swelling in relation to job loss

	Social support			
	High	Med	Low	Total
Two or more joints with observed swelling	1	5	12	18
Other	27	36	17	80
Total	28	41	29	98[a]
Percent with two or more joints swollen	4%	12%	41%	

[a] Two cases have missing data.
$\gamma = 0.732$; $P < 0.0003$.

Bereavement

Everyone acts as though social support were important to those who are bereaved and many authors suggest that this should be appropriate behavior, but hard evidence on the subject seems difficult to come by. Parkes[45] presents some suggestive evidence that opportunities for affiliation and affiliative behavior correlate positively with good psychological state 13 months after bereavement. The most striking data are provided by Burch.[8] Recalculating her data, it is possible to conclude that a married man who lost his mother had no increased probability of suicide. However, if he were single or his marriage had been terminated, his risk of suicide was increased ninefold by the death of his mother. Dr. Burch also showed that those men who had less contact with relatives had a greater probability of suicide than those with more contact. Considering the importance of the question and the potential of the study design, the analyses presented by Gerber[22a] are disappointing. One wishes that the data were more fully presented and more appropriately analyzed. However, on four of the six health dimensions presented, the bereaved subjects who had received professional support were better off during the period 5–8 months after bereavement. Further research in this area is clearly indicated.

Aging and Retirement

In this area, as in hospitalization of children, there are a lot of strong impressions about the importance of social support in protecting people from the consequences of the stress of growing old and infirm. The best data that have come to hand are those of Blau.[5] She supports the view that being married or being employed or having substantial social activity ("participation") is protective against the development of low morale. Similarly, Lowenthal and Haven[36] find in a sample of 280 persons aged 63 and older that 85% of those with low social interaction were depressed, whereas only 42% of those with high social interaction were depressed.

Threat of Death

Life threats are most striking in battle and as life's end approaches. These two situations will be examined in turn. There are many studies of the effects of morale, which is presumably a derivative of social support on the frequency of neuropsychiatric disorders. Rose's[52] rather clean study illustrates the point. He compared two battalions from the same regiment with respect to morale and neuropsychiatric casualties. These battalions were otherwise quite similar. The battalion with high morale had roughly half as high a rate of psychiatric casualties as the battalion with low morale. To the extent that high morale involves high self-esteem and group cohesiveness, mutual esteem support and network support are central to the maintenance of morale.

In a similar vein, Swank[55] found that every soldier in the Normandy campaign who had lost 75% or more of his buddies developed combat exhaustion. Reid[51] reports almost identical findings for bomber crews in the Royal Air Force. Just to clinch the matter firmly, I quote from the military experience of two distinguished psychiatrists. Francis Braceland[6] said, "It became obvious early in the course of the war that the most important prophylactics against psychiatric casualties in the military forces were proper individual motivation and high morale. . . ." William Menninger[40] added, "We seemed to learn anew the importance of group ties in the maintenance of mental health."

It would be improper to close this review without drawing attention to the life sparing effects of anticipated ceremonial occasions. Phillips and Feldman[48] in a truly remarkable paper showed in five different populations that deaths are reduced in the 6 months preceding birthdays and increased in the succeeding 6 months. A summary of their data is presented in Figure 18–1. They went on to hypothesize that, if this were a social support effect, it should be more striking for the most distinguished. This they found to be dramatically confirmed.

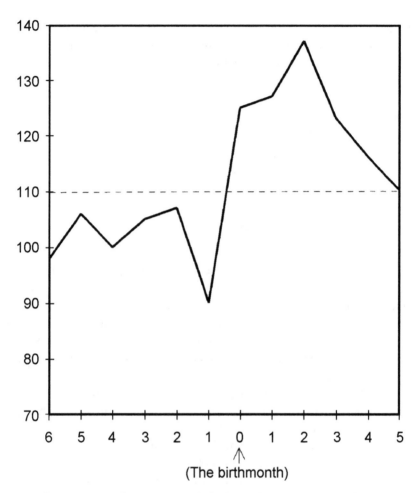

Figure 18–1. Number of deaths before, during, and after birth month (all five samples combined).

Discussion

We have seen strong and often quite hard evidence, repeated over a variety of transitions in the life cycle from birth to death, that social support is protective. The very great diversity of the studies in terms of criteria of support, nature of sample, and method of data collection is further convincing that we are dealing with a common phenomenon. We have, however, seen enough negative findings to make it clear that social support is not a panacea.

The conclusion that supportive interactions among people are important is hardly new. What is new is the assembling of hard evidence that adequate social support can protect people in crisis from a wide variety of pathological states: from low birth weight to death, from arthritis through tuberculosis to depression, alcoholism, and other psychiatric illness. Furthermore, social support can reduce the amount of medication required and accelerate recovery and facilitate compliance with prescribed medical regimens.

In a number of the studies that have been cited, it is possible to suggest alternatives to the social support explanation for the findings. For example, the birth weight findings of Morris et al.,[42] might be due to a reporting artifact, in that high school graduate mothers appreciate the significance of low birth weight and therefore tend to over-report their small babies as unwanted, while the less well-educated mothers do neither. Similarly, the excess of suicides among sons not currently married described by Burch[8] could conceivably be related to unresolved maternal ties, rather than to a lack of social support. At the other extreme, such studies as those of Nuckolls et al.,[44] de Araujo et al.,[16] Egbert et al.,[18] or my own on job termination are considerably less amenable to alternative interpretations because the social support was measured in advance, the stress was defined, and the outcomes were sufficiently specific to avoid major confounding. The crux of the matter seems to be that, although one or two of the studies presented might turn out on further investigation to be truly irrelevant, the series is so long and so diverse that it demands attention.

I may well have missed important findings both positive and negative. I would welcome additions to my files from readers who can identify such omissions. However, it should be clear that I have focused on the interaction of social support with environmental stress and have intentionally omitted a modest volume of studies that demonstrate a simple direct effect of social support on health. These studies are mostly included in the reviews by Gore,[23] Kaplan et al.,[30] and Pinneau.[49] The effect on tuberculosis is noted by Chen and Cobb.[11] The full range of data on coronary heart disease has never been assembled in one place. This deserves attention, for the collective effect of the full set is impressive. These data are not presented here because they are mostly reported as main effects rather than as moderating the effects of social stress.

What remains is to consider possible mechanisms for the observed protective effects. At the present time, the most attractive theory about the nature of this phenomenon involves pathways through facilitation of coping and adaptation. (Coping in my language means manipulation of the environment in the service of self and adaptation means change in the self in an attempt to improve person-environment fit.) It would not be unreasonable to suppose that esteem support would encourage a person to cope, i.e., to go out and attempt to master a problem. Likewise, emotional support and a sense of belonging might provide the climate in which self-identity changes can most readily take place.

As evidence that mastery of a new task takes place best under supportive conditions, I would draw attention to the classical experiment of Coch and French[15] in the pajama factory. They found that "participation" markedly reduced the time needed to get back to full production after a change in the nature of the task. An invitation from management to participate in the planning and implementation of a change is certainly direct esteem support. Participation may incidentally increase other forms of support, but that is not central to the argument that esteem support facilitates coping.

Parsons'[46] study clarified the sick role. Since successful role changes involve identity changes, it is logical to presume that movement in and out of the sick role is assisted by those things that facilitate the relevant identity changes. Clearly, social support facilitated remaining in treatment[3] and may speed recovery.[18] The hypothesis is strong but, as far as I know, untested that social support facilitates identity change, which, in turn, facilitates role change.

Further research on the proposed mechanism through which social support might operate is clearly indicated. In addition, there is an obvious need for further investigation of the moderating effects of social support on the consequences of the following transitions: entry into primary school, entry into college, first job, marriage, residential change, and bereavement. Surely, investigation will proceed on the effect of social support on the outcome of medical treatment because the results are likely to point to methods for reducing the costs of medical care. This review has focused on acute stress. There remains an important question as to whether social support can moderate the effects of chronic stress such as that experienced by air traffic controllers.[14]

There appears to be enough evidence on the importance of social support to warrant action, although, of course, all the details as to the circumstances under which it is effective are not yet worked out. Following the behest of Stephen Smith[53] cited at the beginning of this review, we should start now to teach all our patients, both well and sick, how to give and receive social support. Only in rare instances of clear psychiatric disability should this instruction require a psychiatrist. It seems to me that this is the real function for which Richard Cabot designed the profession of medical social work.

References

1. Angyal A: Neurosis and Treatment: A Holistic Theory. Edited by Hanfmann E, Jones RM. Wiley, New York, 1965

2. Antonovsky A: Conceptual and methodological problems in the study of resistance resources and stressful life events, in Stressful Life Events: Their Nature and Effects. Edited by Dohrenwend BS, Dohrenwend BP. Wiley, New York, 1974, Chapter 15
3. Baekeland F, Lundwall L: Dropping out of treatment: a critical review. Psychol Bull 82:738–783, 1975
4. Berle BB, Pinsky RH, Wolf S, et al: Berle index: a clinical guide to prognosis in stress disease. J Am Med Assoc 149:1624–1628, 1952
5. Blau ZS: Old Age in a Changing Society. New Viewpoints, New York, 1973
6. Braceland FJ: Psychiatric lessons from World War II. Am J Psychiatry 103:587–593, 1947
7. Brown GW, Bhrolchain MN, Harris T: Social class and psychiatric disturbance among women in an urban population. Sociology 9:225–254, 1975
8. Burch J: Recent bereavement in relation to suicide. J Psychosom Res 16:361–366, 1972
9. Caplan G: Support Systems and Community Mental Health. Behavioral Publications, New York, 1974
10. Chambers WN, Reiser MF: Emotional stress in the precipitation of congestive heart failure. Psychosom Med 15:38–60, 1953
11. Chen E, Cobb S: Family structure in relation to health and disease. J Chron Dis 12:544–567, 1960
12. Cobb S: Physiological changes in men whose jobs were abolished. J Psychosom Res 18:245–258, 1974
13. Cobb S, Kasl SV, French JRP Jr, et al: The intrafamilial transmission of rheumatoid arthritis, VII: why do wives with rheumatoid arthritis have husbands with peptic ulcer? J Chron Dis 22:279–293, 1969
14. Cobb S, Rose RM: Hypertension, peptic ulcer and diabetes in air traffic controllers. J Am Med Assoc 224:489–492, 1973
15. Coch L, French JRP Jr: Overcoming resistance to change. Hum Rela 11:512–532, 1948
16. de Araujo G, van Arsdel PP, Holmes TH, et al: Life change, coping ability and chronic intrinsic asthma. J Psychosom Res 17:359–363, 1973
17. Dytrych Z, Matejcek Z, Schüller V, et al: Children born to women denied abortion. Fam Plann Perspect 7:165–171, 1975
18. Egbert LD, Battit GE, Welch CE, et al: Reduction of post-operative pain by encouragement and instruction of patients. N Eng J Med 270:825–827, 1964
19. Engel GL: Psychologic factors in instantaneous cardiac death. N Eng J Med 294:664–665, 1976
20. Forssman H, Thuwe I: One hundred and twenty children born after application for therapeutic abortion refused. Acta Psychiatr Scand 42:71–88, 1966
21. French JRP Jr, Rodgers W, Cobb S: Adjustment as person-environment fit, in Coping and Adaptation. Edited by Coelho GV, Hamburg DA, Adams JE. Basic Books, New York, 1974

22. Fromm E: The Sane Society. Rinehart, New York, 1955
22a. Gerber I, Wiener A, Battin D, et al: Brief therapy to the aged bereaved, in Bereavement: Its Psychosocial Aspects. Edited by Schoenberg B, et al. Columbia University Press, New York, 1975
23. Gore S: The influence of social support and related variables in ameliorating the consequences of job loss. Doctoral dissertation, University of Pennsylvania, 1973
24. Gruenberg E, Snow HB, Bennett CL: Preventing the social breakdown syndrome, in Social Psychiatry, Vol 47. Edited by Redlich FC. ARNMD, Baltimore, MD, 1969
25. Haynes RB, Sackett DL: A Workshop/Symposium: Compliance With Therapeutic Regimens—Annotated Bibliography. Department of Clinical Epidemiology and Biostatistics, McMaster University Medical Centre, Hamilton, Ontario, 1974
26. Holmes TH, Joffe JR, Ketcham JW, et al: Experimental study of prognosis. J Psychosom Res 5:235–252, 1961
27. Hultin M, Ottosson MO: Perinatal conditions of unwanted children. Acta Psychiatr Scand [Suppl] 221:59–76, 1971
28. Jackson JK: The problem of alcoholic tuberculosis patients, in Personality Stress and Tuberculosis. By Sparer PF. International Universities Press, New York, 1954
29. Jessner L, Blom GE, Waldfogel S: Emotional implications of tonsillectomy and adenoidectomy on children. Psychoanal Study Child 7:126–169, 1952
30. Kaplan BH, Cassel JC, Gore S: Social support and health. Paper presented at meetings of American Public Health Association, November 9, 1973
31. Kramer M, Pollack ES, Redick RW, et al: Mental Disorders/Suicide. Harvard University Press, Cambridge, MA, 1972
32. Lambert K: Agapé as a therapeutic factor in analysis. J Anal Psychol 18:25–46, 1973
33. Leigh H, Hofer MA, Cooper J, et al: A psychological comparison of patients in "open" and "closed" coronary care units. J Psychosom Res 16:449–457, 1972
34. Leighton AH: My Name Is Legion. Basic Books, New York, 1959
35. Leighton AH: Come Near. Norton, New York, 1971
36. Lowenthal ME, Haven C: Interaction and adaptation: intimacy as a critical variable. Am Sociol Rev 33:20–30, 1968
37. MacLeod GK, Pressin JA: The continuing evolution of health maintenance organizations. N Eng J Med 228:439–443, 1973
38. Mather HG: Intensive care. Br Med J 2:322, 1974
39. Mather HG, et al: Acute myocardial infarction: home and hospital treatment. Br Med J 3:334–338, 1971
40. Menninger WC: Psychiatric experience in the war 1941–1946. Am J Psychiatry 103:587–593, 1947

41. Moos RM, Insel PM: Issues in Social Ecology. National Press Books, Palo Alto, CA, 1974
42. Morris NM, Udry JR, Chase CL: Reduction of low birth weight rates by prevention of unwanted pregnancies. Am J Pub Health 63:935–938, 1973
43. Murray HA, et al: Explorations in Personality. Oxford, New York, 1938
44. Nuckolls KB, Cassel J, Kaplan BH: Psychosocial assets, life crisis and the prognosis of pregnancy. Am J Epidemiol 95:431–441, 1972
45. Parkes CM: Bereavement: Studies of Grief in Adult Life. International Universities Press, New York, 1972
46. Parsons T: Definition of health and illness in the light of American values and social structure, in Patients, Physicians and Illness. Edited by Jaco EG. Glencoe Free Press, 1958
47. Peabody FW: The care of the patient. J Am Med Assoc 88:877–882, 1927
48. Phillips DP, Feldman KA: A dip in deaths before ceremonial occasions: some new relationships between social integration and mortality. Am Soc Rev 38:678–696, 1973
49. Pinneau SR: Effects of social support on psychological and physiological strains. Dissertation, University of Michigan, 1975
50. Quinn RP: Personal communication, 1973
51. Reid DD: Some measures of the effect of operational stress on bomber crews, in Great Britain Air Ministry, Psychological Disorders in Flying Personnel of the R.A.F. London, His Majesty's Stationery Office, 1947
52. Rose AM: Factors in mental breakdown in combat, in Mental Health and Mental Disorder—A Sociological Approach. Edited by Rose AM. Routledge & Kegan Paul, London, 1956
53. Smith S: On the limitations and modifying conditions of human longevity, the basis of sanitary work, in Public Health Reports and Papers Presented at the Meetings of the American Public Health Association in the year 1873. Riverside, New York, 1874
54. Stein Z, Susser M: Social factors in the development of sphincter control. Dev Med Child Neurol 9:692–706, 1967
55. Swank RL: Combat exhaustion: a descriptive and statistical analysis of causes, symptoms and signs. J Nerv Ment Dis 109:475–508, 1949
56. Weiss RS: The fund of sociability. Transactions 6:36–43, 1969

CHAPTER 19

Natural History of Male Psychological Health, IV

What Kinds of Men Do Not Get Psychosomatic Illness

GEORGE E. VAILLANT, M.D.

Prefatory Remarks

John C. Nemiah, M.D.

By the middle of the twentieth century, psychosomatic medicine had developed a sophisticated concept of symptom formation based on the psychoanalytic model of psychic function, which viewed bodily symptoms as the somatic expression, via autonomic and endocrine pathways, of psychological conflicts aroused by environmental stresses. In the ensuing two decades, the interest of psychosomatic investigators shifted away from central psychodynamic processes to focus on the nature of stress, on the one hand, and on psychophysiological variables on the other. In retrospect, George Vaillant's article (whose initial findings were first presented to the American Psychosomatic Society in 1972) can be seen as a ground-breaking move to refocus attention once again on the psychological processes in bodily illness. In this article, Vaillant reported a quantitative, statistically based relationship of prospectively obtained human developmental and psychological data with the subsequent development of somatic disease. In this context, Vaillant makes clear that psychological variables are indeed significantly related to bodily illness, but that the correlation is with serious, chronic, irreversible somatic illnesses of any kind, not just with those defined as "psychosomatic." The full import of that finding remains to be developed by future psychosomatic investigation.

This article reports on interrelationships between the medical and emotional health of 95 men who were prospectively followed from age 18 to 53. Fifty of these originally healthy men developed illness patterns sometimes called psychosomatic (ulcer, colitis, allergy, hypertension, musculo-skeletal disorders). These men were compared with the other 45 similarly studied men who never developed such illnesses. Although men who developed "psychosomatic" illnesses were more likely to seek medical or psychiatric attention, they exhibited only slightly more psychopathology. Both as children and as adults they had more physical illness of all kinds. They were less likely to indulge in vacations and athletics and more likely to use tranquilizers and excessive alcohol. Men with "psychosomatic" illnesses experienced a greater variety of somatic symptoms under stress, but the loci of these somatic symptoms shifted over time and were not significantly associated with the sites of psychosomatic illness. Premorbidly, the 20 men who were eventually to develop serious irreversible physical illness of any kind reflected far more psychopathology than the 45 men who developed psychosomatic illness.

Introduction

In the past 20 years theories suggesting that duodenal ulcers, asthma, colitis, and hypertension are precipitated by fairly specific emotional conflicts have fallen from favor.[1] The practice of referring individuals with such psychosomatic illnesses to psychiatrists for consultation has become less common. Nevertheless, the majority of theoretical positions derived from psychosomatic research in the period from 1940 to 1960 have remained neither proven nor unproven.

This article will use a 35-year prospective follow-up study of healthy men to examine three of these theoretical positions. The first position is the implicit assumption that psychophysiological symptoms reflect impaired emotional health.[2,3] Many of the psychological screening tests in use today, e.g., the Minnesota Multiphasic Personality Inventory, use multiple physiological symptoms under stress (e.g., headache and stomach pain) as indicators of emotional illness. Some clinicians feel that such somatic symptoms are the price paid by individuals who are inadequately aware of their emotional life.[4,5] Second, since under stress different people experience somatic symptoms in different sites, it has been hypothesized that a given individual may have a characteristic "target organ" for experiencing stress.[3,4] In such theories, the organ affected by *symptoms* under stress should be the same organ that is afflicted by *signs* of psychosomatic illness. Third, there is the implicit assumption that individuals who develop "psychosomatic" illnesses (e.g., colitis, asthma, and hypertension) may reflect more psychopathology than those who develop "somatic" illnesses (e.g., diabetes, myocardial infarction, osteoarthritis).

In general, the evidence for these beliefs has been derived from retrospective data and from patients who repeatedly present themselves for medical attention. The present report, a prospective 35-year study of men who were studied by doctors precisely because they were *not* patients, provides a fresh point of view. As college sophomores these men had been selected for mental and physical health. Over the years, they were systematically asked where in their bodies they experienced emotional stress. Their general health and psychological adjustment were also followed. At age 47, on the basis of almost 30 years of observation, they were ranked for *emotional health.* By this time over half of these men had required medical treatment for hypertension, respiratory allergies, ulcer, colitis, and chronic musculo-skeletal complaints—conditions thought by some physicians to be psychosomatic. At age 53 they were ranked for *physical health.*

A major focus of this article will be the relation of past psychophysiological symptoms to facets of mental health at 47 and to overall physical health at 53. Second, the article will also examine both the stability over time of psychophysiological symptoms under stress (e.g., abdominal pain, headache), and whether such symptoms are associated with signs of physical illness. Third, the article will contrast the mental health of men who develop often transient "psychosomatic" illnesses, both with men who manifest no "psychosomatic illness" and with men who develop chronic physical illnesses. Finally, the article will try to delineate the personality traits that characterize men who go through life without either psychosomatic illness or somatic symptoms under stress—a group of men ignored by prior psychosomatic research.

To harvest life history data, the view must be that from an airplane, not a microscope. Research options are limited. Thus, the research strategy was to dichotomize the sample into men who had and had not required medical attention for complaints thought by some to have a major emotional component.

The arbitrary decision to suggest that ulcer, colitis, hypertension, serious allergy, and musculo-skeletal complaints adequately reflect the universe of psychosomatic disease can please no one. No five disorders ultimately define "psychosomatic illness," but of the many pathological conditions that have been labeled psychosomatic illnesses, the above were those that occurred in this sample.

Methods

Sample

In 1938–42, 268 sophomores from a liberal arts college were selected on the basis of good physical and mental health for a medical study of "normals."[6,7] At an average age of 19 these men were intensively studied by internists, physiologists, anthropologists, psychologists, and psychiatrists. At intervals of roughly every 2 years, with little attrition, their health has been prospectively followed by questionnaire until the present.

In 1968, from the original list of 268 participants, 102 men were randomly chosen for reinterview. Of these men, two had dropped from the study in college, and between 1945 and 1967 five had died. The remaining 95 comprise the present sample. Despite geographic dispersion, all but one man (who died suddenly) were interviewed for 2 hours.

At the time of the original study, each man provided a very complete past medical history; his parents were interviewed with regard to his childhood medical history; each subject was somatotyped by an anthropologist; and autonomic lability was crudely assessed. The study had records of two very complete physical examinations performed while each subject was in college.

Measures

Objective Physical Health

In 1970, when the subjects were aged 45–50, and again in 1975, the study obtained records of a complete physical examination. On 73 men the most recent examination was by an internist and included at least four of the following: electrocardiogram, selected blood chemistries, urinalysis, blood count, and chest film; for 15 men the physical exam was complete, but either it was not done by an internist or less than four of the above studies were performed; for seven men the subject was deceased, or a complete exam had been obtained *and* recent health was alleged to be good still but the exam itself was 5–8 years old. On the basis of these examinations and recent interview data, the men were ranked accordingly:

1. Completely normal health;
2. Almost normal health (e.g., asymptomatic renal stones by x-ray, minimal hypertension);
3. Chronically ill without disability (e.g., diabetes, emphysema, treated hypertension);
4. Ill with physical disability (e.g., myocardial infarction, Parkinsonism, multiple sclerosis); and
5. Dead.

Subjective Physical Health

At five points in time, each man rated his own impression on his general health. These five ratings were averaged.

Somatic Symptoms Under Stress

At initial recruitment into the sample (age 18–19), and three times during follow-up at ages 33, 45, and 50, the men were asked how emotional stress affected them physically. During adult life the question was worded as follows: "When under stress, what do you notice about your physical reactions?"

_____ASTHMA		_____COLD HANDS AND FEET	
_____PALPITATION		_____FREQUENT COLDS	
_____HEADACHE		_____CONSTIPATION	
_____DIARRHEA		_____INABILITY TO CONCENTRATE	

_____INSOMNIA   _____NERVOUSNESS
_____SWEATING   _____IRRITABILITY
_____INDIGESTION OR   _____OTHER (PLEASE SPECIFY)
     ABDOMINAL PAIN
_____SMOKE AND DRINK MORE

At age 19 the same general questions were asked during the course of the physical examination, but in a less rigid format. Six of the physiological symptoms on the list (headache, constipation, diarrhea, indigestion or abdominal pain, palpitation, and sweating) were checked by at least four men.

Several blind ratings with good rater reliability ($r = 0.72$–0.85) were obtained; the methodology is described elsewhere.[6-10] Two raters, blind to other formal assessments, rated 50 of the men on their use or nonuse of 18 mechanisms of defense over 30 years of adult life and on their relative *maturity of defenses*.[8,10] Raters, blind to outcome after age 18, rated the men on their childhood physical health (range 1–5) and *childhood environment*.[6] Another rater, blind to character, health, and defense ratings, rated the men on three 8-item scales reflecting objective evidence of adult *career adjustment,* good *social adjustment,* and sound *psychological adjustment*.[9]

From all available information, including the interview data and questionnaires over 30 years, each man was rated by the author for the behavioral evidence of *hysterical character* (sexual provocativeness, emotionality, egocentricity, exhibitionism, aggression, and oral aggression), *obsessional character* (perseverance, rigidity, emotional constriction, orderliness, strict conscience, and stubbornness), and *oral dependent character* (dependence, pessimism, passivity, self-doubt, fear of sex, and suggestibility). The sheer number of behavioral examples, ranging from 0–20 for each cluster of traits, determined his "score" for that character type. Rater reliability was not obtained [see Lazare et al.[11] for rationale].

Psychosomatic Illness

Only after final ratings on all variables were recorded was any effort made to identify men with psychosomatic illness per se. The prospectively gathered records of each man at age 47 were reviewed for evidence of (a) duodenal ulcer—supported by at least suggestive x-ray evidence; (b) colitis (spastic colon, mucous colitis, irritable bowel disease)—severe enough to require medical attention; (c) hypertension—at least two readings above 140/90. For the purpose of this article, these three conditions will be arbitrarily called psychosomatic illness. Men also were identified who manifested (a) hay fever, vasomotor rhinitis—severe enough to require chronic medication and medical consultation; (b) asthma, and (c) joint diseases—severe enough to result in impaired function for several months (e.g., sciatica, slipped disc, bursitis, low back pain). Other illnesses often perceived as psychosomatic (e.g., neurodermatitis, hyperthyroidism, rheumatoid arthritis) were not observed in this limited sample.

Results

Table 19–1 examines the first hypothesis that psychophysiological symptoms under stress may reflect psychopathology. The average number of the following symptoms (headache, constipation, diarrhea, abdominal pain, palpitation, and sweating) that each man reported under stress at three points in adult life was correlated with several highly intercorrelated measures of mental health at age 47. The number of somatic symptoms under stress correlated only weakly with mental health; in contrast, subsequent physical health at 53 (most chronic illness occurred in these men after age 45) was powerfully correlated with premorbid psychopathology.

Table 19–2 examines the second hypothesis, that target organs should remain stable over time. The table shows the reported frequency of six physiological symptoms that the men in the sample most frequently experienced under stress. Since all men did not return all questionnaires, the total N is only 85. Contrary to the writer's bias, a man who said that he experienced a certain symptom under stress at 19 or 35 or 47 did not usually report experiencing that same symptom at other ages. In fact, the likelihood of men reporting a similar pattern of physical symptoms under stress on subsequent questionnaires was only slightly better than chance.[12] In other words, when the men in this study were followed for 30 years, there did not seem to be consistent "target organs" for experiencing stress.

There was evidence, however, to suggest a natural progression of somatic symptoms over time. Experiencing emotional stress via many *somatic* symptoms in adolescence was associated with experiencing stress via many *mental* symptoms (i.e., nervousness, irritability, and inability to concentrate) in adult life. As these men matured from adolescence to middle age, asthma, hay fever, constipation, diarrhea, and palpitations were reported less often, and the more "cerebral" symptoms of headache, insomnia, and inability to concentrate became more common.[12]

Over the 30-year follow-up period, 25 men experienced one of the three conditions defined above as *psychosomatic*. Eleven men were judged to have

Table 19-1. Strength of correlation among variables theoretically associated with mental health

	Objective physical health (age 53) (1–5)	Oral dependent traits (age 47) (0–20)	Good psychological adjustment (age 47)[a] (0–8)	"Maturity" of defenses (age 47) N = 50 (0–26)	Good social adjustment (age 47) (0–8)	Good career adjustment (age 47) (0–8)
Oral dependent traits	−0.35[b]					
Psychological adjustment[a,9]	0.54[b]	−0.56[b]				
"Maturity" of defenses[9]	0.47[b]	−0.51[b]	0.53[b]			
Good social adjustment[9]	0.43[b]	−0.36[b]	0.49[b]	0.62[b]		
Career adjustment[9]	0.24[c]	−0.56[b]	0.43[b]	0.54[b]	0.33[b]	
Number of somatic symptoms under stress	−0.30[d]	0.29[d]	−0.16	−0.04	−0.24[c]	−0.03

[a] Psychological adjustment was a blind rating based on eight items (presence or absence of inability to take vacations, emotional constriction, lack of clear job satisfaction, clear job dissatisfaction, 10+ psychiatric visits, drug misuse, psychiatric hospitalization, psychiatric diagnosis). See Ref. 9 for detailed definition of career and social adjustment.
[b] $p < 0.001$. Statistic used is Pearson's product-moment correlation coefficient.
[c] $p < 0.05$.
[d] $p < 0.01$.

had an ulcer, 6 to have had colitis, 8 to have had hypertension (but only six were receiving treatment). Forty-five of the 95 men were not known to have suffered from any psychosomatic illness. Of the remaining 25 men, 6 suffered chronic respiratory allergic conditions, 3, mild asthma, and 16 suffered chronic musculoskeletal complaints. For the purpose of this article, these 25 men will be presented separately, but for statistical purposes they will be grouped with the ulcer, hypertension, and colitis patients. Obviously, all these illnesses have multiple determinants; in different men psychological factors played different roles. However, treating the 50 men as a statistical unit permits global comparison with 45 men who over 30 years never developed disorders that by one definition or another could have been labeled "psychosomatic."

There was only weak association between the site of somatic symptoms under stress and the subsequent development of signs of "psychosomatic" illness in the same organ. In adult life, the men who at one point in time developed colitis reported diarrhea under stress at only chance levels over the whole time period. Similarly, the men who developed ulcers did not report significantly more abdominal pain under stress. The five men who in later life were treated for paroxysmal tachycardia or headache had not previously been more likely to report that they had experienced palpitations or headache under stress.

Paradoxically, it was the men with signs of chronic allergy and musculoskeletal disorders who as adults were somewhat more likely to report the symptoms of diarrhea, constipation, and abdominal pain under stress. Indeed, the only significant relationship between psychophysiological symptoms with stress and psychosomatic illness was as follows: men who as adults developed ulcer or colitis were men who at 19 had been twice as likely to have reported diarrhea *or* constipation, *or* abdominal pain under stress ($p < 0.01$).[12] However, there was

Table 19–2. Frequency of somatic symptoms under stress

	Proportion of men reporting symptoms ($N = 85$)		
	Never (%)	On one or two questionnaires (%)	On all questionnaires (%)
Headache	63	35	2
Constipation	85	13	2
Diarrhea	81	15	4
Abdominal pain and indigestion	68	24	8
Palpitation	86	12	2
Sweating	48	41	11

no specificity. Large bowel complaints in youth were not significantly linked to colitis in middle life, or were adolescents who experienced abdominal pain much more likely to develop ulcers when adult.

In comparing the men with psychosomatic illness with those who never developed such illness, no single somatic symptom under stress differentiated the two groups. However, as Figure 19–1 illustrates, the men who seemed least conscious of their physical response to stress were in fact the men least likely to develop psychosomatic illness. On each questionnaire, the men who developed psychosomatic illness reported roughly twice as many somatic symptoms under stress ($p < 0.001$, Student's t-test).

The men who developed psychosomatic illness experienced more illness of other kinds—both subjectively and objectively (Table 19–3). They experienced worse health in childhood. Even excluding their psychosomatic illness, they experienced somewhat worse health as adults. The objective health of men without psychosomatic illness was judged less than excellent in only 27% of cases. The health of men with psychosomatic illness was judged less than excellent in over

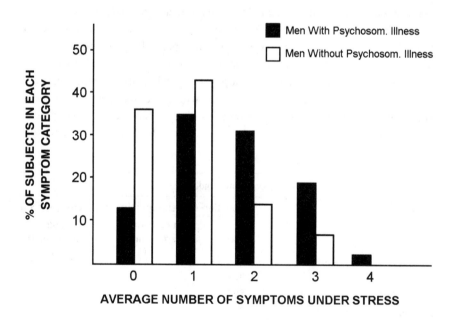

Figure 19–1. Association of psychosomatic illness with the average number of somatic symptoms reported under stress during adult life. [Differences in the number of symptoms experienced by men with and without psychosomatic disease is significant at $p < 0.001$ (Student's t-test).]

half of the cases. By 1975, 4 of the 5 men who died and 11 of the 15 chronically ill fell among the group with psychosomatic illness. (In part, this can be explained by the fact that all 8 of the men with hypertension at 47 were classified on that account as chronically ill at age 53.) From ages 18 to 47, the 50 men with "psychosomatic" illness had spent an average of 7 weeks in the hospital. The 45 men without psychosomatic illness had spent an average of 3 weeks in the hospital ($p < 0.01$, Student's t-test). The psychosomatic illness in question was rarely the cause of the excess hospitalization.

Table 19–4 supports part of the third theoretical position: men with psychosomatic illness exhibited somewhat more psychopathology than men with no psychosomatic illness, but Table 19–5 shows that the men who developed *chronic* physical illness from any cause showed far more psychopathology. Men with psychosomatic illness saw psychiatrists twice as frequently as men without such illness; they took tranquilizers three times as frequently. Although the difference did not attain statistical significance, heavy drinkers were twice as likely, and heavy smokers were 1 ½ times as likely, to exhibit psychosomatic

Table 19–3. Association of physical ill health and psychosomatic illness

Physical factors	Men without psychosomatic illness ($N = 45$) (%)	Men with ulcer, colitis, or hypertension ($N = 25$) (%)	Men with allergy or musculo-skeletal problems ($N = 25$) (%)	Significance
Childhood health *not* excellent	67	80	100	a
Objective health *not* excellent (age 47 excluding "psychosomatic" illness)	22	32	40	NS
Objective health *not* excellent (age 53)	27	60	48	a
Subjective health *not* excellent (age 20–47)[b]	38	68	52	a
Often seeks medical attention (age 20–47)	13	52	48	a

[a]Significant at $p < 0.05$ (chi-square test computed for men without psychosomatic illness vs. all others).
[b]Subjective health (20–47) correlates with objective health at 53 at only 0.10 (Pearson's product-moment correlation coefficient).

illness. On the average, twice as many episodes reflecting the traits of an "oral dependent" personality (i.e., dependence, pessimism, self-doubt, and passivity) had been abstracted from their records [$p < 0.01$, (Student's t-test)]. However, "hysterics" and "obsessive compulsives" were evenly distributed between the groups.

Table 19–4 also suggests that men with psychosomatic illness seemed less able to play. To a statistically significant degree, they were less likely to engage in hobbies and pastimes that involved other people. Subdividing the 50 men with "psychosomatic" illness into those with ulcer, colitis, and hypertension, and those with allergy and musculo-skeletal problems, did not produce significant differences. Good objective adult adjustment[9] (relative success in working and loving) was also twice as common in men who did

Table 19–4. Percentage of 48-year-old men ever experiencing psychosomatic illness manifesting selected mental health variables

Mental health variable (assessed at age 47)	Men without psychosomatic illness (age 20–47) ($N = 45$) (%)	Men with ulcer, colitis, or hypertension (age 20–47) ($N = 25$) (%)	Men with allergy or musculo-skeletal problems (age 20–47) ($N = 25$) (%)	Significance
Adult adjustment in top third	47	16	20	a
10+ psychiatric visits	16	32	36	a
Tranquilizers or sedatives often	9	36	28	a
Ignores vacation	27	64	36	a
No competitive sports	38	64	52	a
Many oral dependent traits	13	24	24	a
No physical symptoms with stress	34	16	12	a
Objectively diagnosed mentally ill[b]	20	40	24	NS
Maturity of defenses in bottom one-third	27	40	36	NS
College soundness in top one-third	35	24	36	NS

[a]Significant at $p < 0.05$ (chi-square test).
[b]Two or more of the following: hospitalized due to emotional distress, given a psychiatric diagnosis at two points in the past, diagnosed emotionally ill at recent interview, lifelong difficulty with anxiety.

not develop psychosomatic illness as in those who did (Table 19–4).

Much more interesting is the fact that 9 of the 10 men with excellent adult adjustment *and* psychosomatic illness are now in good physical health, whereas only half of the 22 men with relatively poor adult adjustment *and* psychosomatic illness are now in good health. In other words, as Tables 19–1 and 19–5 illustrate, it is *chronic* physical illness rather than psychosomatic symptoms per se that appears most strongly correlated with poor mental health. For example, men who were diagnosed as psychologically vulnerable in college and as mentally ill when adult, and men who chronically used immature defenses, were not statistically more likely to develop psychosomatic illness. But, as Table 19–5 illustrates, the presence of these same variables at 45 predicted serious chronic physical illness by age 53, regardless of cause.

When mature (coping) or immature (maladaptive) ego mechanisms were assigned numerical weights by blind raters,[10] use of mature mechanisms correlated powerfully with good physical health ($r = 0.47$) (Table 19–1). In contrast to theory, the defense mechanism of *suppression* was strongly associated with excellent physical health at 53 but was not associated with "psychosomatic" illness. The study did not shed light on whether "immature" defenses facilitated the development of chronic illness, or whether "mature" defenses facilitated recovery.

Table 19–5. Percentage of 53-year-old men with and without chronic physical illness that manifested selected mental health variables

Mental health variable (assessed at age 47)	Men in excellent health (age 53) ($N = 56$) (%)	Men dead or chronically ill (age 53) ($N = 20$) (%)	Significance
Adult adjustment in top third	45	5	a
10+ psychiatric visits	18	55	a
Tranquilizers or sedatives often	12	50	a
Ignores vacation	27	70	a
No competitive sports	39	85	a
Many oral dependent traits	9	50	a
No physical symptoms with stress	29	15	a
Objectively diagnosed mentally ill	13	60	a
Maturity of defenses in bottom one-third	18	65	a
College soundness in top one-third	37	15	a

[a]Significant at $p < 0.05$ (chi-square test). The 19 men with "almost normal health" have been excluded from this table.

A variety of other theoretically relevant childhood and adolescent variables—social class, nail-biting, somatotype, poor childhood environment, even autonomic lability in adolescence—failed to predict future psychosomatic illness.

Discussion

Although the sample was small, and was studied in less depth than in some cross-sectional studies, it had many advantages. It was drawn from a culturally homogeneous sample of nonpatients who, unlike clinic populations, had been studied prospectively and in uniform psychiatric depth. By maintaining the cooperation of subjects for 35 years, it became possible to diagnose personality and psychopathology by overt and redundant behavior rather than by the more impressionistic methods of the clinical interviewer or the psychological test. Throughout their adult life, the men all had access to high-quality medical care. If the sample was biased, it was biased in a way that avoided certain methodological pitfalls. The emotionally ill visit medical doctors far more frequently than do the emotionally healthy.[13, 14] This fact has biased virtually all our knowledge of psychosomatic illness. In many ways, then, the men in this selected sample provide a more, not a less, representative view of psychosomatic illness in the general population than do patients chosen from clinic populations. Nevertheless, even in a sample selected for health, so-called psychosomatic illness is surprisingly common. However, if the observations from this study are to be given credence, they must be confirmed in other population groups and for other so-called psychosomatic illnesses.

To the writer's surprise, this study gave only modest support to the three hypotheses it tested. First, psychophysiological symptoms under stress did not correlate dramatically with emotional dysfunction. Second, over time, *where* in his body a man experienced stress varied considerably. The idea of stable "target organs" was not supported. Third, men without "psychosomatic illness" (as defined here) were only modestly mentally healthier, and their blindly rated childhoods were not superior to those of men with psychosomatic illness.[6] Instead, early onset of *chronic* physical illness from any cause proved far more powerfully correlated with premorbid psychopathology.

The results are in full agreement with those from Hinkle's study of illness in 1,527 men. In that monumental investigation, Hinkle suggested that it was the quantity and not the specificity of illness that identified the psychosomatically ill.[15, 16] In both this study and in Hinkle's, suffering and disability from any physical illness—not just psychosomatic—was highly correlated with emotional illness (Table 19-1).

Perhaps as Ruesch suggested in 1948,[17] the traits of pessimism, self-doubt, passivity, and dependence may be the hallmark of the individual statistically destined to develop and, especially, to complain of psychosomatic illness. Selective emphasis by writers on different traits in this "oral dependent" cluster may account for the wide variety of different personality types that have been reported in the psychosomatic literature. The findings of both Ruesch and this article are supported by another prospective study of adult illness patterns. Stewart[18] contrasted the adolescent personalities of 20 men and women who subsequently developed psychosomatic illness with 25 who did not. Stewart found that it was *subjective* distress (adolescent negative self-image, feelings of inferiority, and multiple-symptom complaints) and not poor objective adjustment that characterized the psychosomatic group.

Put differently, the present study outlines a composite man *unlikely* to develop psychosomatic illness. First, he is less likely to have experienced other illnesses, both in childhood and in adult life. Second, he is less likely to perceive that emotional stress affects him physically. However, he is no less likely to perceive stress in psychological terms; under stress he is just as likely to report irritability, nervousness, or inability to concentrate. Not only is he much less likely to complain of physical ill health, he is also less likely to seek psychotherapy. Although not immune to objective psychological malfunctioning, he tends not to manifest "oral-dependent" or depressive traits like self-doubt, pessimism, passivity, and dependence. He finds comfort in vacations and games with friends, and less often seeks solace in tranquilizers and alcohol.

References

1. Mendelson M, Hirsch S, Webber CS: A critical examination of some recent theoretical models in psychosomatic medicine. Psychosom Med 18:363–373, 1956
2. Dunbar F: Psychosomatic Diagnosis. Hoeber, New York, 1943
3. Gildea EF: Special features of personality which are common to certain psychosomatic disorders. Psychosom Med 11:273–281, 1949
4. Alexander F, French TM, Pollack G: Psychosomatic Specificity: Experimental Study and Results, Vol 1. Chicago University Press, Chicago, IL, 1968
5. Nemiah JC, Sifneos PE: Affect and fantasy in patients with psychosomatic disorders, in Modern Trends in Psychosomatic Medicine, Vol 2. Edited by Hill OW. Appleton-Century-Crofts, New York, 1970, pp 26–34

6. Vaillant GE: Natural history of male psychological health, II: some antecedents of healthy adult adjustment. Arch Gen Psychiatry 31:15–22, 1974
7. Vaillant GE: Adaptation to Life. Little Brown, Boston, MA, 1977
8. Vaillant GE: Theoretical hierarchy of adaptive ego mechanisms: a 30-year follow-up of 30 men selected for psychological health. Arch Gen Psychiatry 24:107–118, 1971
9. Vaillant GE: Natural history of male psychological health, III: empirical dimensions of mental health. Arch Gen Psychiatry 32:420–426, 1975
10. Vaillant GE: Natural history of male psychological health, V: the relation of choice of ego mechanisms of defense to adult adjustment. Arch Gen Psychiatry 33:535–545, 1976
11. Lazare A, Klerman GL, Armor DJ: Oral, obsessive, and hysterical personality patterns. Arch Gen Psychiatry 14:624–630, 1966
12. Vaillant GE, McArthur CC: A 30-year follow-up of somatic symptoms under emotional stress, in Life History Research in Psychopathology, Vol 2. Edited by Roff M, Robins L. University of Minnesota Press, Minneapolis, MN, 1972, pp 199–210
13. McWhinney IR: Beyond diagnosis. N Eng J Med 287:384–387, 1972
14. Dohrenwend BP, Crandell DL: Psychiatric symptoms in community clinic and mental hospital groups. Am J Psychiatry 126:1611–1621, 1970
15. Hinkle LE, Christensen WN, Kane FD, et al: An investigation of the relation between life experience, personality characteristics and general susceptibility to illness. Psychosom Med 20:278–295, 1958
16. Hinkle LE: Ecological observations of the relation of physical illness, mental illness and the social environment. Psychosom Med 23:289–296, 1961
17. Ruesch J: The infantile personality: the core problem of psychosomatic medicine. Psychosom Med 10:134–144, 1948
18. Stewart LH: Social and emotional adjustment during adolescence as related to the development of psychosomatic illness in adulthood. Genet Psychol Monogr 65:175–215, 1962

Index

Page numbers printed in **boldface** *type refer to tables or figures.*

Acne, 33
Ader, Robert, 364
Adrenal cortex. *See also* Adrenaline
   arousal of defense alarm response and, 157
   social stimulation and, 167
   stress and activation of, 47–48, 64, 67
Adrenaline, study of blood pressure and psychosocial stimulation in mice
   interpretation of, 163–167
   methods of, 158–161
   results of, 161–163
Affective disorders, 388
Age. *See also* Children; Elderly; Infants
   obesity and social factors, 313–315, **316**
   race and blood pressure, 262–263
Aggression, 282–283, 284. *See also* Social conflict
Alcoholism, 387–389
Alexander, Franz, 28, 41–42
Anger. *See also* Aggression; Hostility
   race and blood pressure, 255–257, 267, 268
   race and distributions of coping patterns, 257–258
Angina pectoris, 151, 199–200, 204
Animal studies. *See also* Mice; Monkeys; Rats
   anterior pituitary-adrenal cortical activity as response to stress, 47
   depression and, 273–274
   eating behavior of hypothalamic obese animals, 320–321
Anthropology, medical, 225–226
Anticipatory responses
   blood pressure changes in men undergoing job loss, 131–132, **134,** 135, 139, 140
   epinephrine release during, 24
Anxiety, somatic presentation of, 91. *See also* Conditioned fear
Apomorphine, 365
Arrhythmias, cardiac, 193, 385. *See also* Premature ventricular contractions (PVCs)
Arthritis, 389. *See also* Rheumatoid arthritis
Asthma
   attitude as factor in, 30, 33
   role of psychological factors in, 105–106
   social support and treatment of, 386

Asthma *(continued)*
   suggestion and, study of
      interpretation of, 111–115
      methods of, 107–108
      results of, 108–111
Atropine, 113, 195, 198, 216
Attitude
   definition of, 28–29
   study of psychosomatic disease and
      interpretation of, 38–43
      procedures for, 29–34
      results of, 34–36
      statistical methods and, 37–38
Autonomic functions. *See also* Blood pressure; Heart rate
   operant conditioning and, 152
   voluntary control of, 144
Axelrod, Julius, 155–156

Backache, 34
Behavior
   behavioral sink, concept of, 165
   consultation psychiatry on medical wards and grossly disturbed, 94–95
   definition of, 364
   depression in infant monkeys and, 278
   disease and elements of, 363, 364
   endocrine levels during emotional disturbance in monkeys and, 12
   environmental cues and eating, 321–322
   hypothalamic obese animals and eating, 320–321
   and immunosuppression in rats, study of
      development of hypothesis, 365
      methods of, 366–368
      results and interpretation of, 368–375
   obesity treatment and modification of, 322–347
   and social groups in rhesus monkeys, 284–285
   and societal theory of disease, 224, 240, 241–242
   sociological concept of illness behavior, 88
   testosterone levels and determinants of aggressive, 282–283, 284
   type A pattern of, 246
Bereavement. *See* Grief
Berle Index, 386, **386**
Bibliotherapy, treatment of obesity, 340
Blood pressure. *See also* Hypertension
   in men undergoing job loss, study of
      interpretation of, 135–140
      methods of, 120–124
      results of, 124–135
   operant conditioning and heart rate, study of
      development of hypothesis, 145–146
      method of, 146–149
      results and interpretation of, 149–152

Index

and psychosocial stimulation in mice, study of
  interpretation of, 163–167
  methods of, 158–161
  results of, 161–163
race, class, and stress in male residents of Detroit, study of
  development of hypothesis, 248–249
  interpretation of, 263–268
  methods of, 250–253
  results of, 254–263
review of literature on psychological factors in, 119–120
Body, beliefs concerning and theory of disease in Chiapas Highlands of Mexico, 230–232, 236, 241
Body temperature, and depression in infant monkeys, 276, **277**, 278
Body weight, race, and blood pressure, 262–263. *See also* Obesity
Brady, Joseph V., 9–10
Bradycardia, 278
Bronchitis, 113
Brooks, George, 117–118

California Personality Inventory, Flexibility-Rigidity Scale of, 133–134
Cancer, psychological responses to, 87
Caplan, Gerald, 380
Cassel, John, 378
Castration anxiety, 82
Catechol-O-methyl transferase (COMT), 161, 163

Central nervous system
  behavioral conditioning and immunologic processes, 374
  grief and role of, 7
  operant conditioning of heart rate and, 216
Chiapas Highlands (Mexico), study of theory of disease in, 222–223, 226–242
Children. *See also* Infants; Parents
  social support and early development of, 383–384
  social support and hospitalization of, 384–385
Chi-square method, 54
Cholesterol, 139
Class, socioeconomic
  obesity and, 308–319
  patterns of referral in consultation psychiatry and, 79
  race, stress, and blood pressure in male residents of Detroit, study of
    development of hypothesis, 248–249
    interpretation of, 263–268
    methods of, 250–253
    results of, 254–263
Classic study, definition of, 2
Cobb, Sidney, 117–118, 377–378
Coe, Christopher L., 273–274
Cohen, Nicholas, 364
Community mental health movement, 380
Compliance, patient, 387
Conditioned avoidance, 12, 21–22, 23
Conditioned fear, 12–13
Conflict. *See* Social conflict

Congestive heart failure, 212, 213, 214, 385–386
Consistencia, use of term, 228, 229
Constipation, 33
Consultation psychiatry
    challenges for, 71–72
    and diagnostic problems on medical wards, 80–94
    and management problems on medical wards, 94–96
    quantitative aspects of, 73–79
Convalescence, as management problem on medical wards, 95
Conversion hysteria, 82, 89–91
Coping
    and endocrine levels during emotional disturbance in monkeys, 23, 24
    race, blood pressure, and patterns of, 258–259
    race, blood pressure, and skin color, 259–262
    social support and, 381, 393
    suppressed hostility and concept of, 248–249
    measurement of, 253
    race and distributions of, 257–258
Corticosteroids. *See* 17-hydroxycorticosteroid (17-OHCS)
Covert sensitization, 346–347
Culture
    affluence and obesity, 316–319
    cross-cultural studies of medicine, 225–226
    and theory of disease, 221–222, 226, 240–242
    view of illness in Chiapas Highlands of Mexico, study of, 222–223, 226–242
Cushing's syndrome, 89
Cyclophosphamide, 365

Death
    as result of grief, 4–5
    social support and threat of, 391
Defenses, 17-OHCS excretion rates in parents of fatally ill children and psychological, 47–68. *See also* Denial; Suppression
Delirium, as psychological complication of organic disease, 84–86
Denial
    grief and, 8
    race and blood pressure, 266
Depression
    animal studies of, 273–274
    eating and behavioral, 325
    and infant separation in monkeys, study of
    interpretation of, 277–278
    methods of, 274–275
    results of, 275–277
    life events and, 388
    and social support of elderly, 391
    somatic presentation of, 89
Detroit, Michigan
    race riots in 1967, 245–246
    study of race, stress, and blood pressure in male residents of, 248–268
Diabetes mellitus, 214

Index

Diagnosis
    consultation psychiatry in medical settings and referrals, 77–79
    consultation psychiatry and problems of on medical wards, 80–94
Diastolic blood pressure, 139
Diencephalic function, depressive disorders and disturbances in, 278
Digoxin, 196, 197
Dimsdale, Joel E., 171–172
Diphenylhydantoin, 200
Disease, organic. *See also* Psychosomatic disease
    core issues of psychosomatic medicine and theory of, 221–222, 223–225
    grief and concept of, 2–8
    humoral theory of, 239
    psychological complications of, 84–86
    psychological presentation of, 83–84
    psychological reactions to, 86–89
    psychosomatic medicine and behavioral elements in, 363–364
    social support and recovery from, 385–387
    study of theory of in Chiapas Highlands in Mexico, 222–223, 226–242
Double-blind methodology, in psychopharmacology, 331
Dreams, and theory of disease in Chiapas Highlands of Mexico, 235

Drug abuse, delirium and withdrawal states, 85

Eating disorders. *See* Body weight; Obesity
Eczema, 30, 33
Edrophonium, 195, 202–203, 207
Education
    of children and social support, 384
    of mother and birth weight of infants, 382–383
Ego resilience, blood pressure changes and, 129, 130, 132, 138, 140
Elderly, social support and life stress, 390–391
Emotional support, 380
Emotions. *See also* Perception
    disturbance of and endocrine levels in monkeys, study of
        interpretation of, 20–24
        methods for, 11–13
        results of, 15–19
    excessive reactions as management problem on medical wards, 95
    and theory of disease in Chiapas Highlands of Mexico, 228–230
    and treatment of obesity, 303–304
Employment. *See* Workplace
Endocrinology. *See also* Neuroendocrinology
    developments in understanding of, 281–282
    and emotional disturbances in monkeys, study of, 11–24

Endocrinology *(continued)*
   reciprocity between environment and physiology, 282
   testosterone levels and social conflict in monkeys, study of, 283–297
Engel, Bernard T., 155–156, 299–300, 363–364
Engel, George L., 1–2
Enteritis, regional, 34
Epilepsy, 91
Epinephrine, elevations of in monkeys under experimental stress, **14,** 15–24
Esteem support, 380. *See also* Self-esteem
Ethnicity. *See also* Race
   culture and theory of disease, 240
   obesity and social factors, 309–311
Ethnography, research methods of, 226–227

Fabrega, Horacio, 221–222
Family, socioeconomic class and blood pressure in males, 266–267
Films, and research on psychosomatic processes, 172, 173–189
Flexibility-Rigidity Scale (California Personality Inventory), 133–134
Freud, Sigmund, 91, 248

Gender
   obesity and socioeconomic class, 306, 308, 312, 313
   and patterns of referral in consultation psychiatry, 79
   and theory of disease in Chiapas Highlands of Mexico, 230
Graham, David T., 27–28
Grief. *See also* Loss
   and concept of disease, 2–8
   social support and, 390
Guilt, race and blood pressure, 255–258, 267, 268

Harburg, Ernest, 246
Health care
   consequences of obesity and weight reduction, 347–348
   delivery systems for treatment of obesity, 348–356
   folk versus Western systems, 236–239
Health maintenance organizations (HMOs), 379
Heart rate
   depression and infant separation in monkeys, 276, **277,** 278
   operant conditioning and blood pressure, study of
      development of hypothesis, 145–146
      method of, 146–149
      results and interpretation of, 149–152
   operant conditioning and premature ventricular contractions (PVCs), study of
      development of hypothesis, 192–193
      interpretation of, 215–217

Index

materials and methods of, 193–196
results of, 196–215
Henry, James, 155–156
Hepatitis, 89
Hinkle, Lawrence, Jr., 117
Hispanic-Americans. *See* Mexico
Hospitals, medical
    consultation psychiatry and management problems in, 94–96
    prevalence studies of psychiatric morbidity in, 73–76
    social support and hospitalization, 384–385
Hostility. *See also* Aggression; Anger
    hypertensive patients and, 173
    suppressed and coping patterns in Black and White males, 248–249, 253, 267, 268
Humoral theory, of disease, 239
17-Hydroxycorticosteroid (17-OHCS)
    elevated levels of in monkeys under experimental stress, 15–24
    psychological defenses and excretion rates of in parents of fatally ill children, 47–68
Hyperparathyroidism, 4
Hypertension. *See also* Blood pressure
    arousal of defense alarm response and, 157, 266
    attitude and, 30, 33
    hostility and, 131
    operant conditioning and, 145
    perception differences in hypertensive and normotensive patients, study of
        development of hypothesis, 173–174
        interpretation of, 188–189
        methods and materials of, 174–176
        results of, 176–188
    social interaction and role playing, 166
    stressful life events and development of, 138–139
Hyperthyroidism, 30, 33
Hyperventilation, 91
Hypochondriasis, 92–93
Hypothalamus
    defense alarm system and anterolateral, 157
    immune responses and, 372
Hypothermia, 278. *See also* Body temperature
Hysteria, 89–91. *See also* Conversion hysteria

Illness. *See* Disease
Immigration, obesity and socioeconomic class, 309–311
Immunosuppression, study of behaviorally conditioned in rats
    development of hypothesis, 365
    methods of, 366–368
    results and interpretation of, 368–375
Infants. *See also* Children
    birth weight of and social support of mother, 382–383

Infants *(continued)*
   depression and maternal
      separation in monkeys,
      study of
         interpretation of, 277–278
         methods of, 274–275
         results of, 275–277
Instrumental learning. *See* Operant conditioning
Interpersonal relations, and theory of disease in Chiapas Highlands of Mexico, 228–230, 241–242. *See also* Psychosocial stimulation; Social conflict
Interviews
   on attitude and psychosomatic disease, 29–34, 38–41
   on differences in perception of hypertensive and normotensive patients, 182–185
   psychological defenses and 17-OHCS excretion rates in parents of fatally ill children, 50, 52
Irritation, blood pressure changes and, 130, 140
Isoproterenol, 195, 199, 202, 208, 216

Juvenile delinquency, and social support, 383

Kasl, Stanislav, 117–118, 377–378

Ladinos. *See* Mexico
Learning. *See* Operant conditioning
Light, Kathleen C., 245–246
Lipowski, Z. J., 71
Lipsitt, Don R., 143–144

Lithium chloride, 365, 372
Los Angeles, riots in 1990s, 246
Loss, 17-OHCS excretion rates in parents of fatally ill children, study of. *See also* Grief
   case reports, 59–63
   development of hypothesis on, 47–49
   interpretation of, 63–68
   methods for, 49–54
   results of, 54–59
Luparello, Thomas, 105–106
Lupus erythematosus, 89

Malaria, 6
Manning, Peter K., 221–222
Mason, John W., 9–10
Maternal separation, study of depression in monkeys and, 274–278. *See also* Pregnancy
Maya. *See* Mexico
Medical ecology, 225
Medicine. *See also* Disease, organic; Health care; Psychosomatic medicine
   cross-cultural studies of, 225–226
   history of and concepts of disease, 4, 223
Mental illness. *See* Psychiatric disorders
Mestizos. *See* Mexico
Metabolic edema, 30, 33
Mexico, study of theory of disease in Chiapas Highlands, 222–223, 226–242
Mice, blood pressure and psychosocial stimulation in, 158–167. *See also* Animal studies

Index

Migraine, 30, 33
Military, social support and mental health in, 391
Monkeys. *See also* Animal studies
    study of depression and infant separation in, 274–278
    study of endocrine levels during emotional disturbances in, 11–24
    study of testosterone levels and social conflict among, 283–297
Monoamine oxidase (MAO), 161, 163, 166
Multiple schedule program, 13, 24
Multiple sclerosis, 30, 33, 89
Myocardial infarction (MI), 196, 199, 204, 208, 215, 385

Native Americans, acculturation and obesity, 318, **319**. *See also* Mexico
Nemiah, John C., 399–400
Neuroendocrinology, interdisciplinary studies on differentiation of emotional states, 24. *See also* Endocrinology
Noradrenaline, study of blood pressure and psychosocial stimulation in mice, 158–167
Norepinephrine, elevations of in monkeys under experimental stress, 15–24

Obesity
    developments in understanding of psychosomatic approach to, 301–305
    small group environment and, 319–322
    socioeconomic class and, 308–319
    treatment of
        delivery systems for, 348–356
        implications of recent developments in, 347–348
        special therapeutic environments for, 322–347
Object loss, 7
Oken, Donald, 1–2, 46
Operant conditioning
    blood pressure and heart rate, study of
        development of hypothesis, 145–146
        method of, 146–149
        results and interpretation of, 149–152
    heart rate and premature ventricular contractions (PVCs), study of
        development of hypothesis, 192–193
        interpretation of, 215–217
        materials and methods of, 193–196
        results of, 196–215
    significance of for theory of psychosomatic symptoms, 143–144

Pain, experience of and theory of disease in Chiapas Highlands of Mexico, 232
Paranoid schizophrenia, 92

Paraplegia, 82
Parents, of fatally ill children and study of 17-OHCS excretion rates in
  case reports, 59–63
  development of hypothesis on, 47–49
  interpretation of, 63–68
  methods for, 49–54
  results of, 54–59
Pathology, definition of, 3
Patient-personnel conflict, as medical problem on medical ward, 95–96. *See also* Compliance, patient
Perception, study of hypertension and
  development of hypothesis, 173–174
  interpretation of, 188–189
  methods and materials of, 174–176
  results of, 176–188
Personality
  characteristics of men developing psychosomatic illness, study of
    development of hypothesis, 400–402
    interpretation of, 412–413
    measurements of physical and mental health, 403–405
    methods of, 402
    results of, 405–412
  of hypertensive and normotensive patients, 173
Pharmacology
  methodology of double-blind experiment in, 331

operant conditioning of heart rate and, 195, 198–199, 202–204, 207–208
Phentolamine, 195, 208
Phenylephrine, 195, 207–208
Phenylethanolamine *N*-methyltransference (PNMT), **160,** 161, 163, 164, 166
Pheochromocytoma, 91
Plethysmography, whole-body, 106
Porphyria, 89
Positive reinforcement, behavioral treatment of obesity, 345–346
Pregnancy. *See also* Maternal separation
  social support and stress of, 381–382
  view of body and theory of disease in Chiapas Highlands of Mexico, 231–232
Premature ventricular contractions (PVCs), study of operant conditioning and
  development of hypothesis, 192–193
  interpretation of, 215–217
  materials and methods of, 193–196
  results of, 196–215
Prevalence studies, of psychiatric morbidity in medical wards, 73–79
Propranolol, 195, 202–203, 207
Psoriasis, 33
Psychiatric disorders
  obesity and, 305, **306, 307**
  patients with history of as management problem on medical ward, 96

prevalence of on medical wards, 73–79
somatic presentation of, 89–94
and theory of disease in Chiapas Highlands of Mexico, 235–236
Psychoneuroimmunology, 118
Psychopharmacology. *See* Pharmacology
Psychosocial stimulation, study of blood pressure in mice and
interpretation of, 163–167
methods of, 158–161
results of, 161–163
Psychosomatic disease. *See also* Psychosomatic medicine
characteristics of men developing, study of
development of hypothesis, 400–402
interpretation of, 412–413
measurements of physical and mental health, 403–405
methods of, 402
results of, 405–412
films and research on processes of, 172
specificity-of-attitude hypothesis of, 27–43
Psychosomatic medicine. *See also* Psychosomatic disease
asthma and role of suggestion, study of, 107–115
and behavioral elements in disease, 363–364
behaviorally conditioned immunosuppression in rats, study of, 365–375
blood pressure and changes in men undergoing job loss, study of, 120–140
psychosocial stimulation in mice, study of, 158–167
race, class, and stress in male residents of Detroit, study of, 248–268
consultation psychiatry and, 71–97
contributions of to health science, 1–2
depression and infant separation in monkeys, study of, 274–278
developments and redirections in until mid-1970s, 377–378
endocrine levels during emotional disturbances in monkeys, study of, 11–24
grief and concept of disease, 2–8
male psychological health, study of, 400–413
obesity and, 301–357
operant conditioning and heart rate, study of, 145–152, 192–217
Selye's concept of stress and research on, 46
social conflict and testosterone levels in monkeys, study of, 283–297
as social movement, 301
stress and differences in perceptions of hypertensive and normotensive patients, study of, 173–189

Psychosomatic medicine *(continued)*
   stress and social support, study of, 379–394
   symptom formation, concept of, 399–400
   theory of disease in Chiapas Highlands of Mexico, 223–242
   workplace and research on, 117–118
Psychosomatic Medicine (journal), 301

Questionnaires, study of differences of perception and hypertension, 185–188
Quinidine, 196, 204, 209

Race. *See also* Ethnicity
   and blood pressure changes in men undergoing job loss, 136
   class, stress, and blood pressure in male residents of Detroit, study of
     development of hypothesis, 248–249
     interpretation of, 263–268
     methods of, 250–253
     results of, 254–263
     riots and social violence, 245–246
Rahe, Richard H., 117–118
Rats, study of behaviorally conditioned immunosuppression in, 365–375. *See also* Animal studies
Raynaud's disease, 33–34
Record-keeping, and behavioral treatment of obesity, 341, 344–345
Referrals, psychiatric consultation for medical inpatients, 76–79
Reite, Martin, 273–274
Religion, obesity and social factors, 310–311
Renal disease, 164
Reparation, in grief, 5
Respiration, influence on blood pressure and heart rate, 151. *See also* Asthma
Rewards, and behavioral treatment of obesity, 343–344, 345–346
Rheumatoid arthritis, 30, 33
Rose, Robert M., 282–283
Rubin, Robert T., 281–283

Saccharin, 365
Sapira, Joseph, 27–28
Schilder, Paul, 84, 97
Schizoaffective disorder, 93
Schizophrenia
   hypochondriasis and, 92
   psychological defenses and 17-OHCS excretion rates, 65
   socioeconomic class and, 308
   somatic presentation of, 91–92
Self-esteem, blood pressure changes and, 130, 140. *See also* Esteem support
Self-help groups, for treatment of obesity, 351–356
Self-monitoring, and behavioral treatment of obesity, 341, 344–345
Shapiro, David, 191–192

Index

Skin color
   measurement of, 252–253
   race, blood pressure, and coping responses, 259–262, 267, 268
   socioeconomic status and blood pressure, 267
Slavery, and oppression of Black males in contemporary society, 249
Sleep disturbance, 275, 278
Smith, Stephen, 379
Smoking, behavior therapy for, 326
Social breakdown syndrome, 384
Social conflict, and testosterone levels in monkeys, study of
   development of hypothesis, 283–285
   interpretation of, 293–297
   methods of, 285–286
   results of, 286–293
Social deprivation, 165, 166
Social psychology, treatment of obesity, 321–322
Social situation. *See also* Class, socioeconomic; Interpersonal relations; Psychosocial stimulation; Social conflict; Social support
   small group environment and obesity, 319–322
   and special therapeutic environments for treatment of obesity, 322–347
Social support
   implications of research on, 392–394
   life stress and, 387–389
   aging and retirement, 390–391
   bereavement, 390
   birth weight of infants, 382–383
   early development of children, 383–384
   employment termination, 389, **390**
   hospitalization, 384–385
   pregnancy, 381–382
   threat of death, 391
   understanding of concept of, 379–381
Socioeconomic status. *See* Class, socioeconomic
Somatic illness. *See* Disease, organic
Specificity hypothesis, of psychosomatic disease, 27–28
Statistical methods
   asthma and suggestion, study of, 108–109
   attitudes and psychosomatic disease, study of, 34–38
   blood pressure changes in men undergoing job loss, study of, 127
   17-OHCS excretion in parents of fatally ill children, study of, 54–59
Stein, Marvin, 106
Steroids. *See also* 17-hydroxycorticosteroid (17-OHCS); Testosterone
   immune response and elevation in levels of, 372–374, 375
   psychiatric side effects of, 96
Stimulus control, behavioral treatment of obesity, 342, 345
Streltzer, Jon, 221–222

Stress
  blood pressure and
    review of literature on psychological factors in, 119–120
    study of changes in men undergoing job loss, 120–140
    study of changes in mice exposed to psychosocial stimulation, 158–167
    study of race and class in male residents of Detroit, 248–268
  grief and
    concept of psychological, 7
    concepts of health and disease, 5
    object loss, 7
  immune processes and, 372
  multiple hormone responses to, 282
  parents of fatally ill children, study of 17-OHCS excretion in, 47–68
  perception differences in hypertensive and normotensive patients, study of, 173–189
  Selye's concept of, 46
  social conflict and testosterone levels in monkeys, study of, 283–297
  social support and life events, 379–394
  somatic symptoms in men undergoing, 403–404, 405–412
  variability of responses to, 118

Stunkard, Albert J., 299–300
Suggestion, study of asthma and
  interpretation of, 111–115
  methods of, 107–108
  results of, 108–111
Suicide
  consultation psychiatry on medical wards and, 94
  social support and, 393
Suppression, defense mechanism of, 411. *See also* Hostility
Systolic blood pressure, 139
Szent-Gyorgyi, Albert, 8

Tachycardia, operant conditioning and, 145
Taste aversion, 365
Testosterone, social conflict and levels of in monkeys, 283–297
Therapist, role in behavioral treatment of obesity, 335–341
Toilet training, and social support, 383
TOPS (Take Off Pounds Sensibly), 351–356
Tuberculosis, 387–388
Tyrosine hydroxylase, **160,** 161, 163, 164, 166

Ulcer, duodenal, 30, 33
Ulcerative colitis, 30, 32
Uncertainty, epinephrine release and, 24
Uncomplicated grief, 3, 5
Unemployment. *See* Workplace
Urticaria, 32

Vachon, Louis, 105–106

Index

Vaillant, George, 400
Visceral responses, operant conditioning of, 193
Vomiting, 33, 193

Weight reduction, commercial enterprises for, 356
Weight Watchers, 356
Weiner, Herbert, 9–10
Wise, Thomas N., 71–72
Witchcraft, and theory of disease in Chiapas Highlands of Mexico, 233

Workplace
    blood pressure changes in men undergoing job loss, study of
        interpretation of, 135–140
        methods of, 120–124
        results of, 124–135
    psychosomatic research in, 117–118
    social support and employment termination, 389, **390**
    social support and retirement, 390–391